Oral Lipid-Based Formulations

DRUGS AND THE PHARMACEUTICAL SCIENCES
A Series of Textbooks and Monographs

Executive Editor
James Swarbrick
PharmaceuTech, Inc.
Pinehurst, North Carolina

Advisory Board

Larry L. Augsburger
University of Maryland
Baltimore, Maryland

Harry G. Brittain
Center for Pharmaceutical Physics
Milford, New Jersey

Jennifer B. Dressman
Johann Wolfgang Goethe University
Frankfurt, Germany

Anthony J. Hickey
University of North Carolina School of
Pharmacy
Chapel Hill, North Carolina

Jeffrey A. Hughes
University of Florida College of
Pharmacy
Gainesville, Florida

Ajaz Hussain
Sandoz
Princeton, New Jersey

Trevor M. Jones
The Association of the
British Pharmaceutical Industry
London, United Kingdom

Stephen G. Schulman
University of Florida
Gainesville, Florida

Elizabeth M. Topp
University of Kansas School of
Pharmacy
Lawrence, Kansas

Vincent H. L. Lee
University of Southern California
Los Angeles, California

Jerome P. Skelly
Alexandria, Virginia

Peter York
University of Bradford School of
Pharmacy
Bradford, United Kingdom

Geoffrey T. Tucker
University of Sheffield
Royal Hallamshire Hospital
Sheffield, United Kingdom

Oral Lipid-Based Formulations

Enhancing the Bioavailability of Poorly Water-Soluble Drugs

Edited by

David J. Hauss

Bristol-Myers Squibb Company
Princeton, New Jersey, USA

informa

healthcare

New York   London

Informa Healthcare USA, Inc.
52 Vanderbilt Avenue
New York, NY 10017

© 2007 by Informa Healthcare USA, Inc.
Informa Healthcare is an Informa business

No claim to original U.S. Government works
Printed in the United States of America on acid-free paper
10 9 8 7 6 5 4 3 2 1

International Standard Book Number-10: 0-8247-2945-5 (Hardcover)
International Standard Book Number-13: 978-0-8247-2945-5 (Hardcover)

Library of Congress Cataloging-in-Publication Data

Oral lipid-based formulations : enhancing the bioavailability of poorly
    water-soluble drugs / [edited by] David J. Hauss.
        p. ; cm. -- (Drugs and the pharmaceutical sciences; v. 170)
    Includes bibliographical references and index.
    ISBN-13: 978-0-8247-2945-5 (hb : alk. paper)
    ISBN-10: 0-8247-2945-5 (hb : alk. paper)
    1. Lipids--Therapeutic use. 2. Drugs--Solubility. 3. Solutions (Pharmacy)
4. Drugs--Dosage forms. I. Hauss, David J. II. Series.
    [DNLM: 1. Biological Availability. 2. Solubility--drug effects. 3. Dosage
Forms. 4. Drug Administration Routes. 5. Drug Delivery Systems--methods.
W1 DR893B v.170 2007 / QV 38 O635 2007]
    RS201.E87O7377 2007
    615'.1--dc22   2007008964

Visit the Informa Web site at
www.informa.com

and the Informa Healthcare Web site at
www.informahealthcare.com

The editor wishes to express his sincere gratitude to Professor Jennifer B. Dressman, to whom this book is dedicated, for her guidance, mentorship, and unfaltering support.

"The significant problems we face cannot be solved at the same level of thinking we were at when we created them."

—*Albert Einstein*

Preface

It has been estimated that between 40% and 70% of all new chemical entities identified in drug discovery programs are insufficiently soluble in aqueous media to allow for their adequate and reproducible absorption from the gastrointestinal tract following oral administration. Many individuals maintain that reliance on combinatorial chemistry is responsible for creating this solubility problem. However, one need only review the literature to be reminded of the relationship between pharmacophore lipophilicity and biological activity that has surfaced repeatedly throughout the recorded history of pharmacology. So, have we not perhaps been negligent in our failure to anticipate the biopharmaceutical properties of contemporary drug candidates that were previously shown to be characteristic of many highly potent pharmacophores? Our inability to efficiently develop oral dosage forms for the majority of these poorly soluble compounds could certainly be construed as evidence of negligence.

Oral lipid-based formulations, which are by no means a recent technological innovation, have not only proven their utility for mitigating the poor and variable gastrointestinal absorption of poorly soluble, lipophilic drugs, but in many cases have shown the ability to reduce or eliminate the influence of food on the absorption of these drugs. A cursory review of the literature will clearly underscore not only the scientific interest in oral lipid-based formulations, but will reinforce the promise and versatility that this technology holds for addressing the constant and growing problems surrounding the oral delivery of many poorly soluble drug candidates. Despite these realities, marketed oral drug products employing lipid-based formulations are currently outnumbered 25 to 1 by conventional formulations. As with any drug delivery technology, there are practical limitations to the successful application of oral lipid-based formulations. However, considerable inertia and reluctance to embrace necessary change appears to be fueling our failure to fund the research that would allow us to push past these limitations.

Currently, lipid-based formulations occupy a small but successful niche for dealing with oral delivery of poorly soluble drugs. The majority of application and manufacturing expertise for these formulations is, not surprisingly, limited to smaller specialty companies. However, the services of these organizations are being leveraged with increasing frequency, which bodes well for more widespread acceptance of oral lipid-based formulations by the industry at large. Greater demand for this technology should drive increased research efforts directed at solving solubility and stability issues and refinement of in vitro and in vivo models for more reliable projection of formulation performance in humans. Increased regulatory acceptance of oral lipid-based formulations is expected to follow these anticipated developments. This book seeks to provide a balanced and comprehensive summary of both the theoretical and practical aspects of oral lipid-based formulations to formulators wishing to employ the technology as well as scientific and marketing executives who wish to gain a greater understanding of a developing technology that is expected to assume increasing prominence in the years to come.

The first two chapters provide a thorough review of currently marketed drug products formulated with lipids and a comprehensive summary of the excipients used to prepare these formulations. Next, the reader is guided through the initial stages of lipid-based formulation development, beginning with feasibility assessment and prototype formulation design and followed by process scale-up and manufacturing considerations. The development and characterization of liquid, semi-solid, and self-emulsifying formulations is covered in detail and many illustrative examples are included. Subesequent chapters provide detailed treatises on the in vitro and in vivo evaluation of these formulations, including an excellent review on the physiology of gastrointestinal lipid absorption, which is key to understanding the mechanisms by which lipid-based formulations enhance drug bioavailability. Finally, two case studies detailing oral lipid-based formulation development in an industrial pharmaceutical company setting are presented, providing an appreciation for the challenges encountered in applying this technology as well as practical examples of how these challenges were surmounted.

The editor wishes to acknowledge the many fine women and men, all experts in their fields, who willingly contributed their precious time and knowledge to make this book possible and who persevered through the tedious, and at times challenging, process of authorship.

The editor also wishes to acknowledge Professor Gordon L. Amidon for his encouragement and for valuable discussions during the conceptualization and planning of this book.

David J. Hauss

Contents

Contributors

Hashim Ahmed   Pharmaceutical and Analytical Research and Development, Roche, Nutley, New Jersey, U.S.A.

Jochem Alsenz   Preformulation F. Hofmann-LaRoche Grenzacherstrasse, Basel, Switzerland

Karen Beltz   Institute of Pharmaceutical Technology, Johann Wolfgang Goethe University, Frankfurt am Main, Germany

William J. Bowtle   Department of Research and Development, Encap Drug Delivery, Livingston, U.K.

William N. Charman   Department of Pharmaceutics, Victorian College of Pharmacy, Monash University, Parkville, Victoria, Australia

Jennifer Dressman   Institute of Pharmaceutical Technology, Johann Wolfgang Goethe University, Frankfurt am Main, Germany

Dimitris G. Fatouros   Department of Pharmaceutics and Analytical Chemistry, The Danish University of Pharmaceutical Sciences, Copenhagen, Denmark

Rachna Gajjar   Department of Pathology, University of Cincinnati Medical Center, Cincinnati, Ohio, U.S.A.

Ping Gao   Small Molecule Pharmaceutics, Amgen, Inc., Thousand Oaks, California, U.S.A.

Lowell Gibson   Eli Lilly and Company, Indianapolis, Indiana, U.S.A.

Mette Grove   LEO Pharma A/S, Ballerup, Denmark

A. Waseem Malick   Pharmaceutical and Analytical Research and Development, Roche, Nutley, New Jersey, U.S.A.

Chun-Min Lo   Department of Pathology, University of Cincinnati Medical Center, Cincinnati, Ohio, U.S.A.

Walter Morozowich   Prodrug/Formulation Consultant, Kalamazoo, Michigan, U.S.A.

Anette Müllertz   Department of Pharmaceutics and Analytical Chemistry, The Danish University of Pharmaceutical Sciences, Copenhagen, Denmark

Wantanee Phuapradit   Pharmaceutical and Analytical Research and Development, Roche, Nutley, New Jersey, U.S.A.

Christopher J. H. Porter   Department of Pharmaceutics, Victorian College of Pharmacy, Monash University, Parkville, Victoria, Australia

Karen Schamp   Institute of Pharmaceutical Technology, Johann Wolfgang Goethe University, Frankfurt am Main, Germany

Abu T. M. Serajuddin   Novartis Pharmaceuticals Corporation, East Hanover, New Jersey, U.S.A.

Navnit H. Shah   Pharmaceutical and Analytical Research and Development, Roche, Nutley, New Jersey, U.S.A.

Paul Sirois   Eli Lilly and Company, Indianapolis, Indiana, U.S.A.

Robert G. Strickley   Formulation and Process Development, Gilead Sciences, Inc., Foster City, California, U.S.A.

Patrick Tso   Department of Pathology, University of Cincinnati Medical Center, Cincinnati, Ohio, U.S.A.

Madhav Vasanthavada   Novartis Pharmaceuticals Corporation, East Hanover, New Jersey, U.S.A.

Yu-E Zhang   Pharmaceutical and Analytical Research and Development, Roche, Nutley, New Jersey, U.S.A.

1

Currently Marketed Oral Lipid-Based Dosage Forms: Drug Products and Excipients

Robert G. Strickley

Formulation and Process Development, Gilead Sciences, Inc., Foster City, California, U.S.A.

INTRODUCTION

This chapter focuses on the commercially available lipid-based formulations for oral delivery, along with the lipid excipients in the formulations. The geographical focus is the United States, the United Kingdom, and Japan since formulation information of commercial pharmaceutical products is available for these countries (1–3), but not so readily with other locations (4). The lipid excipients employed in lipid-based oral formulations have been reviewed (5) and include oils composed of medium-chain triglycerides or long-chain triglycerides, lipid soluble solvents, and surfactants. The published information on oral formulations usually includes only the qualitative list of most excipients (1–5); thus determining the exact amounts of excipients in a particular formulation is not possible. In certain cases, more quantitative formulation information is provided, thus allowing for estimates of the amount administered of a specific excipient.

A lipid-based oral formulation is used for water-insoluble drugs in cases where typical formulation approaches (i.e., solid wet granulation, solid dry granulation, water-soluble liquid in a capsule) do not provide the required bioavailability, or when the drug itself is an oil (i.e., dronabinol, ethyl icosapentate, indometacin farnesil, teprenone, and tocopherol nicotinate). Tables 1 to 3 are lists of selected commercially available lipid-based oral formulations in the United States, the United Kingdom and Japan, respectively, arranged alphabetically by drug name and also showing the drug's chemical structure, indication, dose, the marketed formulation, list of excipients, and storage conditions. Tables 2 and 3 also have the year that the commercial drug product was first introduced into the marketplace in Japan or the United Kingdom.

The majority of commercially available oral formulations are solid dosage forms such as tablets or capsules, but there are also many solubilized oral formulations including bulk oral solutions, syrups, elixirs, or solutions filled into soft or hard capsules. The commercially available lipid-based oral formulations are either in capsules or bulk oral solutions. Although the estimates that follow are approximate (2,3), for exact accounting is difficult, it appears that lipid-based oral products account for at least 2% to 4% of the commercially available drugs products in each market surveyed, with approximately 2% in the United Kingdom (total marketed drug products include 864 tablets, 303 capsules, 87 oral solutions, of which at least 21 are lipid based), 3% in the United States (total marketed drug products include 556 tablets, 264 capsules, and 19 oral solutions, of which at least 27 are lipid-based), and 4% in Japan (total marketed drug products include 157 tablets, and 43 capsules, of which 8 at least are lipid based).

Table 4 is a list of the lipid and surfactant excipients used in lipid-based oral formulations, and these excipients include oils composed of medium-chain triglycerides (coconut oil and palm seed oil) or long-chain triglycerides (e.g., corn oil, olive oil, peanut oil, rapeseed oil, sesame oil, soybean oil, hydrogenated soybean oil, and hydrogenated vegetable oil), beeswax, oleic acid, soy fatty acids, d-α-tocopherol, corn oil mono-di-triglycerides, medium-chain mono- and diglycerides, and many surfactants (e.g., cremophor EL, cremophor RH40, cremophor RH60, Polysorbate 20, Polysorbate 80, d-α-tocopherol polyethylene glycol 1000 succinate (TPGS), Span 20, Labrafils®, Labrasol®, and Gelucires®). The lipid excipient d-α-tocopherol also has antioxidant properties, and is in such products as indometacin farnesil 100 mg hard gelatin capsules, and teprenone hard gelatin capsules and fine granules.

This chapter is organized into two main sections, comprising either capsule or oral solution formulations, with each section beginning with simple one-excipient formulations and progressing to more complex formulations.

CAPSULES: SOFT AND HARD

Both soft and hard gelatin capsules are used for lipid-based oral formulations. Liquid formulations can be filled into either soft or hard capsules, whereas semisolids or solid formulations are filled into hard capsules.

(*Text continues on page 16*)

Table 1 List of Selected Commercially Available Lipid-Based Formulations for Oral Administration in the United States in 2005

Molecule/trade name/company/ date of initial marketing	Chemical structure	Indication	Dose	Type of formulation, strength	Lipid excipients and surfactants	Nonlipid excipients	Storage
Amprenavir/ Agenerase®/ GlaxoSmithKline/ 2000 in the U.K.		HIV antiviral	1200 mg (8 capsules) b.i.d.	Soft gelatin capsule, 50, 150 mg	TPGS (280 mg in the 150 mg capsule)	PEG 400 (247, 740 mg), propylene glycol (19, 57 mg)	RT
			Pediatrics: >4 years old, <50 kg at 17 mg/kg (1.1 mL/kg) t.i.d.; >50 kg at 1400 mg (~93 mL) b.i.d.	Oral solution, 15 mg/mL	TPGS (~12%)	PEG 400 (~17%), propylene glycol (~5%), sodium chloride, sodium citrate, citric acid, flavors/ sweeteners	RT
Bexarotene/ Targretin®/Ligand/ 2001 in the U.K.		Antineo plastic	300–750 mg (4–10 capsules) q.d.	Soft gelatin capsule, 75 mg	Polysorbate 20	PEG 400, povidone, BHA	RT, avoid high temperature, humidity and light

(*Continued*)

Table 1 List of Selected Commercially Available Lipid-Based Formulations for Oral Administration in the United States in 2005 (*Continued*)

Molecule/trade name/company/ date of initial marketing	Chemical structure	Indication	Dose	Type of formulation, strength	Lipid excipients and surfactants	Nonlipid excipients	Storage
Calcitriol/ Rocaltrol®/Roche/ 1996 in the U.K. (capsules only)		Calcium regulator	Adults: 0.25–0.5 µg (1 capsule) q.d.	Soft gelatin capsule, 0.25, 0.5 µg	Fractionated triglyceride of coconut oil (medium-chain triglyceride)	BHA, BHT	15–30°C protect from light
			Pediatrics: 10–15 ng/kg (0.01–0.015 mL/kg) q.d.	Oral solution, 1 µg/mL	Fractionated triglyceride of palm seed oil	BHA, BHT	15–30°C protect from light
Ciprofloxacin/ Cipro®/Bayer		Antibiotic	15 mg/kg b.i.d., not to exceed the adult dose of 500 mg per dose	Microcapsules for constitution to a suspension, 5% or 10% in solid, 50 or 100 mg/mL in suspension	Bottle 1— solid: polyvinyl-pyrrolidone, methacrylic acid copolymer, hydroxypropyl methylcellulose, magnesium stearate, and polysorbate 20 Bottle 2— diluent: medium-chain triglycerides, sucrose, lecithin, water, and strawberry flavor		Store below 30°C but not frozen

Drug/Manufacturer/Year	Structure	Indication	Dose	Dosage form	Composition	Solvent	Storage
Cyclosporin A/I. Neoral® Novartis/1995 in the U.K.	$C_{62}H_{117}N_{11}O_{12}$; MW = 1202.64	Immuno-suppressant, prophylaxis for organ transplant rejection	2–10 mg/kg/ day, b.i.d. (1–7 capsules)	Soft gelatin capsule, 10, 25, 50, 100 mg	dl-α-tocopherol, corn oil-mono-di-triglycerides, polyoxyl 40 hydrogenated castor oil (cremophor RH 40)	Ethanol 11.9%, glycerol, propylene glycol	RT
			2–10 mg/kg/day, b.i.d. (1–7 mL)	Oral solution, 100 mg/mL	dl-α-tocopherol, corn oil-mono-di-triglycerides, polyoxyl 40 hydrogenated castor oil	Ethanol 11.9%, propylene glycol	RT, do not store in the refrigerator
CyclosporinA/II. Sandimmune® Novartis			2–10 mg/kg/day, b.i.d. (1–7 capsules)	Soft gelatin capsule, 25, 100 mg	Corn oil, polyoxy-ethylated linoleic glycerides (Labrafil M-2125CS)	Ethanol 12.7%, glycerol	RT
			2–10 mg/kg/day, b.i.d. (1–7 mL)	Oral solution, 100 mg/mL	Olive oil, polyoxy-ethylated oleic glycerides (Labrafil M-1944CS)	Ethanol 12.5%	RT

(Continued)

Table 1 List of Selected Commercially Available Lipid-Based Formulations for Oral Administration in the United States in 2005 (*Continued*)

Molecule/trade name/company/ date of initial marketing	Chemical structure	Indication	Dose	Type of formulation, strength	Lipid excipients and surfactants	Nonlipid excipients	Storage
Cyclosporin A/III Gengraf®/Abbott			2–10 mg/kg/day, b.i.d. (1–7 capsules)	Hard gelatin capsule, 25, 100 mg	Polyoxyl 35 castor oil (cremophor EL), polysorbate 80	Ethanol 12.8%, propylene glycol	RT
Cyclosporin A/IV Cyclosporin capsules/Sidmak			1–9 mg/kg/day 70–700 mg, (1–7 capsules)	Soft gelatin capsule, 100 mg	Caprylic/capric triglycerides (Labrafac), dl-α-tocopherol, glyceryl caprylate, PEG-8 caprylic/ capric glycerides (Labrasol), PEG-35 castor oil (cremophor EL)		RT
Doxercalciferol/ Hectorol®/ Bone care		Management of secondary hyperpara-thyroidism associated with chronic renal dialysis	10–20 μg, three times weekly (4–8 capsules)	Soft gelatin capsule, 0.5, 2.5 μg	Fractionated triglyceride of coconut oil (medium-chain triglyceride)	BHA, ethanol	RT

Drug/Brand/Manufacturer	Structure	Indication	Dose	Dosage form	Vehicle/oil	Other excipients	Storage
Dronabinol/Marinol®/Roxane and Unimed		Anorexia or nausea	2.5–10 mg (1 capsule) b.i.d.	Soft gelatin capsule, 2.5, 5, 10 mg	Sesame oil	None	8–15°C, protect from freezing
Dutasteride/Avodart™/GlaxoSmith Kline/2003 in the U.K. (capsules only)		Treatment of benign prostrate hyperplasia	0.5 mg q.d (1 capsule)	Soft gelatin capsule, 0.5 mg	Mixture of mono- and diglycerides of caprylic/capric acid	BHT	RT
Isotretinoin/Accutane®/Roche/1983 in the U.K.		Anti-comedogenic	0.5–1.0 mg/kg/day subdivided in two doses (1–2 capsules)	Soft gelatin capsule, 10, 20, 40 mg	Beeswax, hydrogenated soybean oil flakes, hydrogenated vegetable oils, soybean oil	BHA, EDTA	RT, protect from light
Lopinavir and ritonavir/Kaletra®/Abbott/2001 in the U.K.		HIV antiviral	400/100 mg b.i.d. (2 tablets) or 800/200 mg q.d. (4 tablets) / 400/100 mg b.i.d. (3 capsules)	Tablet 200 mg lopinavir and 50 mg ritonavir / Soft gelatin capsule, 133.3 mg lopinavir and 33.3 mg ritonavir	Sorbitan monolaurate (Span 20) / Oleic acid, polyoxyl 35 castor oil (cremophor EL)	Sodium stearyl fumarate, copovidone, silicon dioxide / Propylene glycol	RT / 2–8°C, or at room temperature for <2 months

(Continued)

Table 1 List of Selected Commercially Available Lipid-Based Formulations for Oral Administration in the United States in 2005 (*Continued*)

Molecule/trade name/company/ date of initial marketing	Chemical structure	Indication	Dose	Type of formulation, strength	Lipid excipients and surfactants	Nonlipid excipients	Storage
			400/100 mg b.i.d. (5 mL)	Oral solution, 80 mg/mL lopinavir and 20 mg/mL ritonavir	Polyoxyl 40 hydrogenated castor oil (cremophor RH 40), peppermint oil	Alcohol (42.2% v/v), glycerin, propylene glycol, sodium chloride, sodium citrate, citric acid, water, and flavors/ sweeteners	2–8°C, or at room temperature for <2 months
Progesterone/ Prometrium®/ Solvay		Hormone replacement therapy	200–400 mg q.d. (2–4 capsules)	Soft gelatin capsule, 100, 200 mg micronized	Peanut oil	None	RT, protect from light and excessive moisture
Ritonavir/ Norvir®/ Abbott/1999 in the U.K.		HIV antiviral	Adults 600 mg (6 capsules) b.i.d.	Soft gelatin capsule, 100 mg	Oleic acid, polyoxyl 35 castor oil (cremophor EL)	BHT, ethanol	2–8°C, or at room Temperature for <1 month

Drug/Brand/Company	Structure	Indication	Dosage	Dosage form	Composition	Excipient	Storage
Saquinavir/ Fortovase™/ Roche/1998 in the U.K. Discontinued in 2006 (14)			Pediatrics 250–450 mg/m² up to a maximum of 600 mg (<7.5 mL) b.i.d.	Oral solution, 80 mg/mL	Polyoxyl 35 castor oil (cremophor EL) sweetener, dye	Ethanol (43%), water, propylene glycol, citric acid, flavors,	RT
		HIV antiviral	1200 mg (6 capsules) t.i.d. without ritonavir; 1000 mg (5 capsules) b.i.d. with ritonavir	Soft gelatin capsule, 200 mg	Medium-chain mono- and diglycerides, dl-α-tocopherol	Povidone	2–8°C, or at room temperature for <3 months
Sirolimus/ Rapamune®/ Wyeth-Ayerst/ 2001 in the U.K.		Immuno-suppressant	6 mg (6 mL) loading dose followed by 2 mg (2 mL) q.d.	Oral solution, 1 mg/mL	Phosal 50 PG® (phosphatidyl-choline, mono- and diglycerides, soy fatty acids, ascorbyl palmitate), polysorbate 80	Phosal 50 PG® (propylene glycol, ethanol 1.5–2.5%)	2–8°C, or at room temperature for <15 days
Tipranavir/ Aptivus®/ Boehringer Ingelheim/		HIV antiviral	500 mg (2 capsules) with ritonavir 200 mg b.i.d.	Soft gelatin capsule, 200 mg	Polyoxyl 35 castor oil (cremophor EL), medium-chain mono-and diglycerides	Ethanol (7% w/w or 0.1 g per capsule), propylene glycol	2–8°C prior to opening the bottle, room temperature for <60 days

(Continued)

Table 1 List of Selected Commercially Available Lipid-Based Formulations for Oral Administration in the United States in 2005 (*Continued*)

Molecule/trade name/company/date of initial marketing	Chemical structure	Indication	Dose	Type of formulation, strength	Lipid excipients and surfactants	Nonlipid excipients	Storage
Tolterodine tartrate/Detrol® LA/Pharmacia & UpJohn/2001 in the U.K.		Overactive bladder—muscarinic receptor antagonist	2–4 mg q.d. (1 capsule)	Extended release hard gelatin capsules, 2, 4 mg	Medium-chain triglycerides, oleic acid	Sucrose, hypromellose, ethylcellulose	RT
Tretinoin/Vesanoid®/Roche/2001 in the U.K.		Antineo-plastic	45 mg/m² subdivided (8 capsules) b.i.d.	Soft gelatin capsule, 10 mg	Beeswax, hydrogenated soybean oil flakes, hydrogenated vegetable oils, soybean oil	BHA, EDTA	RT
Valproic acid/Depakene®/Abbott		Antiepileptic	10–60 mg/kg/day (3–15 capsules)	Soft gelatin capsule, 250 mg	Corn oil	None	RT

Abbreviations: BHA, butylatedhydroxyanisole; b.i.d., twice daily; BHT, butylatedhydroxytoluene; EDTA, ethylenediamine tetraacetic acid; PEG, polyethyelene glycol; q.d., once daily; q.i.d., four times daily; RT, room temperature; t.i.d., three time daily; TPGS, tocopherol polyethylenenglycol succinate.

Table 2 List of Selected Commercially Available[a] Lipid-Based Formulations for Oral Administration in the United Kingdom in 2005

Molecule/trade name/company/date of initial marketing	Chemical structure	Indication	Dose	Commercial oral formulation	Lipid excipients and surfactants	Nonlipid excipients	Storage
Alfacalcidol/ One-Alpha® capsules/Leo Laboratories/ 2000		Calcium regulator	0.5–1 μg q.d. (1 capsule)	Soft gelatin capsule, 0.25, 0.5, 1.0 μg	Sesame oil dl-α-tocopherol	None	RT
Clofazimine/ Lamprene® capsules 100 mg/ Alliance Pharmaceuticals/ 1998		Treatment of leprosy in combination with dapsone and rifampicin	Maximum 300 mg q.d. for up to 3 mo (3 capsules)	Soft gelatin capsule, 100 mg (micronized suspension in an oil-wax base)	Rapseed oil, wax blend (beeswax, hydrogenated soybean oil, partially hydrogenated plant oils)	BHT, citric acid, PG	Below 25°C
Clomethiazole edisilate/ Heminevrin® capsules/ AstraZeneca/ 2002		Sedative	1–4 capsules as needed	Soft gelatin capsule, 192 mg	Medium-chain triglycerides from fractionated coconut oil	None	RT

(Continued)

Table 2 List of Selected Commercially Available[a] Lipid-Based Formulations for Oral Administration in the United Kingdom in 2005 (*Continued*)

Molecule/trade name/ company/date of initial marketing	Chemical structure	Indication	Dose	Commercial oral formulation	Lipid excipients and surfactants	Nonlipid excipients	Storage
Efavirenz/ Sustiva® oral solution/ Bristol-Meyers Squibb/1999		HIV antiviral	Adults: 600 mg q.d. (up to 20 mL); pediatrics: 270–600 mg (9–20 mL)	Oral solution, 30 mg/mL	Medium-chain triglycerides	Benzoic acid, strawberry/ mint flavor	RT
Fenofibrate/ Fenogal®/ Genus/2002		Antihyper-lipoproteinemic	200 mg (1 capsule) q.d.	Hard gelatin capsule, 200 mg	Lauryl macrogel-glycerides (Gelucire 44/14)	Macrogel 20,000 (PEG 20,000), HPC	RT
Morphine sulfate/MXL® capsules/Napp Pharmaceuticals/ 1996		Analgesic	30–200 mg q.d. (1 capsule)	Hard gelatin capsules containing multiparticulates, 30, 60, 90, 120, 150, and 300 mg	Hydrogenated vegetable oil	PEG 6000, talc, magnesium stearate	RT

Drug/trade name/dose/manufacturer/year	Structure	Indication	Dosage	Formulation	Excipients	Coating	Storage
Testosterone undecanoate/Restandol® 40 mg/Organon Laboratories/1981		Hormone replacement therapy	40–160 mg q.d. (1–4 capsules) (swallow entire capsule or sprinkled onto soft cold food)	Soft gelatin capsules, 40 mg HSE (equivalents of testosterone, 61 mg of testosterone undecanoate)	Oleic acid	None	Store under refrigeration (2–8°C) until dispensed, then at RT after dispensing. Protect from light and heat.
Valproic acid/Convulex® 100 mg, 200 mg, 500 mg/Pharmacia/1991	$H_3C-\underset{H_2}{C}-\underset{H_2}{CH_2}-CH-\underset{}{C}\overset{O}{\underset{}{}}-OH$ $H_3C-\underset{H_2}{C}-\underset{H_2}{C}$	Antiepileptic	10–60 mg/kg/day up to 2500 mg per day (1–5 capsules)	Soft gelatin capsule, 100, 200, and 500 mg	Medium-chain triglycerides	Coating is hydroxypropyl-methyl-cellulose phthalate, and dibutyl-phthalate	RT

aSome of the products available in the United Kingdom are also available in the United States (see Table 1).

Abbreviations: PEG, polyethylene glycol; RT, room temperature; HPC, hydroxypropyl cellulose.

Table 3 List of Selected Commercially Available Lipid-Based Formulations for Oral Administration in Japan in 2005

Molecule/tradename/ company/date of initial marketing	Chemical structure	Indication	Dose	Commercial oral formulation	Lipid excipients and surfactants	Nonlipid excipients	Storage
Ethyl icosapentate/ Epadel® capsules 300/Mochida Pharmaceuticals/ 1990		Hyperlipidemia	600 mg (2 capsules) t.i.d.	Soft gelatin capsules, 300 mg	α-tocopherol	None	RT
Ibudilast/Ketas® capsules 10 mg/ Kyorin Pharmaceutical/ 1989		Asthma, and cerebovascular disorders	10 mg (1–2 capsules) b.i.d. or t.i.d.	Extended release, hard gelatin capsules, 10 mg white sustained release granules and enteric coated sustained release granules	Polyoxyl 60 hydrogenated castor oil (cremophor RH 60)	Lactose, MCC, povidone, aminoalkyl-methacrylate-copolymer RS, PEG 6000, sodium chloride, and silicon dioxide, magnesium stearate	RT
Indometacin farnesil/Infree® capsules/Eisai Co./1991		Anti-inflammatory and analgesic	200 mg (1–2 capsules) b.i.d.	Hard gelatin capsule, 100 mg (solid)	α-tocopherol	Hydrated silicon dioxide, MCC, tartaric acid, PEG 6000	RT
				Soft gelatin capsules, 200 mg (liquid)	Polyoxyl 60 hydrogenated castor oil (cremophor RH 60),	Aspartic acid	RT

Drug/brand/manufacturer/year	Indication	Dose	Dosage form	Oily vehicle	Active/lipid component	Excipients	Storage
Menatetrenone/Glakay® capsules 15 mg/Eisai Co./1995	Osteoporosis	45 mg (3 capsules) t.i.d.	Soft gelatin capsule, 15 mg (contents of capsule are a viscous liquid or semisolid)	hydrogenated oil, glyceryl monooleate	Propylene glycol esters of fatty acid, glyceryl monooleate		RT, protect from light
Teprenone/Selbex® capsules 50 mg and fine granules 10%/Eisai Co./1984	Acute gastritis	150 mg (3 capsules) t.i.d	Hard capsule, 50 mg (contents of capsule are granules or powder)		α-tocopherol	Hydrated silicon dioxide, talc, mannitol, PEG 6000, lactose	RT
		150 mg (1.5 grams of granules) t.i.d.	Fine granules, 10% w/w		α-tocopherol	Hydrated silicon dioxide, talc, hydroxy-propylcellulose, mannitol, lactose	RT
Tocopherol nicotinate/Juvela® N Soft capsules/Eisai Co./1984	Hypertension, hyperlipidemia	200 mg (1 capsule) t.i.d.	Soft gelatin capsule, 200 mg (contents of capsule are a viscous suspension or semisolid)	Medium-chain triglycerides, glycol esters of fatty acid	Aspartic acid		RT

Abbreviations: MCC, microcrystalline cellulose; PEG, polyethylene glycol; RT, room temperature.

Table 4   Solubilizing Excipients Used in Commercially Available Lipid-Based Oral Formulations

Water-insoluble excipients	Triglycerides	Surfactants
Beeswax	*Long-chain triglycerides*	Glyceryl monooleate
Oleic acid	Corn oil	Polyoxyl 35 castor oil
Soy fatty acids	Olive oil	(cremophor EL)
d-α-tocopherol	Peanut oil	Polyoxyl 40
(vitamin E)	Rapseed oil	hydrogenated castor
Corn oil mono-di-	Sesame oil	oil (cremophor RH40)
triglycerides	Soybean oil	Polyoxyl 60
Medium-chain	Hydrogenated	hydrogenated castor
(C_8/C_{10}) mono- and	soybean oil	oil (cremophor RH60)
diglycerides	Hydrogenated	Polysorbate 20
Propylene	vegetable oils	(tween 20)
glycol esters of		Polysorbate 80
fatty acids		(tween 80)
	Medium-chain triglycerides	d-α-tocopheryl
	Caprylic/capric	polyethylene glycol
	triglycerides derived	1000 succinate (TPGS)
	from coconut oil or	Sorbitan monolaurate
	palm seed oil	(Span 20)
		PEG 300 oleic
		glycerides (Labrafil®
		M-1944CS)
		PEG 300 linoleic
		glycerides (Labrafil®
		M-2125CS)
		PEG 400
		caprylic/capric
		glycerides
		(Labrasol®)
		PEG 1500 lauric
		glycerides
		(Gelucire® 44/14)

Abbreviations: PEG, polyethyelene glycol; TPGS, tocopherol polyethylenenglycol succinate.

One-Lipid Excipient Formulations

The simplest lipid-based formulations contain only one excipient such as oleic acid, α-tocopherol, corn oil, peanut oil, sesame oil, medium-chain triglyceride, or medium-chain mono- and diglycerides. There are at least 10 commercially available (by prescription) one-lipid excipient oral formulations, and all are marketed in soft capsules. Many of the over-the-counter soft gelatin capsules use polyethylene glycol or medium-chain triglycerides as the solubilizing excipient.

1. Clomethiazole edisilate is the ethanedisulfonate salt of clomethiazole, which is an oily viscous liquid as the free base, but the edisilate salt is a solid with a melting point of 124°C (6) and is the commercial form in Heminevrin® capsules, with 192 mg (60 mg equivalent of clomethiazole) dissolved in medium-chain triglycerides and filled into soft gelatin capsules. Clomethiazole is a short acting hypnotic and sedative with anticonvulsant effects, and Heminevrin is indicated for treatment of the restlessness and insomnia that accompany alcohol withdrawal. Clomethiazole has a short half-life and low bioavailability due to extensive hepatic first-pass metabolism (3). The dose of Heminevrin is one to four capsules as needed, and the capsules are stored at room temperature. Heminevrin capsules have been available in the United Kingdom since 1998.

2. Dronabinol, also known as Δ-9-tetrahydrocannabinol, is the principal psychoactive component of cannabis and finds therapeutic application as an antiemetic for treatment of the nausea and vomiting associated with cancer chemotherapy or as an appetite stimulant to treat AIDS wasting syndrome. Dronabinol is highly hydrophobic oil at ambient room temperature and after oral administration, is almost completely absorbed (90% to 95%). However, the bioavailability is only about 10% to 20% due to extensive hepatic first-pass hepatic metabolism (2). Dronabinol is formulated as a solution in sesame oil in 2.5 mg, 5 mg, and 10 mg Marinol® soft gelatin capsules. The dose is 2.5 to 10 mg (one capsule) twice daily. Marinol should be stored at 8 to 15°C and must be protected from freezing. Marinol is available in the United States.

3. Ethyl icosapentate exists as a liquid at ambient room temperature and is formulated as a solution in α-tocopherol in 300 mg Epadel® soft gelatin capsules. Ethyl icosapentate is used in the treatment of hyperlipidemia and arteriosclerosis obliterans. The dose of ethyl icosapentate is 600 mg (two capsules) three times daily and the product should be stored at controlled room temperature in moisture-proof containers protected from light. Epadel has been available in Japan since 1990.

4. Progesterone is a water-insoluble steroid that is sparingly soluble in vegetable oils. Progesterone is formulated as a partially solubilized, micronized suspension in peanut oil in 100 mg Prometrium® soft gelatin capsules, which is available in the United States. The absolute oral bioavailability of progesterone has not been determined, but the systemic exposure is increased following micronization (2). The dose of progesterone is 200 to 400 mg (two to four capsules) once daily and Prometrium® should be stored at controlled room temperature in moisture-proof containers protected from light. Progesterone, formulated in vegetable fat, is available in the United Kingdom as Cyclogest® 200 mg and 400 mg pessaries and is indicated for the treatment of premenstrual syndrome.

5. Testosterone undecanoate is an ester prodrug of testosterone intended for oral administration in hormone replacement therapy. Free testosterone is inactive following oral administration due to virtually complete hepatic first-pass extraction. However, the undecanoate ester prodrug is transported via the intestinal lymphatic system, thereby circumventing the hepatic portal circulation and the associated presystemic first pass metabolism (3). Testosterone undecanoate is solubilized in oleic acid in Restandol® 40 mg soft gelatin capsules that contain 61 mg of testosterone undecanoate, which is equivalent to 40 mg of testosterone. The oral daily dose of testosterone undecanoate (one to four capsules) is equivalent to 40 to 160 mg of free testosterone. Restandol must be stored refrigerated prior to dispensing, after which it may be stored at controlled room temperature. Restandol has been available in the United Kingdom since 1981.

6. Valproic acid, an anticonvulsant with an intrinsic water solubility of 1.3 mg/mL (2), is formulated as a solution in corn oil and is available in the United States as 250 mg Depakene® soft gelatin capsules. In the United Kingdom, valproic acid is formulated as a solution in medium-chain triglycerides as 100 mg, 200 mg and 500 mg Convulex® enteric coated soft gelatin capsules, where it has been available since 1991. The dose of valproic acid is 600 to 2500 mg daily, and both products should be stored at controlled room temperature.

7. Calcitriol is a nonionizable and water-insoluble synthetic vitamin D analog which is active in the regulation of the absorption of calcium and its utilization in the body and is intended for the treatment of hypocalcemia. Calcitriol is formulated as a solution in a fractionated medium-chain triglyceride of coconut oil, along with the antioxidants butylated hydroxyanisole (BHA) and butylated hydroxytoluene (BHT), as 0.25 and 0.5 μg Rocaltrol® soft gelatin capsules, which have been available in the United Kingdom since 1996, and are also available in the United States. Rocaltrol is also available (U.S. only) as a 1 μg/mL oral solution formulated in a fractionated triglyceride of palm seed oil. Calcitriol is not available in Japan but a similar molecule, falecalcitriol, is available and marketed as a conventional solid tablet formulation. The dose of calcitriol is 0.25 to 0.5 μg (one capsule) and Rocaltrol should be stored at controlled room temperature.

8. Dutasteride, a water-insoluble steroid derivative used in the treatment of benign prostatic hyperplasia, is formulated as a solution in capric and caprylic mono- and diglycerides (medium-chain mono- and diglycerides) as 0.5 mg Avodart® soft gelatin capsules. The average bioavailability of dutasteride from Avodart is 60%, with a range of 40% to 94% (2,3). The dose of dutasteride is 0.5 mg (one capsule) once daily and the product should be stored at controlled room temperature. Avodart has been available in the United Kingdom since 2003, and is also available in the United States.

9. Various nutritional supplements available by prescription are formulated in soft gelatin capsules using, as solubilizing excipients, linoleic acid, vitamin E (dl-alpha-tocopherol acetate), or soybean oil. Encora® is a nutritional supplement with essential fatty acids and is available in a blister package with two tablets and two capsules on each blister card designated for AM and PM oral administration. The Encora capsules are pink, liquid-filled soft gelatin containing 650 mg of omega-3 fatty acid (equivalent to approximately 180 mg of docosahexaenoic acid and 360 mg of eicosapentaenoic), 10 mg of linoleic acid, and 50 IU of vitamin E. Chromagen® soft gelatin capsules, indicated in the treatment of anemia, contain 70 mg of iron and 150 mg of calcium ascorbate dissolved in soybean oil.

Two-Excipient Formulations

The next level of complexity in lipid-based formulations is those that contain two excipients. Some typical combinations are sesame oil with α-tocopherol, medium-chain triglyceride with ethanol, and propylene glycol esters of fatty acids with glyceryl mono-oleate. There are at least three commercially available two-lipid excipient oral formulations, all of which are delivered in soft gelatin capsules.

1. Alfacalcidol, a dehydroxy derivative of calcitriol, is formulated as a solution in a mixture of sesame oil and α-tocopherol in 0.25 μg, 0.5 μg, and 1.0 μg One-Alpha®soft gelatin capsules which have been available in the United Kingdom since 2000. The dose of alfacalcidol is 0.25 to 1.0 μg (one capsule) daily and One-Alpha soft gelatin capsules should be stored at controlled room temperature. In Japan, alfacalcidol (Alfarol®) is available in capsule, solution, and powder formulations that employ potassium sorbate as the major excipient.

2. Doxercalciferol is similar to calcitriol and alfacalcidol in chemical structure, clinical application, and formulation, and is formulated as a solution in ethanol and a fractionated medium-chain triglyceride of coconut oil as 2.5 μg Hectorol® soft gelatin capsules. The dose of doxercalciferol is 10 to 20 μg (four to eight capsules) three times weekly and Hectorol should be stored at controlled room temperature. Hectorol is available in the United States.

3. Menatetrenone (also known as vitamin K_2), a practically water insoluble prenylated napththoquinone used in the treatment of osteoporosis, is formulated as a solution in propylene glycol esters of fatty acids and glyceryl mono-oleate as 15 mg Glakay® soft gelatin capsules. The bioavailability of menatetrenone is highly dependent on the dietary status of the patient at the time of dosing, with an approximate seven-fold increase in the systemic exposure (as determined from the plasma concentration area-under-the-curve) being observed following postprandial dosing as compared to the fasted state (3). The influence

of dietary fat on the bioavailability of menatetrenone is dependent upon the quantity of fat consumed at the time of dosing, with a three-fold increase in exposure occurring when the amount of ingested fat was increased from 9 g to 35–54 g. The dose of menatetrenone is 45 mg (three capsules) three times daily after meals and Glakay should be stored at ambient room temperature protected from light. Glakay has been available in Japan since 1995.

Three-Excipient Formulations

Ascending the scale of complexity of lipid-based formulations are those that contain mixtures of three excipients. Typical examples of such combinations include: (*i*) TPGS, polyethylene glycol (PEG) 400, and PG; (*ii*) oleic acid, cremophor EL, and ethanol or PG; (*iii*) polysorbate 20, PEG 400, and povidone; (*iv*) medium-chain mono- and diglycerides, α-tocopherol, and povidone; (*v*) medium-chain triglycerides, glycol esters of fatty acids, and aspartic acid. There are at least five commercially available, three-excipient lipid-based oral formulations, and all are delivered in soft gelatin capsules.

1.   Amprenavir, a poorly water-soluble HIV protease inhibitor, is formulated as a solution in a combination of (approximate proportions) 23% TPGS, 60% PEG 400 and 5% propylene glycol as 50 mg and 150 mg Agenerase® soft gelatin capsules. The micelle-forming excipient, TPGS, was first synthesized in 1950 by the Eastman Chemical Company as a water-dispersible form of vitamin E with improved gastrointestinal absorption (7). TPGS is currently recognized by formulators as "an effective oral absorption enhancer for improving the bioavailability of poorly absorbed drugs and as a vehicle for lipid-based drug delivery" (8). TPGS forms micelles at concentrations ≥ 0.2 mg/mL in water and improves the aqueous solubility of amprenavir from 36 to 720 μg/mL (8). It was also shown, by directional transport studies employing caco-2 cell monolayers, that TPGS is a potent inhibitor of active efflux even at concentrations 10-fold below the critical micelle concentration (9), suggesting that monomeric TPGS is capable of inhibiting the efflux mechanism. Therefore, TPGS not only improves the gastrointestinal absorption of amprenavir by improving its aqueous solubility but also by increasing its permeability through inhibition of intestinal efflux. The bioavailability of amprenavir in conventional capsule or tablet formulations is near zero, but has been shown to increase to 69% $\pm$ 8% following oral administration of 25 mg/kg to beagle dogs in formulations containing 20% TPGS, with a further increase in bioavailability to 80% $\pm$ 16% occurring when the content of TPGS was increased to 50% (9). The dose of amprenavir is 1200 mg (eight capsules) twice daily and Agenerase® soft gelatin capsules should be stored at controlled room temperature. Agenerase soft gelatin capsules and oral solution have been

available in the United Kingdom since 2000 and are also available in the United States.

2. Bexarotene, a benzoic acid derivative, is a selective activator of the retinoid X receptor indicated for the treatment of T-cell lymphoma. The free acid form of bexarotene is solubilized in a mixture of polysorbate 20 and PEG 400 in combination with povidone and BHA as an antioxidant in 75 mg Targretin® soft gelatin capsules. The dose of bexarotene is 300 to 750 mg (4 to 10 capsules) once daily and Targretin soft gelatin capsules should be stored at controlled room temperature. Targretin has been available in the United Kingdom since 2001, and is also available in the United States.

3. Ritonavir, an HIV protease inhibitor with a peptide-like structure, has an intrinsic water solubility of $1.0\,\mu g/mL$ and two weakly basic thiazole groups with pKa's of 1.8 and 2.6, which preclude the possibility of solubilization through manipulation of the formulation pH (10). The initial hard gelatin capsule formulation of ritonavir (Norvir®) was marketed as an amorphous, semi-solid dispersion containing 100 mg of ritonavir solubilized in a mixture of caprylic/capric medium-chain triglycerides, polyoxyl 35 castor oil, citric acid, ethanol, polyglycolyzed glycerides, polysorbate 80 and propylene glycol (11). However, unexpected precipitation of amorphous ritonavir as a less soluble crystalline form in the excipient matrix negatively impacted both the drug dissolution rate and bioavailability, leading to a temporary withdrawal of the product from the market in 1998 (12,13). Norvir was reintroduced in 1999 after reformulation as a thermodynamically stable solution containing 100 mg of ritonavir solubilized in a mixture of oleic acid, cremophor EL, ethanol and the antioxidant, BHT, delivered in soft gelatin capsules. The dose of ritonavir is 600 mg (six capsules) twice daily and Norvir soft gelatin capsules must be stored refrigerated at 2 to 8°C, or at room temperature for no more than one month. Norvir is available in the United Kingdom and the United States, and also in the fixed-dose combination product, Kaletra® (see next paragraph).

4. Lopinavir and ritonavir are water-insoluble HIV protease inhibitors used in the treatment of HIV infection. Kaletra, the combination formulation of lopinavir and ritonavir is replacing Norvir (ritonavir; see previous paragraph). Kaletra soft gelatin capsules are a fixed-dose combination product containing 133.3 mg of lopinavir and 33.3 mg ritonavir, solubilized in a mixture of oleic acid, cremophor EL, and propylene glycol. The dose of Kaletra is three capsules twice daily and Kaletra soft gelatin must be stored refrigerated at 2 to 8°C or at controlled room temperature for no more than two months. In part due to this storage restriction, in 2005/2006 a lipid-containing solid tablet of kaletra was introduced that is stored at room temperature and is made by a melt extrusion process. Kaletra tablets contain 200 mg lopinavir and 50 mg

ritonavir in a matrix of sorbitan monolaurate (Span 20), povidone, sodium stearyl fumarate and silicon dioxide. The dose of Kaletra tablets is 2 tablets twice daily or 4 tablets once daily. Ritonavir inhibits hepatic cytochrome P450 3A (CYP3A) and the intestinal P-glycoprotein (P-gp) efflux pump and increases the oral bioavailability of lopinavir. The oral bioavailability of lopinavir is increased when coadministered with ritonavir. Kaletra has been available in the United Kingdom since 2001, and is also available in the United States.

5. Saquinavir is a water-insoluble HIV protease inhibitor that was first introduced in 1996 as a solid oral dosage form (Invirase®) and subsequently, as a lipid-based formulation in a soft gelatin capsule (Fortovase®) containing 200 mg of saquinavir solubilized in a mixture of α-tocopherol and medium-chain mono- and diglycerides in combination with povidone. However, in 2006 Fortovase was removed from the market due to lack of demand (14); however, but saquinavir is still available as 200 mg and 500 mg Invirase hard gelatin capsules. The dose of Fortovase was 1200 mg (six capsules) three times daily or, if taken in combination with ritonavir (which is known to increase the bioavailability of saquinavir), 1000 mg (five capsules) twice daily. Fortovase capsules were stored refrigerated at 2 to 8°C, or at room temperature for no more than three months.

6. Tocopherol nicotinate is the nicotinic acid ester of α-tocopherol and is indicated in the treatment of hypertension, hyperlipidemia, and peripheral circulatory disturbances. The bioavailability of tocopherol nicotinate is subject to considerable food effect, increasing approximately 30-fold following postprandial administration, as compared to the fasted state. Tocopherol nicotinate, which exists as an orange-yellow liquid or solid that is practically insoluble in water, is formulated as a viscous suspension or semisolid in a mixture of medium-chain triglycerides and glycol esters of fatty acids, in combination with aspartic acid, in 200 mg Juvela®N soft gelatin capsules. The dose of tocopherol nicotinate is 200 mg (one capsule) three times daily and Juvela N may be stored at controlled room temperature. Juvela N has been available in Japan since 1984.

Four-Excipient Formulations

The most complex lipid-based formulations currently marketed contain mixtures of four excipients such as (*i*) ethanol, cremophor EL, propylene glycol, and mono/diglycerides of caprylic/capric acid; (*ii*) rapeseed oil, beeswax, hydrogenated soybean oil, and partially hydrogenated plant oils; and (*iii*) cremophor RH 60, hydrogenated oil, and glyceryl mono-oleate in combination with aspartic acid. There are at least five commercially available four-excipient lipid-based oral formulations and all are delivered in soft gelatin capsules.

1. Tipranavir is a water-insoluble HIV protease inhibitor that was approved in 2005 and is formulated as a solution in a combination of ethanol (7% w/w or 0.1 g per capsule), cremophor EL, propylene glycol, and mono/diglycerides of caprylic/capric acid as 250 mg Aptivus® soft gelatin capsules (15). The dose of Aptivus is two capsules per day coadministered with 200 mg of ritonavir, twice daily. Tipranavir has limited absorption in humans because it is a substrate and a potent inducer of the intestinal P-gp efflux pump, as well as a substrate for CYP3A4 metabolism. The oral bioavailability of tipranavir is not published, but coadministration with ritonavir is essential in order to achieve effective tipranavir plasma concentrations since ritonavir inhibits the intestinal P-gp efflux pump and CYP3A. There was a 29-fold increase in the trough plasma concentrations of tipranavir when 500 mg was coadministered with 200 mg of ritonavir in healthy adults (15). Aptivus capsules coadministered with ritonavir should be give with food since the bioavailability of tipranavir was increased approximately 30% by a high fat diet. Aptivus capsules must be stored refrigerated at 2 to 8°C prior to opening the bottle and after opening the bottle, at room temperature for less than 60 days.

2. Clofazimine, used in the treatment of leprosy, is practically insoluble in water. It is formulated as a suspension in an oil-wax matrix composed of rapeseed oil, beeswax, hydrogenated soybean oil, and partially hydrogenated plant oils in 100 mg Lamprene® soft gelatin capsules. The oral bioavailability of clofazimine from Lamprene is 70%, increasing substantially when administered with food (3). The dose of clofazimine is up to 300 mg (three capsules) daily and Lamprene must be stored below 25°C and protected from moisture. Clofazimine has been available in the United Kingdom since 1998.

3. Indometacin farnesil is an ester prodrug of the active moiety, indometacin, which finds therapeutic application as an anti-inflammatory and analgesic. Indometacin farnesil exists as an oily liquid that is practically insoluble in water. Indometacin farnesil is formulated as a viscous solution in a mixture of cremophor RH 60, hydrogenated oil, and glyceryl mono-oleate in combination with aspartic acid in 200 mg Infree® soft gelatin capsules. The oral bioavailability of indometacin farnesil is decreased when administered in the fasted state, but absorption is improved following a standard meal containing only 10 g of fat (3). The dose of indometacin farnesil is 200 mg (one capsule) twice daily and Infree may be stored at controlled room temperature. Indometacin farnesil has been available in the Japan since 1991.

4. Isotretinoin, an isomer of tretinoin, is an anticomedogenic indicated in the treatment of severe cystic acne. Isotretinoin demonstrates rapid

but erratic absorption that is approximately doubled following post-prandial administration, as compared to the fasted state (2). The absolute bioavailability of isotretinoin has not been reported. Isotretinoin is formulated as a solution in a combination of beeswax, soybean oil, hydrogenated vegetable oils, and hydrogenated soybean oil as 10, 20, and 40 mg Accutane® soft gelatin capsules. The dose of isotretinoin is 0.5 to 1.0 mg/kg/day (one to two capsules) and Accutane should be stored at controlled room temperature protected from light. Isotretinoin is available in the United States, and has been available in the United Kingdom since 1983. There are currently available two generic versions of this product, both having formulations nearly identical to that of Accutane.

5.   Tretinoin is a water-insoluble antineoplastic agent that is formulated as a solution in a combination of beeswax, soybean oil, and hydrogenated vegetable and soybean oils as 10 mg Vesanoid® soft gelatin capsules. The oral bioavailability of tretinoin has been reported to be >60% based on recovery of approximately two-third of an administered dose in the urine (2). The dose of tretinoin is 45 mg/m²/day (eight capsules twice daily) and Vesanoid should be stored at room temperature protected from light. Tretinoin is available in the United States, and has been available in the United Kingdom since 2001.

Extended Release Formulations

There are at least three commercially available extended release formulations that contain lipid excipient(s), and all are delivered in hard gelatin capsules.

1.   Ibudilast is used in the treatment of asthma and cerebrovascular disorders. Ibudilast is very slightly soluble in water and is formulated in a controlled release matrix with the surfactant, cremophor RH60, in combination with several other excipients to prepare sustained release granules and enteric coated sustained release granules that are filled into hard gelatin capsules and marketed as Ketas® 10 mg capsules. The usual dose of Ketas is one capsule (10 mg) three times daily and the product should be stored at room temperature. Ketas has been available in Japan since 1989.

2.   Tolterodine tartrate is indicated in the treatment of overactive urinary bladder, is soluble in water to the extent of 12 mg/mL and is available as both immediate-release tablets and prolonged-release capsules (2) in which the compound is formulated with the lipid excipients, oleic acid, and medium-chain triglycerides, in combination with sucrose spheres, hydroxymethylcellulose, and ethylcellulose as 2 mg and 4 mg Detrol® LA (Detrusitol® XL in the United Kingdom) hard gelatin capsules. The systemic exposures from the immediate-release tablets and prolonged-release capsules are bioequivalent in terms of

areas under the plasma concentration versus time profiles (AUC). However, the rates of exposure differ, with the prolonged-release capsules producing a t_{max} of four hours, as compared to one to two hours for the immediate-release tablets, and C_{max} and C_{min} values that are respectively, 75% and 150% that of the immediate-release tablets (2). There is no effect of food on the pharmacokinetics of either formulation of tolterodine tartrate. The dose of Detrol LA is 2 to 4 mg (one capsule) daily and the product should be stored at controlled room temperature. Tolterodine tartrate immediate -release tablets have been available in the United Kingdom since 1998 with the prolonged-release capsules being introduced in 2001. The products are also available in the United States.

3.   Morphine sulfate is a water-soluble analgesic that is available in many dosage forms, including one lipid-containing, extended release formulation. MXL® hard gelatin capsules contain 30, 60, or 90 mg of morphine sulfate in a semi-solid matrix of hydrogenated vegetable oil in combination with PEG6000, talc, and magnesium stearate. The oral bioavailability of morphine, delivered from a solution or other immediate-release formulation, is approximately 40% and patient-dependent due to extensive glucuronidation (2), but increases to 100% when delivered from the MXL extended-release formulation (3). The dose of morphine ranges from 30 to 200 mg once a day, which is one to two capsules. The MXL hard gelatin capsules can be swallowed whole or the capsule opened and the contents sprinkled onto soft, cold food, and the product should be stored at controlled room temperature. MXL hard gelatin capsules have been available in the United Kingdom since 1996.

Microemulsion Formulations

Microemulsions (discussed in greater detail elsewhere in this book) are thermodynamically stable, isotropically clear dispersions composed of a polar solvent, an oil, a surfactant, and a cosurfactant. Microemulsions have demonstrated considerable potential for drug delivery due to their ability to solubilize highly hydrophobic drugs in both oral (16) and parenteral intravenous formulations (17–20). A microemulsion preconcentrate is a formulation in which the polar solvent, which is normally water, is replaced by one with greater solubilizing power. Ethanol is a typical example of such a solvent as it is frequently capable of solubilizing many drugs to concentrations in excess of 100 mg/mL. Upon contact with aqueous media (e.g., gastrointestinal fluids), microemulsion preconcentrates spontaneously form oil-in-water microemulsions. There are currently at least three marketed microemulsion preconcentrate formulations, all of which are cyclosporin A products.

Cyclosporin A is a sparingly water-soluble, lipophilic, cyclic peptide with a molecular weight of 1201 Da indicated for the prevention of organ transplant rejection that was originally formulated in a mixture of 12.7% ethanol (12.7%), corn oil, glycerol, and Labrafil M-2125CS as 25 mg, 50 mg, and 100 mg Sandimmune® soft gelatin capsules. The absolute oral bioavailability of cyclosporin A as Sandimmune is erratic, being <10% in liver transplant patients or as high as 89% in some renal transplant patients (2). To improve and normalize the oral bioavailability of cyclosporin A, a microemulsion preconcentrate was developed that contains ethanol (11.9%), dl-α-tocopherol, corn oil-mono-di-triglycerides, polyoxyl 40 hydrogenated castor oil (cremophor RH 40), and propylene glycol in 10 mg, 25 mg, 50 mg, and 100 mg Neoral® soft gelatin capsules. The bioavailability of cyclosporine from the Neoral formulation is 20% to 50% greater than that of the original Sandimmune formulation (2). In addition, the Neoral cyclosporine A peak plasma concentrations are 40% to 106% higher than those of the Sandimmune formulation. The dose of cyclosporin A is 2 to 10 mg/kg/day (one to seven capsules) and Neoral capsules are to be stored at room temperature. Neoral has been available in the United Kingdom since 1995, and is also available in the United States.

Cyclosporin A is also available in another proprietary formulation that upon dilution with water forms a dispersion similar to a microemulsion (2). This hard gelatin capsule product, marketed in the United States under the trade name of Gengraf®, is composed of a solution of cyclosporin A in ethanol (12.8%), polyethylene glycol, polyoxyl 35 castor oil (cremophor EL), polysorbate 80, and propylene glycol and is available in 25 mg or 100 mg dosage strengths. Gengraf and Neoral are bioequivalent, with virtually identical pharmacokinetic profiles. Gengraf capsules should be stored at room temperature.

Labrasol and Gelucire 44/14 are spontaneously self-emulsifying surfactants contained in many oral drug products throughout the world. Solufen®-Gé capsules, marketed in Europe, contain 200 mg of ibuprofen solubilized in 244 mg of Gelucire 44/14. Up to six capsules per day may be administered, which corresponds to a maximum daily intake of 1464 mg of Gelucire 44/14 (Table 5). The lipid-lowering agent fenofibrate, which is a water insoluble prodrug of fenofibric acid, is available in Europe as hard gelatin capsules containing 200 mg of the fenofibrate solubilized in Gelucire 44/14 and PEG 20,000 and is marketed as Fenogal®, Lipirex®, CiL® Kapselin, and Fenofibrat AZU® Kapselin. Cyclosporin A is marketed by Sidmak as soft gelatin capsules containing 100 mg of the drug solubilized in a mixture of medium-chain triglycerides (Labrafac®), dl-α-tocopherol, Labrasol, and cremophor EL. Each capsule contains approximately 250 mg of Labrasol and up to seven capsules per day are administered, which corresponds to an estimated maximum daily intake of approximately 1.8 grams of Labrasol (Table 5).

ORAL SOLUTIONS

Oral solutions are normally intended for pediatric patients or for those patients who cannot swallow a tablet or capsule. Most oral solutions contain coloring or

Table 5 Estimated Maximum Amount of Selected Excipients Administered from Oral Formulations

Excipient	Estimated maximum amount administered orally	Product (drug)
Ethanol	3.2 mL, b.i.d.	Norvir® oral solution (ritonavir)
Gelucire 44/14	1464 mg/day	Solufen 200 mg (ibuprofen)
Labrasol®	1800 mg/day	Cyclosporin A (generic)
Medium-chain triglyceride	20 mL, q.d.	Sustiva 30 mg/mL oral solution (efavirenz)
PEG 400	15,640 mg, b.i.d.	Agenerase® oral solution (amprenavir)
Propylene glycol	50,600 mg, b.i.d.	Agenerase® oral solution (amprenavir)
TPGS	11,000 mg, b.i.d.	Agenerase® oral solution (amprenavir)

Abbreviations: b.i.d., twice daily; PEG, polyethyelene glycol; q.d., once daily; TPGS, tocopherol polyethylenenglycol succinate.

flavoring agents and are dispensed in multi-dose containers which must either be preserved or demonstrated incapable of supporting microbial proliferation. Some lipid-containing oral solutions are relatively simple formulations, containing a single excipient (e.g., medium-chain triglycerides), while others are complex mixtures of surfactants, solvents, flavors, sweeteners, and salts. While the majority of oral solutions are aqueous based, at least seven are lipid-based or contain a significant amount of a lipid as a critical formulation component.

1. Calcitriol, in addition to being available as Rocaltrol soft gelatin capsules, is available in the United States as a 1 μg/mL oral solution in a fractionated triglyceride of palm seed oil to which have been added the antioxidants, BHA, and BHT. The pediatric dose in patients over three years of age is 0.25 to 0.5 μg (0.25 to 0.5 mL) daily. For children less than three years of age, the dose is 10 to 15 ng/kg (0.01 to 0.15 mL/kg) daily. Rocaltrol oral solution is dispensed in a 15 mL multi-dose container and is supplied with 20 single-use graduated oral dispensers. Rocaltrol oral solution should be stored at controlled room temperature protected from light.

2. Efavirenz is a water-insoluble non-nucleoside reverse transcriptase inhibitor widely used in the treatment of HIV infection. Efavirenz is available as Sustiva® 600 mg tablets in the United Kingdom and the United States but has also been available in the United Kingdom since 1999 as a 30 mg/mL oral solution in medium-chain triglycerides in

combination with benzoic acid and strawberry/mint flavor. The daily dose of efavirenz is 600 mg (20 mL) for adults and for children is 270 to 600 mg (9 to 20 mL). These dosing regimens deliver the maximum amount of medium-chain triglycerides per unit dose of any currently marketed oral lipid-based formulation (Table 5). The colorless Sustiva oral solution is packaged in a 180 mL multi-dose container that should be stored at controlled room temperature.

3. Sirolimus is a nonionizable and water-insoluble immunosuppressant that is formulated in Rapamune® as a 1 mg/mL solution in polysorbate 80 and the proprietary excipient combination, Phosal 50 PG®, which is composed of phosphatidylcholine, propylene glycol, mono- and diglycerides, 1.5% to 2.5% ethanol, soy fatty acids and ascorbyl palmitate. The oral bioavailability of sirolimus from Rapamune oral solution is approximately 14% when dosed in the fasted state, increasing to approximately 20% when given with a high-fat meal (2). Rapamune is also available in a nanoparticulate tablet formulation from which the highest bioavailability of 27% is achieved (2). The loading dose of sirolimus is 6 mg (6 mL) followed by a maintenance dose of 2 mg (2 mL) daily. Rapamune is supplied in a 60 mL multi-dose container and should be stored refrigerated at 2 to 8°C and used within 30 days of opening. Alternatively, Rapamune may be stored at controlled room temperature for up to 15 days. Rapamune is available in the United States and has been available in the United Kingdom since 2001.

4. Amprenavir is available as both Agenerase® soft gelatin capsules (see previously) or as Agenerase oral solution. As an oral solution, amprenavir is solubilized to the extent of 15 mg/mL in a combination of (approximate percentages) 12% TPGS, approximately 17% PEG 400 and approximately 55% propylene glycol and flavored with grape, bubblegum, and peppermint. In children over four years of age, the dose of amprenavir is 17 mg/kg (1.1 mL/kg) three times daily, which delivers a total daily amount of 8 g of TPGS, 36 g of propylene glycol, and 11 g of PEG 400 assuming a total patient body weight of 20 kg. Due to the potential toxicity of the large dose of coadministered propylene glycol (approximately 1650 mg/kg per day), Agenerase oral solution is contraindicated in infants and children below the age of four years. The oral bioavailability of amprenavir from the oral solution is approximately 14% less than that from the capsule formulation (2), thus requiring the maximum adult dose of the oral solution to be adjusted to 1400 mg, which is approximately 92 mL, twice daily. The total excipient amounts coadministered in conjunction with a daily adult dose of amprenavir is 22 g of TPGS, 102 g of propylene glycol, and 32 g of PEG 400, representing the estimated highest amounts of TPGS, PEG 400, and propylene glycol given orally (Table 5). Agenerase oral solution is packaged in

a 240 mL multi-dose container and should be stored at room temperature. The product has been available in the United Kingdom since 2000, and is also available in the United States.

5. Ritonavir is formulated as both Norvir® soft gelatin capsules (see previously) and Norvir oral solution, which contains 80 mg/mL of ritonavir solubilized in a mixture of cremophor EL, propylene glycol, 43% ethanol, water, and peppermint oil. The pediatric dose of ritonavir is 250 to 450 mg/m^2, or up to a maximum of 600 mg (7.5 mL) twice daily. The total amount of ethanol administered in conjunction with a daily adult dose of ritonavir as the oral solution is 3.2 mL twice daily, representing the estimated highest amount of ethanol given orally (Table 5). The Norvir oral solution is packaged in a 240 mL multi-dose container and should be stored at room temperature. Although it is being replaced by Kaletra, Norvir oral solution has been available in the United Kingdom since 1996 and is also available in the United States.

6. Lopinavir and ritonavir are coformulated as both Kaletra tablets (see previously) and Kaletra oral solution. This fixed-dose combination product contains 80 mg/mL of lopinavir and 20 mg/mL of ritonavir solubilized in propylene glycol, 42% ethanol, water, glycerin, the surfactant cremophor RH 40, and peppermint oil. The dose of Kaletra oral solution is 5 mL twice daily. Kaletra oral solution is packaged in a 160 mL multi-dose container and should be stored refrigerated at 2 to 8°C or at room temperature for no more than two months. Kaletra oral solution has been available in the United Kingdom since 2001 and is also available in the United States.

7. Cyclosporin A is available as Neoral and Sandimmune oral solutions, as well as Neoral, Sandimmune, and Gengraf soft gelatin capsules (see previously). Sandimmune solution contains 100 mg/mL of cyclosporin A dissolved in ethanol (12.5%), olive oil, and Labrafil M-1944CS. The dose of Sandimmune oral solution ranges from 1 to 7 mL daily and is to be administered after dilution with milk or orange juice. Sandimmune oral solution is packaged in a 50 mL multi-dose container and should be stored at room temperature. Neoral oral solution is a microemulsion preconcentrate containing 100 mg/mL of cyclosporin A dissolved in ethanol (11.9%), dl-α-tocopherol, corn oil-mono-di-triglycerides, polyoxyl 40 hydrogenated castor oil (cremophor RH 40), and propylene glycol. The dose of Neoral oral solution ranges from 1 to 7 mL daily and should be further diluted with orange or apple juice at room temperature and administered immediately. Neoral oral solution is packaged in a 50 mL multi-dose container and should be stored at room temperature. Neoral has been available in the United Kingdom since 1995, and both Neoral and Sandimmune oral solutions are available in the United States.

ORAL SUSPENSIONS

Similar to oral solutions, oral suspensions are normally intended for pediatric patients or for those patients who cannot swallow a tablet or capsule. Most oral suspensions contain coloring or flavoring agents and are dispensed in multi-dose containers. There is at least one lipid-based oral suspension commercially available. Ciprofloxacin is available as Cipro™ Oral Suspension that is packaged with two bottles. One bottle contains 5% or 10% w/w ciprofloxacin that is encapsulated into solid microcapsules containing povidone, methacrylic acid copolymer, hypromellose, magnesium stearate, and polysorbate 20. The second bottle contains the diluent composed of medium-chain triglycerides, sucrose, lecithin, water, and strawberry flavor. The contents of the two bottles are mixed to generate suspensions of 50 or 100 mg/mL ciprofloxacin. The dose of ciprofloxacin is 15 mg/kg, but not to exceed the adult dose of 500 mg. Cipro oral suspension should be stored below 30°C, and not frozen.

CONCLUSIONS

As of 2005, at least 31 drugs in 41 lipid-based formulations intended for oral delivery are commercially available in the United States, the United Kingdom, and Japan. Oral lipid-based products began entering the marketplace in 1981 and currently account for at approximately 3% of the commercially available oral formulations. The total daily dose of active drug substance administered in these formulations ranges from 0.25 μg to 2000 mg. For capsule products, the amount of active drug substance contained in a unit dose ranges from 0.25 μg to 500 mg, and for oral solution products from 1 μg/mL to 100 mg/mL. The total amount of lipid excipient administered in a single dose of a capsule formulation ranges from 0.5 to 5 g, but can range from as low as 0.1 mL to as high as 20 mL for oral solution products. Lipid-based formulations range in complexity from simple, one-excipient solutions (e.g., sesame or corn oil) to multi-excipient, self-emulsifying drug delivery systems (SEDDS). The excipients in lipid-based oral formulations include water-insoluble triglycerides (e.g., corn oil, olive oil, peanut oil, rapeseed oil, sesame oil, soybean oil, hydrogenated vegetable oils, hydrogenated soybean oil, and medium-chain triglycerides of coconut oil and palm seed oil), organic liquids/semi-solids (e.g., beeswax, DL-α-tocopherol, oleic acid, medium-chain mono- and diglycerides, propylene glycol esters of fatty acids), nonionic surfactants (e.g., cremophor EL, cremophor RH 40, cremophor RH 60, d-α-tocopherol polyethylene glycol 1000 succinate, glyceryl monooleate, polysorbate 20, polysorbate 80, sorbitan monolaurate, Labrafil M-1944CS, Labrafil M-2125CS, and Labrasol), a phospholipid (phosphatidylcholine), and water-miscible organic solvents (e.g., polyethylene glycol 400, ethanol, propylene glycol, glycerin). Some oral lipid-based products tolerate room temperature storage for only brief periods of time and require long-term storage at 2 to 8°C due to chemical and/or physical stability issues.

REFERENCES

1. Liu R. Water-Insoluble Drug Formulation. Denver, Colorado: Interpharm Press, 2000.
2. Physician's Desk Reference. 59th ed. Montvale, NJ: Thomson Healthcare, Inc, 2005.
3. For the United States of America: www.rxlist.com, www.fda.gov/cder, www.access-data.fda.gov/scripts/cder/iig/index.cfm; For the United Kingdom: http://emc.medicines. org.uk/; For Japan: http://www.e-search.ne.jp/~jpr/jprdb/eindex.html (accessed March 12, 2007).
4. For the European Union: http://www.emea.eu.int/index/indexh1.htm; for Sweden: http://www.mpa.se/eng/spc/index.shtml; for New Zealand: http://www.medsafe. govt.nz/DatasheetPage.htm; for South Africa: http://home. intekom.com/pharm/ (March 12, 2007).
5. Strickley RG. Solubilizing excipients in oral and injectable formulations. Pharm Res 2004; 21(2): 201–230.
6. O'Neil MJ. The Merck Index. 13th ed. Whitehouse Station, NJ: Merck Research Laboratories Division of Merck & Co., Inc., 2001.
7. Cawley JD, Stern MH. Water-Soluble Tocopherol Derivatives, US Patent 2,680,749 (1954).
8. H-W S, Wu, Hopkins WK. Characteristics of d-α-tocopheryl PEG 1000 succinate for applications as an absorption enhancer in drug delivery systems. Pharm Tech 1999; 23:10.
9. Yu L, Bridgers A, Polli J, et al. Vitamin-E-TPGS increases absorption flux of an HIV protease inhibitor by enhancing its solubility and permeability. Pharm Res 1999; 16:1812–1817.
10. Law D, Krill SL, Schmitt EA, et al. Physicochemical considerations in the preparation of amorphous ritonavir-polyethylene glycol 8000 solid dispersions. J Pharm Sci 2001; 90:1015–1025.
11. Physician's Desk Reference. 51st ed. Montvale, NJ: Medical Economics Company, Inc., 1997.
12. Abu TM Serajuddin. Solid dispersion of poorly water-soluble drugs: early promises, subsequent problems, and recent breakthroughs. J Pharm Sci 1999; 88:1058–1066.
13. Pharmacy Today. An Official Publication of the American Pharmaceutical Association, 1999; 5:10.
14. http://www.rocheusa.com/products/FTVDearDoctorFINAL.pdf (March 12, 2007).
15. Physician's Desk Reference. 60th ed. Montvale, NJ: Thomson Healthcare, Inc., 2006.
16. Tenjarla S. Microemulsions: an overview and pharmaceutical applications. Crit Rev Ther Drug Carrier Syst 1999; 16:461–521.
17. Constantinides PP, Tustian A, Kessler DR. Toco emulsions for drug solubilization and parenteral delivery. Adv Drug Del Rev 2004; 56:1243–1255.
18. Hwang SR, Lim S-J, Park J-S, Kim C-K. Phospholipid-based microemulsion formulation of all-trans-retinoic acid for parenteral administration, Intl J Pharm 2004; 276:175–183.
19. Kang BK, Khang G. Controlled release of paclitaxel from microemulsion containing PLGA and evaluation of anti-tumor activity in vitro and in vivo. Intl J Pharm 2004; 286:147–156.
20. Corswant CV, Thore P, Engstrom S. Triglyceride-based microemulsion for intravenous administration of sparingly soluble substances. J Pharm Sci 1998; 87(2):200.

2

Lipid-Based Excipients for Oral Drug Delivery

Lowell Gibson

Eli Lilly and Company, Indianapolis, Indiana, U.S.A.

INTRODUCTION

The goal of an oral lipid based formulation is to improve the bioavailability of a poorly water soluble drug to an extent greater than that achievable with a conventional oral solid dosage form. The primary mechanism by which lipid-based formulations enhance bioavailability is through solubilization of the drug, although other mechanisms of absorption enhancement have been implicated and include reduction of P-glycoprotein-mediated efflux, mitigation of hepatic first pass metabolism through enhanced lymphatic transport (1–3), prolongation of gastrointestinal (GI) transit time, or protection from degradation in the GI tract.

The formulator has hundreds of potential excipients from which to choose for the preparation of lipid-based formulations and the number of possibilities can seem overwhelming. In addition, it is not uncommon for a given excipient to be marketed by multiple suppliers, each of whom assigns their own unique trade name, thereby adding to the confusion. Despite the number of possibilities, only a relatively small subset of lipids has found application in clinical formulation development due to a limited or nonexistent history of pharmaceutical application or, more commonly, a lack of regulatory approval. This chapter will describe the pharmaceutically relevant properties of the following, currently marketed classes of lipid excipients:

- Fatty acids
- Natural oils and fats

- Semi-synthetic mono-, di-,and triglycerides
- Semi-synthetic polyethylene glycol (PEG) derivatives of glycerides and fatty acids
- Polyglyceryl fatty acid esters
- Cholesterol and phospholipids

In addition, the product trade names and suppliers of these excipients will be provided.

FATTY ACIDS

Fatty acids are monocarboxylic acid derivatives of saturated or unsaturated aliphatic hydrocarbons (Fig. 1) (4,5). The individual carbon atoms comprising the hydrocarbon chains are numbered sequentially, beginning with the carboxyl carbon, which is assigned the number "1." However, less frequently applied numbering conventions have been described in the literature (6). Since the molecular structures of fatty acids are often large and potentially complex, various

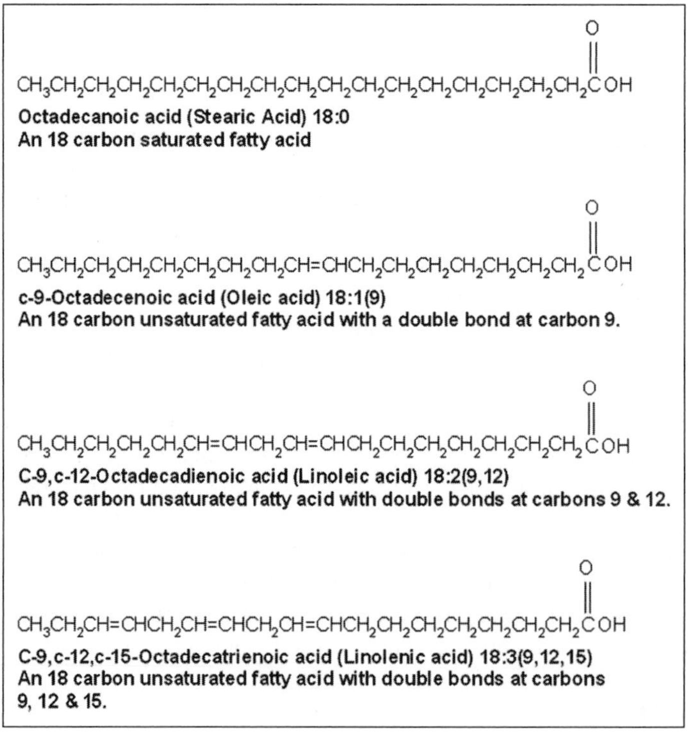

$$CH_3CH_2CH_2CH_2CH_2CH_2CH_2CH_2CH_2CH_2CH_2CH_2CH_2CH_2CH_2CH_2\overset{\displaystyle O}{\overset{\|}{C}}OH$$

Octadecanoic acid (Stearic Acid) 18:0
An 18 carbon saturated fatty acid

$$CH_3CH_2CH_2CH_2CH_2CH_2CH_2CH_2CH=CHCH_2CH_2CH_2CH_2CH_2CH_2CH_2\overset{\displaystyle O}{\overset{\|}{C}}OH$$

c-9-Octadecenoic acid (Oleic acid) 18:1(9)
An 18 carbon unsaturated fatty acid with a double bond at carbon 9.

$$CH_3CH_2CH_2CH_2CH_2CH=CHCH_2CH=CHCH_2CH_2CH_2CH_2CH_2CH_2CH_2\overset{\displaystyle O}{\overset{\|}{C}}OH$$

C-9,c-12-Octadecadienoic acid (Linoleic acid) 18:2(9,12)
An 18 carbon unsaturated fatty acid with double bonds at carbons 9 & 12.

$$CH_3CH_2CH=CHCH_2CH=CHCH_2CH=CHCH_2CH_2CH_2CH_2CH_2CH_2\overset{\displaystyle O}{\overset{\|}{C}}OH$$

C-9,c-12,c-15-Octadecatrienoic acid (Linolenic acid) 18:3(9,12,15)
An 18 carbon unsaturated fatty acid with double bonds at carbons 9, 12 & 15.

Figure 1 Examples illustrating the nomenclature used to describe the positions of unsaturated carbon–carbon double bonds in long chain fatty acids.

abbreviated forms of nomenclature have been developed. One common method for describing the hydrocarbon chain length and the number and relative positions of unsaturated carbon–carbon double bonds is illustrated using linoleic acid as an example (Fig. 1) (6). The abbreviated name for linoleic acid is 18:2 (9,12), which describes a fatty acid of 18 carbons in chain length, which possesses two carbon–carbon double bonds at positions 9 and 12 on the chain (i.e., there are carbon–carbon double bonds between carbons numbered 9 and 10 and also between carbons 12 and 13). The letter "c" preceding the name of a fatty acid is used to denote the "*cis*" configuration of the molecule, and indicates that the hydrogen atoms attached to the nonrotatable double-bonded carbons of an unsaturated fatty acid lie on the same side of the double bond while the hydrocarbon chains comprising the remainder of the molecule occupy similar positions on the opposite side of the molecule (Fig. 2). The majority of naturally-occurring fatty acids possess the *cis* configuration (7). The "*trans*" (abbreviated 't') designation describes the molecular configuration in which two hydrogen atoms occupy positions on opposite sides of the carbon–carbon double bond of an unsaturated fatty acid; the two hydrocarbon chains comprising the remainder of the molecule are similarly opposed in their positions of attachment about the point of unsaturation (Fig. 2). *Trans* fatty acids are more linear in shape than their corresponding *cis* forms, which allows closer alignment of, and greater attractive interaction between, the individual fatty acid molecules. This in turn results in higher melting points for the *trans* form of the fatty acid as compared to its *cis* form. Naturally occurring *cis* fatty acids are partially converted to *trans* fatty acids during purification of the natural product sources and subsequent to hydrogenation processes. As such, the typical western diet contains a significant amount of *trans* fatty acids.

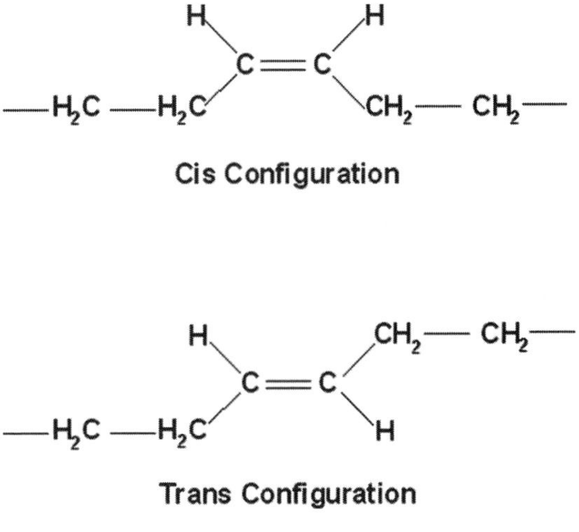

Figure 2 Examples of *cis* and *trans* configurations encountered in unsaturated fatty acids.

Table 1 lists some common saturated and unsaturated fatty acids that may be used in pharmaceutical lipid formulations (4–6,8–11). Saturated fatty acids with eight or fewer carbons are flowable liquids at room temperature; those fatty acids of 10 or more carbons in chain length are semi-solids at room temperature and possess melting points that increase in proportion to the hydrocarbon chain length but decrease with increasing degree of unsaturation. As an example, the

Table 1 Common and Systematic Names, Shorthand, Melting Points, and Water Solubility for Some Saturated and Unsaturated Fatty Acids

Common name	Systematic name	Shorthand	Melting point (°C)	Water solubility
Formic	Methanoic	1:0	8.3	Miscible
Acetic	Ethanoic	2:0	16.6	Miscible
Propionic	Propanoic	3:0	−21.5	Miscible
Butyric	Butanoic	4:0	−7.9	Miscible
Valeric	Pentanoic	5:0	−34.5	37 mg/g
Caproic	Hexanoic	6:0	−3.4	10 mg/g
Caprylic	Octanoic	8:0	16	7 mg/g
Capric	Decanoic	10:0	31.5	2 mg/g
Lauric	Dodecanoic	12:0	44.2	Insoluble
Myristic	Tetradecanoic	14:0	53.9	Insoluble
Myristoleic	c-9-Tetradecenoic	14:1 (9)	−4	Insoluble
—	Pentadecanoic	15:0	52.3	Insoluble
Palmitic	Hexadecanoic	16:0	63.1	Insoluble
Palmitoleic	c-9-Hexadecenoic	16:1 (9)	−0.5	Insoluble
Margaric	Heptadecanoic	17:0	61	Insoluble
Margaroleic	c-10-Heptadecenoic	17:1 (10)	12.5	Insoluble
Stearic	Octadecanoic	18:0	69.6	Insoluble
Oleic	c-9-Octadecenoic	18:1 (9)	13.4	Insoluble
Ricinoleic	12-Hydroxy-c-9-octadecenoic	18:1 (9) OH (12)[a]	5.5	Insoluble
Linoleic	c-9, c-12-Octadecadienoic	18:2 (9,12)	−5	Insoluble
Linolenic	c-9, c-12, c-15-Octadecatrienoic	18:3 (9,12,15)	−11	Insoluble
Arachidic	Eicosanoic	20:0	76.5	Insoluble
Gadoleic	c-9-Eicosenoic	20:1 (9)	23	Insoluble
Gondoic	c-11-Eicosenoic	20:1 (11)	24	Insoluble
—	c-11, c-14-Eicosadienoic	20:2 (11,14)	—	Insoluble
Behenic	Docosanoic	22:0	79.9	Insoluble
Erucic	c-13-Docosenoic	22:1 (13)	33.8	Insoluble
Lignoceric	Tetracosanoic	24:0	86	Insoluble

[a]Does not follow shorthand rules.

fatty acids stearic, oleic, linoleic, and linolenic, are all 18 carbons in chain length, differing only in the number of unsaturated carbon–carbon double bonds. Stearic acid, which is fully saturated, possesses a melting point of 69.6°C; oleic acid, which possesses a single unsaturated carbon–carbon double bond, possesses a significantly lower melting point of 13.4°C; linoleic acid, which has two unsaturated bonds, melts at −5°C and linolenic acid, which has three unsaturated bonds, melts at −11°C. Saturated fatty acids of four or fewer carbons in chain length are water-miscible; water miscibility declines rapidly as the hydrocarbon chain increases in length, with fatty acids comprised of 12 or more carbons being practically insoluble in water.

Fatty acids find pharmaceutical application primarily as solubilizing vehicles for poorly water-soluble drugs whereas the semi-synthetic PEG fatty acid esters (discussed later) find application not only as solubilizers, but as surfactants and emulsifiers, as well (Table 2) (12–18). Excipients from both of these classes are compatible with either soft or hard gelatin capsules.

Hydrophile–Lipophile Balance

The "hydrophile–lipophile balance" (HLB) is a measure of the relative hydrophilicity and lipophilicity of amphiphilic molecules (e.g., surfactants and emulsifiers), which possess both a hydrophilic and a lipophilic region. HLB values can be calculated from the relative size and strength of hydrophilic and lipophilic portions of the molecule or determined experimentally by various methods (12,19). Relative hydrophilicity increases with increasing HLB value; excipients with HLB values <9 are considered to be hydrophobic, whereas those with values >11 are considered hydrophilic (19).

Preparation of an oil-in-water emulsion of a particular lipophilic excipient requires that the HLB value of the surfactant be matched to the requirements of the excipient. Table 3 shows the required surfactant HLB values for several lipid excipients commonly used to prepare oil-in-water emulsion formulations of poorly water-soluble drugs (12,19,20). The required surfactant HLB value for emulsifying a particular excipient can be determined empirically by preparing several emulsions of the excipient over a range of surfactant HLB values produced by mixtures of various proportions of a hydrophobic and a hydrophilic surfactant of the same chemical type [e.g., hydrophobic SPAN 80 (HLB = 4.3) and hydrophilic TWEEN 80 (HLB = 15), both of which are oleates]. The required HLB is that producing the best quality emulsion (e.g., resistance to phase separation and high degree of dispersion) (19). The relative proportions of the surfactants required to prepare a two-component mixture of a specific HLB may be calculated from the following relationships:

$$\text{Percentage of surfactant A} = \frac{100(\text{Desired HLB} - \text{HLB of surfactant B})}{\text{HLB of surfactant A} - \text{HLB of surfactant B}}$$

$$\text{Percentage of surfactant B} = 100 - \text{Percentage of surfactant A}$$

Table 2 Fatty Acids and Fatty Acid Esters

Excipient	Chemical name or composition	Trade name/supplier	Physical state at 25°C or melting point	Hydrophile–lipophile balance	Uses
Ethyl oleate	Ethyl ester of oleic acid [18:1 (9)]	Crodamol EO/Croda Estol ETO 3660/Uniqema	Liquid		Vehicle, solubilizer
Isopropyl myristate	Isopropyl ester of myristic (14:0) acid	Estol 1512 IPM/Uniqema Estol 1514 IPM/Uniqema Crodamol IPM/Croda	Liquid		Vehicle, solubilizer, lubricant, emulsifier
Isopropyl palmitate	Isopropyl ester of palmitic (16:0) acid	Estol 1517 IPP/Uniqema Stepan IPP/Stepan	Liquid		Vehicle, solubilizer, lubricant, emulsifier
Linoleic acid	c-9, c-12-Octadecadienoic acid [18:2 (9,12)]	Crossential L99/Croda	Liquid		Vehicle, solubilizer
Oleic acid	c-9-Octadecenoic acid [18:1 (9)]	Priolene 6929/Uniqema Crossential O94/Croda Super Refined Oleic Acid NF/Croda	Liquid	1	Vehicle, solubilizer
PEG-6 propylene glycol di caprylate/ caprate	Dicaprylic acid (8:0) and capric acid (10:0) esters of propylene glycol and PEG 300	Acconon 200 E6/Abitec	Liquid	12	Vehicle, surfactant, solubilizer
Propylene glycol dicaprate	Capric acid (10:0) diester of propylene glycol	Captex 100/Abitec	Liquid		Vehicle, solubilizer
Propylene glycol monocaprylate	Caprylic acid (8:0) monoester of propylene glycol	Capryol 90/Gattefosse Capmul PG-8/Abitec	Liquid	6	Vehicle, solubilizer, absorption enhancer, coemulsifier

Propylene glycol mono/dicaprylate	Caprylic acid (8:0) mono and diesters of propylene glycol	Capryol PGMC/Gattefosse Imwitor 408/Sasol	Liquid	5	Vehicle, solubilizer, absorption enhancer, coemulsifier
Propylene glycol dicaprylate/ dicaprate	Caprylic acid (8:0) and capric acid (10:0) diesters of propylene glycol	Captex 200/Abitec Captex 200P/Abitec Miglyol 840/Sasol Estol PDCC 1526/Uniqema Neobee M-20/Stepan	Liquid		Vehicle, solubilizer, vehicle for capsules
Propylene glycol di (2-ethylhexanoate)	2-Ethylhexanoic acid diesters of propylene glycol	Captex 800/Abitec	Liquid		Vehicle, solubilizer
Propylene glycol monolaurate	Monolauric acid ester (12:0) of propylene glycol	Lauroglycol 90/Gattefosse Capmul PG-12/Abitec	Liquid	5	Vehicle, solubilizer, cosurfactant in microemulsions
Propylene glycol mono/dilaurate	Lauric acid (12:0) mono and di esters of propylene glycol	Imwitor 412/Sasol Lauroglycol FCC/ Gattefosse	Liquid	4	Vehicle, solubilizer, absorption enhancer, coemulsifier
Propylene glycol monostearate	Stearic acid (18:0) mono ester of propylene glycol	Stepan PGMS Pure/Stepan Monosteol/Gattefosse	34–38	3–4	Solubilizer, surfactant, emulsifier, lubricant
Stearic acid	Octadecanoic acid (18:0)	Pristerene 9559/Uniqema	54–56		Lubricant

Abbreviation: PEG, polyethylene glycol.

Table 3 Required Surfactant Hydrophile–Lipophile Balance for
Oil-in-Water Emulsification of Various Lipids

Material	Required hydrophile–lipophile balance
Caprylic/capric triglycerides (medium chain triglycerides)	5 (11[a])
Castor oil	14
Cholesterol	10–11
Coconut oil	5
Corn oil	8
Cottonseed oil	6
Ethyl oleate	11
Hydrogenated castor oil	8
Isopropyl myristate	12
Isopropyl palmitate	12
Isostearic acid	15–16
Lauric acid	16
Linoleic acid	16
Oleic acid	17
Olive oil	7–8
Palm oil	7
Rapeseed oil	7
Ricinoleic acid	16
Safflower oil	7
Sesame oil	7–8
Soybean oil	6

[a]Required hydrophile–lipophile balance for Croda, Inc., Crodamol GTCC PN.

Note that the chosen surfactant pair must include one surfactant with an HLB higher, and the other with an HLB lower, than the desired HLB of the surfactant blend (19).

   The chemical type of the surfactants used to make an emulsion also affects the quality of the emulsion. After the required HLB for emulsification of the excipient is determined, emulsions of the excipient are prepared with several binary mixtures of hydrophobic and hydrophilic surfactants mixed in the ratio which produces the required HLB. Each surfactant of a given pair is of the same chemical type, but each pair of surfactants should be of different chemical types. The surfactant pair that produces the best quality emulsion (as defined previously) is identified and used to prepare the final emulsion formulation (19). For example, if the required HLB for emulsification of an excipient is 12, emulsions containing mixtures of the surfactants, SPAN 20 and TWEEN 20 (laurates), SPAN 40 and TWEEN 40 (palmitates), SPAN 60 and TWEEN 60 (stearates), or SPAN 80 and TWEEN 80 (oleates), in proportions yielding an HLB of 12, can be prepared and the best emulsion selected as the final formulation. Screening for the ideal surfactant pair is empiric, with the ultimate selection being determined by the quality of the resulting emulsion (12,19).

Oxidation

Fatty acids and lipids containing fatty acids (fatty acid esters, mono-, di-, and triglycerides, phospholipids) can undergo autocatalytic chain reaction oxidation (autoxidation). In addition, any oxygen-sensitive drug formulated in the lipid may oxidize as well. Lipid oxidation is catalyzed by impurities including peroxides, metal ions, and photochemical sensitizers, such as chlorophyll and riboflavin, which interact with light to produce triplet or singlet oxygen. These highly reactive oxygen species catalyze the peroxidation of many types of lipids resulting in subsequent degradation to alcohols, furans, aldehydes, ketones, and acids, which give oxidized or "rancid" lipids their unpleasant tastes and odors (6).

The rate of oxidative degradation is proportional to the degree of unsaturation or number of carbon–carbon double bonds in the fatty acid molecule and since oxidation is an autocatalytic reaction, the rate of oxidation increases as the reaction progresses (6).

Oxidation of lipids can usually be controlled by various methods, including reduction of oxygen in the lipid and in the container head space, protection from light and purification to remove peroxides and metal ions. Addition of free radical quenching agents such as α-tocopherol, β-carotene, ascorbic acid, butylated hydroxyanisole (BHA), butylated hydroxytoluene (BHT), propyl gallate or nordihydroguaiaretic acid (NDGA), or the addition of metal chelators such as diethylenetriaminepentaacetate (DTPA) or ethylenediaminetetraacetate (EDTA) have also been proven effective for controlling lipid oxidation (21–23).

NATURAL OILS AND FATS

Naturally occurring oils and fats are comprised of mixtures of various triglycerides (TG) which are more correctly (but rarely) referred to as triacylglycerols, since chemically they are fatty acid tri-esters of glycerol (Fig. 3). Table 4 lists trade names and suppliers of several common natural oils, including some that have been hydrogenated to decrease the number of double bonds, thereby conferring resistance to oxidative degradation (4,13–15,24,25).

Naturally occurring triglycerides contain fatty acids of varying chain lengths and degrees of unsaturation (Tables 5 and 6). Based on the hydrocarbon chain

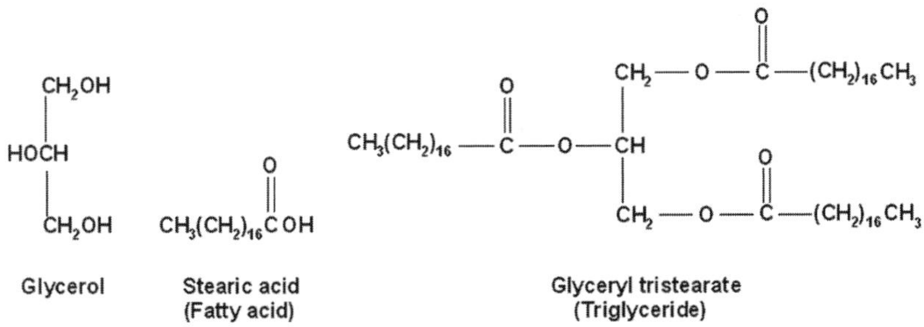

Figure 3   Structural components of a triglyceride (e.g., glyceryl tristearate).

Table 4 Natural and Hydrogenated Oils

Excipient	Trade name/supplier	Physical state at 25°C or melting point
Canola oil	Pureco Canola/Abitec	Liquid
Coconut oil	Pureco 76/Abitec Coconut Oil EP/Karlshamns	Liquid
Corn oil	Super Refined Corn Oil NF/Croda Super Refined Corn Oil NF-NP/Croda Corn oil/Karlshamns	Liquid
Cottonseed oil	Super Refined Cottonseed Oil NF/Croda Super Refined Cottonseed Oil NF-NP/Croda	Liquid
Olive oil	Super Refined Olive Oil NF/Croda Super Refined Olive Oil NF-NP/Croda	Liquid
Palm oil	Palm oil/Welch, Holme & Clark	Liquid
Peanut (Arachis) oil	Super Refined Peanut Oil NF/Croda Super Refined Peanut Oil NF-NP/Croda Lipex 101 Arachis Oil/Karlshamns	Liquid
Rapeseed oil	Rapeseed oil/Welch, Holme & Clark Rapeseed Oil Refined EP/Karlshamns	Liquid
Safflower oil	Super Refined Safflower Oil USP/Croda Super Refined Safflower Oil USP-NP/Croda	Liquid
Sesame oil	Super Refined Sesame Oil NF/Croda Super Refined Sesame Oil NF-BB/Croda Super Refined Sesame Oil NF-NP/Croda	Liquid
Soybean oil	Pureco Soybean/Abitec Super Refined Soybean Oil USP/Croda Super Refined Soybean Oil USP-NP/Croda Soybean Oil Refined EP/Karlshamns	Liquid
Hydrogenated soybean oil	Akosol 405/Karlshamns	Solid
Sunflower oil	Sunflower Oil Refined EP/Karlshamns	Liquid
High oleic sunflower oil	Pureco HOS/Abitec	Liquid
Hydrogenated vegetable oil	Wecobee M/Stepan Wecobee FS/Stepan Wecobee S/Stepan	35 39.8 44
Partially hydrogenated vegetable oil	Pureco HSC-1/Abitec	Solid

Note: Croda oils designated NP contain no preservatives.

length of their component fatty acids, triglycerides can be classified as short (less than five carbons), medium (6 to 12 carbons), or long chain (more than 12 carbons).

SEMI-SYNTHETIC MONO-, DI-, AND TRIGLYCERIDES

In addition to the naturally occurring triglycerides, there are several commercially available semi-synthetic glycerides that offer more uniform compositions (Table 7) (4,14–18,24,25). These excipients which are compatible with both soft and hard gelatin capsules, find application as solubilizing vehicles, emulsifiers, suspending, and wetting agents and in various controlled release dosage forms.

Lipid Heterogeneity

Although the fatty acid content and composition of the semi-synthetic glycerides are more uniform than that of naturally occurring glycerides, a certain amount of variability in these parameters, as well as in the relative positions on the glycerol backbone to which the individual fatty acids are esterified, can be expected. This compositional variability is a function of the excipient brand as well as the particular manufacturing lot of a given excipient, for which the composition will vary within ranges defined by the manufacturer. For example, Table 8 shows the fatty acid compositions for different brands of medium chain triglycerides, which are comprised of a mixture of glyceryl tricaprylate and tricaprate. The manufacturers (Abitec®, Sasol®, and Stepan®) each produce two different brands, distinguished by the relative content of caprylic and capric acids, as well as by the acceptable ranges for each of these fatty acids and the content of caproic, lauric, and myristic acids (15,16,18).

Similarly, mono- or diglyceride excipients are not single component materials and often contain several different fatty acids as well as varying amounts of higher or lower order glycerides. For example, the product data sheet for the Capmul GMO-50, EP brand of glyceryl monooleate (Abitec), describes the following fatty acid composition of this excipient: palmitic acid (12% maximum), stearic acid (6% maximum), oleic acid (60% minimum), linoleic acid (2% maximum), arachidic acid (2% maximum), and eicosenoic acid (2% maximum). In addition, it states that the mono-, di-, and triglyceride contents are 55% to 65%, 15% to 35%, and 2% to 10%, respectively. Therefore, although this excipient is considered to be glyceryl monooleate, its content of fatty acids other than oleic may range as high as 40% and the content of di- and triglycerides may range as high as 45% (16). Variable composition is typical of most lipid excipients and has the potential to cause differences in formulation performance, both in vitro and in vivo.

From the foregoing discussion, it should be apparent that the formulator must recognize the potential for compositional variability of lipid excipients between different brands of the "same" excipient as well as between different lots of the same brand. Fortunately, this information is readily available from the excipient manufacturer in the form of product data sheets and certificates of analysis. In particular, it must never be assumed that different brands of a particular excipient are equivalent. Finally, the formulator must gain an understanding of which excipient properties or compositional characteristics are critical to the formulation's performance and ensure that each excipient lot falls within the specified range of acceptability.

Table 5 Percent Fatty Acid Content of Selected Fats and Oils

Fat or oil	Melting point (°C)	Caproic	Caprylic	Capric	Lauric	Myristic	Myristoleic	Pentadecanoic	Palmitic	Palmitoleic	Margaric	Margaroleic	Stearic	Oleic	Ricinoleic[a]	Linoleic	Linolenic	Eicosanoic	Eicosenoic	Eicosadienoic	Behenic	Erucic	Tetracosanoic
No. of carbons: no. of double bonds		6:0	8:0	10:0	12:0	14:0	14:1	15:0	16:0	16:1	17:0	17:1	18:0	18:1	18:1	18:2	18:3	20:0	20:1	20:2	22:0	22:1	24:0
Sunflower oil	−18					0.1			7	0.1	0.1		5	19		68	0.8	0.4	0.1		0.7		
Castor oil	−12								2				1	7	87	3							
Corn oil	−10					0.1			11	0.2	0.1		2	25		60	1	0.4					
Olive oil (virgin)	−6								9	0.6	0.1		3	80		6	0.7	0.4			0.1		
Peanut oil	−5					0.1			11	0.2	0.1	0.1	2	47		32		1	2		3		1
Cottonseed oil	0–5				0.1	0.7			22	0.6	0.1	0.1	3	19		54	0.7	0.3			0.2		
Canola oil	17–22					0.1			4	0.3	0.1		2	61		21	9	0.7	1		0.3	0.7	0.2
Rapeseed oil	17–22					0.1			4	0.3			1	19		14	11	0.7	7	0.7	0.5	41	1
Coconut oil	21–27	0.5	7	6	47	19			9				3	7		2	0.1	0.1					
Soybean oil	22–31					0.1			11	0.1	0.1		4	23		54	8	0.3			0.3		
Palm oil	26–30				0.1	1			44	0.2	0.1		4	39		10	0.4	0.3			0.1		
Palm kernel oil	26–30	0.2	3	3	48	16			8				3	15		2		0.1	0.1				
Cocoa butter	30–35					0.1			26	0.4	0.3		34	34		3		1	0.1		0.2		
Lard	36–42			0.1	0.1	2		0.1	26	3	0.4	0.2	14	44		10	0.4	0.2	0.7	0.1			
Tallow	40–46				0.1	3	0.9	0.5	24	4	2	0.8	19	43		3	0.7	0.2	0.3				

[a]Ricinoleic acid is monohydroxylated on carbon number 12.

Table 6 Distributions of Fatty Acids on the Three Positions of Glycerol in Selected Oils

Positional distributions of fatty acids (mol. %) in triacyl-*sn*-glycerols of seed oils

Oil	Position	\multicolumn{7}{c}{Fatty acids (no. of carbons:no. of double bonds)}

Oil	Position	16:0	18:0	18:1	18:2	18:3	C20-C24
Peanut	1	14	5	59	19		4
	2	2	tr	59	39		1
	3	11	5	57	10		15
Rapeseed[a]	1	4	2	23	11	6	53
	2	1		37	36	20	6
	3	4	3	17	4	3	70
Soybean	1	14	6	23	48	9	
	2	1	tr	22	70	7	
	3	13	6	28	45	9	
Linseed	1	10	6	15	16	53	
	2	2	1	16	21	60	
	3	6	4	17	13	59	
Maize	1	8	3	28	50	1	
	2	2	tr	27	70	1	
	3	14	3	31	52	1	
Olive	1	13	3	72	10	1	
	2	1		83	14	1	
	3	17	4	74	5		
Cocoa butter	1	34	50	12	1	1	1
	2	2	2	87	9		
	3	37	53	9	tr		2

[a]High erucic acid rapeseed oil.
Abbreviation: tr, trace (<0.5%).

SEMI-SYNTHETIC POLYETHYLENE GLYCOL (PEG) DERIVATIVES OF GLYCERIDES AND FATTY ACIDS

Table 9 lists several excipients that are mixtures of mono-, di-, and triglycerides with fatty acid esters of PEG, along with their respective trade names and suppliers, key physical properties and common pharmaceutical applications (4,13,16–18,26). These excipients find application as fluid or thermo-softening semi-solid solubilizing vehicles, surfactants and wetting agents, and as emulsifiers and coemulsifiers in self-emulsifying drug delivery systems (SEDDS) and self-microemulsifying drug delivery systems (SMEDDS). These excipients are compatible with both soft and hard gelatin capsules, can be inherently self-emulsifying and span the range of HLB values, from highly lipophilic (PEG-6 glyceryl oleate, HLB 3-4) to water soluble (PEG-40 hydrogenated castor oil, HLB 14–16) (17–19).

(*Text continues on page 51.*)

Table 7 Mono-, Di-, and Triglycerides

Excipient	Chemical name or composition	Trade name/supplier	Melting point	Hydrophile–lipophile balance	Uses
Glyceryl triacetate (triacetin)	Triacetic acid (2:0) esters of glycerol	Captex 500 P/Abitec Triacetin/Sigma-Aldrich	−78		Solubilizer, vehicle
Glyceryl mono-, di-, tribehenate	Mono-, di-, and tri-docosanoic acid (22:0) esters of glycerol	Compritol 888/ATO/Gattefosse	69–74	2	Controlled release, tablet lubricant, and binder
Glyceryl tribehenate (tribehenin)	Tridocosanoic acid (22:0) esters of glycerol	Syncrowax HR-C/Croda Tribehenin/Sigma-Aldrich	78		Suspending agent, lubricant, and controlled release
Glyceryl tributyrate (tributyrin)	Tributyric acid (4:0) esters of glycerol	Tributyrin/Sigma-Aldrich	−75		Solubilizer, vehicle
Glyceryl mono- and dicaprate	Mono- and dicapric acid (10:0) esters of glycerol	Capmul MCM C-10/Abitec	40–41		Solubilizer, emulsifier, coemulsifier
Glyceryl tricaprate (tricaprin)	Tricapric acid (10:0) esters of glycerol	Captex 1000/Abitec Tricaprin/Sigma-Aldrich	31–32		Solubilizer, vehicle
Glyceryl mono- and dicaprylate	Mono- and dicaprylic acid (8:0) esters of glycerol	Capmul MCM C-8/Abitec Imwitor 308/Sasol Imwitor 988/Sasol	— 30–34 20–25	6 3–4	Solubilizer, emulsifier, coemulsifier
Glyceryl tricaprylate (tricaprylin)	Tricaprylic acid (8:0) esters of glycerol	Captex 8000/Abitec Neobee 895/Stepan Tricaprylin/Sigma-Aldrich	9–10		Solubilizer, vehicle

Glyceryl mono- and dicaprylate/caprate	Mono- and dicaprylic acid (8:0) and capric acid (10:0) esters of glycerol	25–30	3–4	Capmul MCM/Abitec Imwitor 742/Sasol	Solubilizer, vehicle, emulsifier, coemulsifier
Glyceryl tricaprylate/caprate (medium chain triglycerides)	Tricaprylic (8:0) and capric acid (10:0) esters of glycerol	−5	1	Miglyol 810/Sasol Miglyol 812N/Sasol Neobee 1053/Stepan Neobee M5/Stepan Captex 300/Abitec Captex 355/Abitec Crodamol GTCC/Croda Labrafac CC/Gattefosse Labrafac Lipophile/Gattefosse Estasan GT8-60 3575/ Uniqema Estasan GT8-65 3577/ Uniqema Estasan GT8-70 3579/ Uniqema	Solubilizer, vehicle for capsule formulations
Glyceryl tricaprylate/caprate/laurate	Tricaprylic acid (8:0), capric acid (10:0), and lauric acid (12:0) esters of glycerol	Liquid		Captex 350/Abitec	Solubilizer, vehicle
Glyceryl tricaprylate/caprate/linoleate	Tricaprylic acid (8:0), capric acid (10:0), and linoleic acid (18:2) esters of glycerol	Liquid		Captex 810D/Abitec Miglyol 818/Sasol	Solubilizer, vehicle for capsule formulations

(Continued)

Table 7 Mono-, Di-, and Triglycerides (*Continued*)

Excipient	Chemical name or composition	Trade name/supplier	Melting point	Hydrophile–lipophile balance	Uses
Glyceryl tricaprylate/caprate/stearate	Tricaprylic acid (8:0), capric acid (10:0), and stearic acid (18:0) esters of glycerol	Softisan 378/Sasol	39–42		Solubilizer, vehicle for capsule formulations
Glyceryl tricaprylate/caprate/succinate	Tricaprylic acid (8:0), capric acid (10:0), and succinic acid esters of glycerol	Miglyol 829/Sasol	Liquid		Solubilizer, vehicle for capsule formulations
Glyceryl monolaurate	Monolauric acid (12:0) ester of glycerol	Stepan GML/Stepan Imwitor 312/Sasol	56–60	3–4	Solubilizer, emulsifier for w/o emulsions
Glyceryl dilaurate	Dodecanoic acid (12:0) diester of glycerol	Stepan GDL/Stepan	30	4	Solubilizer, emulsifier
Glyceryl trilaurate (trilaurin)	Trilauric acid (12:0) esters of glycerol	Dynasan 112/Sasol Trilaurin/Sigma-Aldrich	45–47		Solubilizer, vehicle, lubricant, controlled release agent
Glyceryl monolinoleate	Monooctadecadienoic (18:2) acid ester of glycerol	Maisine 35-1/Gattefosse	Liquid	3	Solubilizer, vehicle for capsule formulations

Name	Chemical description	Trade name/Supplier	Melting point	HLB	Applications
Glyceryl trimyristate (trimyristin)	Trimyristic acid (14:0) esters of glycerol	Dynasan 114/Sasol; Trimyristin/Sigma-Aldrich	56–57		Solubilizer, vehicle, lubricant, controlled release agent
Glyceryl monooleate	Monooleic acid (18:1) ester of glycerol	Capmul GMO/Abitec; Peceol/Gattefosse; Drewmulse GMO/Stepan	24	3	Emulsifier, solubilizer, wetting agent, vehicle for capsule formulations
Glyceryl mono- and dioleate	Mono- and dioleic acid (18:1) esters of glycerol	Capmul GMO-50/Abitec; Capmul GMO-K/Abitec	14–19		Solubilizer, emulsifier
Glyceryl trioleate (triolein)	Trioleic acid (18:1) esters of glycerol	Emerest 2423/Cognis; Triolein/Sigma-Aldrich	−4 to −5		Solubilizer, lubricant
Glyceryl tripalmitate (tripalmitin)	Tripalmitic acid (16:0) esters of glycerol	Dynasan 116/Sasol; Tripalmitin/Sigma-Aldrich	66		Solubilizer, lubricant, controlled release
Glyceryl palmitostearate	Mixture of mono-, di-, and tripalmitic acid (16:0) and stearic acid (18:0) esters of glycerol	Precirol ATO 5/Gattefosse	53–57	2	Lubricant, controlled release, thickener, suspending agent
Glyceryl monostearate	Mono stearic acid (18:0) ester of glycerol	Capmul GMS-50K/Abitec; Imwitor 491/Sasol; Geleol/Gattefosse; Stepan GMS 63F/Stepan	57	3–4	Solubilizer, emulsifier, controlled release, lubricant

(Continued)

Table 7 Mono-, Di-, and Triglycerides (*Continued*)

Excipient	Chemical name or composition	Trade name/supplier	Melting point	Hydrophile–lipophile balance	Uses
Glyceryl distearate	Octadecanoic acid (18:0) diester of glycerol	Stepan GDS 386F/Stepan	54	2	Emulsifier, coemulsifier, wetting agent, lubricant
Glyceryl mono-, di-, and tristearate	Mono-, di-, and tristearic acid (18:0) esters of glycerol	Imwitor 900/Sasol	54–64	3	Solubilizer, emulsifier, coemulsifier, lubricant
Glyceryl tristearate (tristearin)	Tristearic acid (18:0) esters of glycerol 72	Dynasan 118/Sasol Tristearin/Sigma-Aldrich	72		Lubricant, controlled release
Glyceryl tri-undecanoate (triundecanoin)	Triundecanoic acid (11:1) esters of glycerol	Captex 8227/Abitec Tri-undecanoin/Sigma-Aldrich	25–29		Solubilizer, vehicle, lubricant
Hard fat	Glycerol esters of saturated C8-C18 fatty acids Glycerol esters of saturated C12-C18 fatty acids	Gelucire 33/01/Gattefosse Gelucire 39/01/Gattefosse Gelucire 43/01/Gattefosse	33–37 37–42 42–46	1	Vehicle for capsule formulations, controlled release

Table 8 Composition of Some Medium Chain Triglycerides

Fatty acid	Captex 300 (Abitec)	Captex 355 (Abitec)	Miglyol 810 (Sasol)	Miglyol 812N (Sasol)	Neobee 1053[a] (Stepan)	Neobee M5[a] (Stepan)
Caproic (C6:0)	Max. 4	Max. 6	Max. 2	Max. 2	0	2
Caprylic (C8:0)	60–70	50–75	65–80	50–65	56	68
Capric (C10:0)	25–35	22–45	20–35	30–45	44	29
Lauric (C12:0)	Max. 1	Max. 4	Max. 2	Max. 2	0	1
Myristic (C14:0)	—	—	Max. 1	Max. 1	—	—

[a]Typical composition.

The thermo-softening excipients, such as the Gelucire product line (Gattefosse S.A.), must be melted in order to (preferably) solubilize or, alternatively, suspend the drug in the excipient matrix which is subsequently filled into hard gelatin capsules in the molten state; the relatively low melting temperature of soft gelatin capsules (40°C) usually precludes the use of these capsules with thermo-softening excipients. Additional excipients, such as glyceryl monostearate and PEG esters, may be incorporated into the molten excipient matrix to prevent uncontrolled polymorphic changes subsequent to congealing of the matrix, which can adversely affect the dissolution profile and potentially reduce drug absorption in vivo (27).

It should also be noted that colloidal silicon dioxide may be added to fluid lipid excipients to yield thixotropic formulations useful for preparing lipid suspensions of solid drug substances. For this purpose, hydrophilic colloidal silicon dioxide is used for preparing immediate release formulations, whereas the hydrophobic form finds application in the preparation of controlled release formulations (27).

POLYGLYCERYL FATTY ACID ESTERS

The polyglyceryl fatty acid esters are composed of a chain of glycerol molecules, linked together by ether linkages, which are esterified with one or more fatty acid molecules (Table 10). For example, polyglyceryl-6 dioleate is a chain of six glycerol molecules esterified with two molecules of oleic acid. Hydrophilicity increases as the polyglycerol chain length and number of free hydroxyl groups increases and decreases with increasing number or chain length of the esterified fatty acids. Therefore, the hydrophilicity can range from low, approaching that of the triglycerides (polyglyceryl-6 octastearate, HLB 2.5) to high (polyglyceryl-10 mono, dioleate, HLB 11). These excipients find application as surfactants, solubilizers, vehicles, emulsifiers, and drug crystallization inhibitors (4,16,17).

(*Text continues on page 55.*)

Table 9 Mixtures of Mono-, Di-, and Triglycerides with Fatty Acid Esters of Polyethylene Glycols

Excipient	Chemical name or composition	Trade name/supplier	Physical state at 25°C or melting point	Hydrophile–lipophile balance	Uses
PEG-4 glyceryl caprylate/caprate	Caprylic acid (C8:0) and capric acid (C10:0) esters of glycerol and PEG 200	Labrafac Hydro WL 1219/Gattefosse	Liquid	5	Vehicle, surfactant, solubilizer
PEG-6 glyceryl caprylate/caprate	Caprylic acid (C8:0) and capric acid (C10:0) esters of glycerol and PEG 300	Softigen 767/Sasol Acconon CC-6/Abitec	Liquid	18	Vehicle, water soluble surfactant, solubilizer, coemulsifier
PEG-6 glyceryl linoleate	Mono-, di-, and trilinoleic acid (C18:2) esters of glycerol and mono and diesters of PEG 300	Labrafil M 2125 CS/ Gattefosse	Liquid	3–4	Vehicle, solubilizer, vehicle for softgels, coemulsifier, lipid phase or cosurfactant in microemulsions.
PEG-6 glyceryl oleate	Mono-, di-, and trioleic acid (C18:1) esters of glycerol and mono- and diesters of PEG 300	Labrafil M 1944 CS/ Gattefosse	Liquid	3–4	Vehicle, solubilizer, vehicle for softgels, coemulsifier, lipid phase or cosurfactant in microemulsions.
PEG-8 glyceryl caprylate/caprate	Mono-, di-, and tricaprylic acid (C8:0) and capric acid (C10:0) esters of glycerol and mono- and diesters of PEG 400	Labrasol/Gattefosse Acconon MC-8/Abitec	Liquid	14	Vehicle, solubilizer, surfactant for microemulsions

Name	Trade name/Supplier	Composition	Melting point (°C)	HLB	Applications
PEG-32 glyceryl laurate	Gelucire 44/14/Gattefosse Acconon C-44/Abitec	Mono-, di-, and trilauric acid (C12:0) esters of glycerol plus mono- and difatty acid esters of PEG-1500. May contain some free PEG and glycerol.	42–48	14	Solubilizer, semisolid matrix capsule vehicle, emulsifier for semisolid SMEDDS
PEG-32 glyceryl palmitostearate	Gelucire 50/13/ Gattefosse	Mono-, di-, and tripalmitic acid (C16:0) and stearic acid (C18:0) esters of glycerol plus mono- and difatty acid esters of PEG-1500. May contain some free PEG and glycerol.	46–51	13	Solubilizer, semisolid matrix capsule vehicle, emulsifier for semisolid SMEDDS
PEG-35 castor oil (polyoxyl 35 castor oil, USP/NF)	Cremophor EL/BASF Etocas 35 NF/Croda	Mixture of glyceryl PEG ricinoleate (35 moles of ethylene oxide per mole of castor oil) with fatty acid esters of PEG, free PEGs and ethoxylated glycerol.	Liquid	12–14	Water soluble nonionic surfactant, vehicle, solubilizer, emulsifier
PEG-40 castor oil	Marlowet R 40/Sasol	Glyceryl PEG ricinoleate with 40 moles of ethylene oxide per mole of castor oil	Liquid	13	Vehicle, solubilizer, emulsifier
PEG-40 hydrogenated castor oil	Cremophor RH-40/BASF	Hydrogenated glyceryl PEG ricinoleate with 40 moles of ethylene oxide per mole of castor oil	16–26	14–16	Solubilizer, water soluble nonionic surfactant, emulsifier, wetting agent

Abbreviations: PEG, polyethylene glycol; SMEDDS, self-microemulsifying drug delivery systems.

Table 10 Polyglycerol Fatty Acid Esters

Excipient	Chemical name or composition	Trade name/supplier	Physical state at 25°C or melting point	Hydrophile–lipophile balance	Uses
Polyglyceryl-3 oleate	Monooleic acid [18:1 (9)] ester of a 3 glycerol unit chain	Caprol 3GO/Abitec	Liquid	6.5	Surfactant, solubilizer, vehicle, emulsifier
Polyglyceryl-3 dioleate	Dioleic acid [18:1 (9)] ester of a 3 glycerol unit chain	Plurol Oleique CC497/Gattefosse	Liquid	6	Surfactant, solubilizer, vehicle, emulsifier, vehicle for capsules
Polyglyceryl-3 stearate	Monostearic acid (18:0) ester of a 3 glycerol unit chain	Caprol 3GS/Abitec	Solid	7	Surfactant, solubilizer, emulsifier
Polyglyceryl-3 diisostearate	Diisostearic acid (18:0) ester of a 3 glycerol unit chain	Plurol Diisostearique/Gattefosse	Liquid	6–7	Surfactant, solubilizer, vehicle, emulsifier
Polyglyceryl-6 dioleate	Dioleic acid [18:1 (9)] ester of a 6 glycerol unit chain	Caprol MPGO/Abitec Plurol Oleique/Gattefosse	Liquid	10	Surfactant, solubilizer, vehicle, emulsifier, lubricant, crystallization inhibitor
Polyglyceryl-6 octastearate	Octastearic acid (18:0) ester of a 6 glycerol unit chain	Caprol ET/Abitec	38	2.5	Surfactant, solubilizer, crystallization inhibitor
Polyglyceryl-10 mono, dioleate	Mono- and dioleic acid [18:1 (9)] esters of a 10 glyceryl unit chain	Caprol PGE 860/Abitec	Liquid	11	Surfactant, solubilizer, vehicle, emulsifier
Polyglyceryl-10 decaoleate	Decaoleic acid [18:1 (9)] ester of a 10 glycerol unit chain	Caprol 10G10O/Abitec	Liquid	3	Surfactant, solubilizer, vehicle, emulsifier, lubricant, crystallization inhibitor

CHOLESTEROL AND THE PHOSPHOLIPIDS

Cholesterol and phospholipids find pharmaceutical application as solubilizers, surfactants, and emulsifiers in mixed micelles and emulsions (Fig. 4, Table 11) (28,29). In addition, phospholipids have been used as antioxidants for triglycerides (6) and are the primary constituents of liposomes, which have found only limited application in oral drug delivery due to instability in the GI tract. However, liposomes composed of a 7:2 molar ratio of distearoylphosphatidylcholine/cholesterol were found to be stable to pancreatic lipase and bile salts in vitro, suggesting potential application of these formulations in oral drug delivery (30).

Oxidation and Hydrolysis

As previously discussed for free fatty acids and glycerides, the fatty acids of phospholipids are also prone to oxidation (21–23). In addition, phospholipids are subject to hydrolysis. Phosphatidylcholine, a phospholipid commonly used in formulations, has four hydrolyzable ester bonds, specifically, two fatty acid esters of glycerol, a glycerophosphate ester and a phosphocholine ester (Fig. 4).

(Text continues on page 59.)

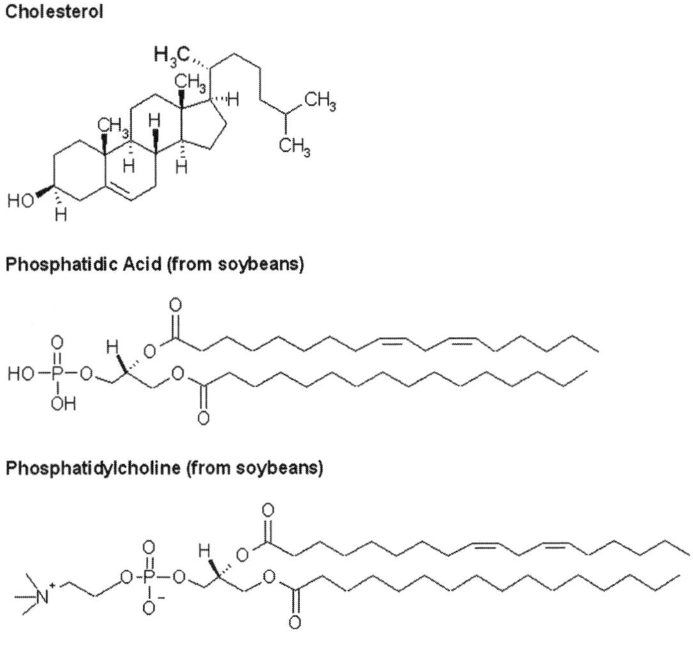

Cholesterol

Phosphatidic Acid (from soybeans)

Phosphatidylcholine (from soybeans)

Figure 4 Chemical structures of cholesterol and some phospholipids commonly employed in pharmaceutical formulations.

Table 11 Cholesterol and Phospholipids

Excipient	Chemical name or composition	Trade name/supplier	Charge
Cholesterol	Cholest-5-en-3β-ol	Avanti Polar Lipids	Neutral
Sodium cholesteryl sulfate	Cholest-5-en-3β-ol sulfate sodium salt	Sigma-Aldrich	Negative
L-α-Lecithin	Mixture of phosphatidylcholine, phosphatidylethanolamine, phosphatidylinositol, phosphatidic acid, and lysophatidylcholine. May also contain triglycerides, sterols, fatty acids, carbohydrates, and sphingolipids	Avanti Polar Lipids	Mixture of negative and zwitterionic
Egg lecithin	Similar to L-α-lecithin.	Avanti Polar Lipids	Mixture of negative and zwitterionic
Phosphatidic acid	Mixture of fatty acid diesters of glycerophosphoric acid	Avanti Polar Lipids	Negative
Dioleoylphosphatidic acid	1,2-Dioleoyl-sn-glycero-3-phosphate (DOPA)	Avanti Polar Lipids	Negative
Dipalmitoylphosphatidic acid	1,2-Palmitoyl-sn-glycero-3-phosphate (DPPA)	Avanti Polar Lipids	Negative
Phosphatidylcholine	A mixture of 1,2-diacyl-sn-glycero-3-phosphocholines with the composition varying with the source.	Avanti Polar Lipids Phospholipon 90G/ American Lecithin Phospholipon 80/ American Lecithin	Zwitterion
Dierucoylphosphatidylcholine	1,2-Dierucoyl-sn-glycero-3-phosphocholine	Avanti Polar Lipids	Zwitterion
Dilauroylphosphatidylcholine	1,2-Dilauroyl-sn-glycero-3-phosphocholine (DLPC)	Avanti Polar Lipids	Zwitterion
Dilinoleoylphosphatidylcholine	1,2-Dilinoleoyl-sn-glycero-3-phosphocholine	Avanti Polar Lipids	Zwitterion
Dimyristoylphosphatidylcholine	1,2-Dimyristoyl-sn-glycero-3-phosphocholine (DMPC)	Avanti Polar Lipids	Zwitterion
Dioleoylphosphatidylcholine	1,2-Dioleoyl-sn-glycero-3-phosphocholine (DOPC)	Avanti Polar Lipids	Zwitterion
Dipalmitoylphosphatidylcholine	1,2-Dipalmitoyl-sn-glycero-3-phosphocholine (DPPC)	Avanti Polar Lipids	Zwitterion

Name	Description	Source	Charge
Palmitoyl-oleoylphosphatidylcholine	1-Palmitoyl-2-oleoyl-*sn*-glycero-3-phosphocholine (POPC)	Avanti Polar Lipids	Zwitterion
Disteroylphosphatidylcholine	1,2-Distearoyl-*sn*-glycero-3-phosphocholine (DSPC)	Avanti Polar Lipids	Zwitterion
Hydrogenated egg phosphatidylcholine	A mixture of 1,2-hydrogenated diacyl-*sn*-glycero-3-phosphocholines from eggs.	Avanti Polar Lipids	Zwitterion
Hydrogenated soy phosphatidylcholine	A mixture of 1,2-hydrogenated diacyl-*sn*-glycero-3-phosphocholines from soybeans.	Avanti Polar Lipids Phospholipon 100H/American Lecithin Phospholipon 90H/American Lecithin Phospholipon 80H/American Lecithin	Zwitterion
Phosphatidylcholine and lyso-phosphatidylcholine	Phosphatidylcholine 68–84% and lyso-phosphatidylcholine NMT 15% with negatively charged lipids.	NAT 8729/American Lecithin	Negative
Phosphatidylethanolamine	A mixture of 1,2-diacyl-*sn*-glycero-3-phosphoethanolamines with the composition varying with the source.	Avanti Polar Lipids	Zwitterion
Dioleoylphosphatidylethanolamine	1,2-Dioleoyl-*sn*-glycero-3-phosphoethanolamine (DOPE)	Avanti Polar Lipids	Zwitterion
Distearoylphosphatidylethanolamine	1,2-Distearoyl-*sn*-glycero-3-phosphoethanolamine (DSPE)	Avanti Polar Lipids	Zwitterion
Phosphatidylglycerol	A mixture of 1,2-diacyl-*sn*-glycero-3-[phospho-*rac*-(1-glycerol)]s with the composition varying with the source.	Avanti Polar Lipids	Negative
Dimyristoylphosphatidylglycerol	1,2-Dimyristoyl-*sn*-glycero-3-[phospho-*rac*-(1-glycerol)] (DMPG)	Avanti Polar Lipids	Negative
Dioleoylphosphatidylglycerol	1,2-Dioleoyl-*sn*-glycero-3-[phospho-*rac*-(1-glycerol)] (DOPG)	Avanti Polar Lipids	Negative
Dipalmitoylphosphatidylglycerol	1,2-Dipalmitoyl-*sn*-glycero-3-[phospho-*rac*-(1-glycerol)] (DPPG)	Avanti Polar Lipids	Negative
Distearoylphosphatidylglycerol	1,2-Distearoyl-*sn*-glycero-3-[phospho-*rac*-(1-glycerol)] (DSPG)	Avanti Polar Lipids	Negative

(Continued)

Table 11 Cholesterol and Phospholipids (*Continued*)

Excipient	Chemical name or composition	Trade name/supplier	Charge
Palmitoyl-oleoylphosphatidylglycerol	1-Palmitoyl-2-oleoyl-*sn*-glycero-3-[phospho-*rac*-(1-glycerol)] (POPG)	Avanti Polar Lipids	Negative
Phosphatidylinositol	A mixture of 1,2-diacyl-*sn*-glycero-3-phosphoinositols with the composition varying with the source.	Avanti Polar Lipids	Negative
Phosphatidylserine	A mixture of 1,2-diacyl-*sn*-glycero-3-phospho-L-serines with the composition varying with the source.	Avanti Polar Lipids Alcolec PS 90P/ American Lecithin	Zwitterion
Dioleoylphosphatidylserine	1,2-Dioleoyl-*sn*-glycero-3-phospho-L-serine (DOPS)	Avanti Polar Lipids	Zwitterion
Palmitoyl-oleoylphosphatidylserine	1-Palmitoyl-2-oleoyl-*sn*-glycero-3-phospho-L-serine (POPS)	Avanti Polar Lipids	Zwitterion
Sphingomyelin	(2S,3R,4E)-2-Acylaminooctadec-4-ene-3-hydroxy-1-phosphocholine. Also called ceramide-1-phosphocholine.	Avanti Polar Lipids	Zwitterion
Proprietary vehicle	Empty liposomes for addition of drugs containing: NLT 20% phospholipids from soybeans (primarily phosphatidylcholine), 14–18% ethanol, water to 100%	Natipide II/American Lecithin	
Proprietary vehicle	NLT 34% phosphatidylcholine and other phospholipids in sunflower oil	Phosal 35 SB/American Lecithin	
Proprietary vehicle	NLT 50% phosphatidylcholine NMT 6% lysophosphatidylcholine 33.8–41.2% propylene glycol	Phosal 50 PG/American Lecithin	
Proprietary vehicle	NLT 50% phosphatidylcholine NMT 6% lysophosphatidylcholine in safflower oil, glycerin, caprylic/capric triglycerides, alcohol, glyceryl stearate, and ascorbyl palmitate	Phosal 50 SA+/American Lecithin	
Proprietary vehicle	NLT 53% phosphatidylcholine, NMT 6% lysophosphatidylcholine, 3–6% ethanol in caprylic/capric triglycerides, glyceryl stearate, oleic acid, and ascorbyl palmitate	Phosal 53 MCT/American Lecithin	
Proprietary vehicle	72–78% Phosphatidylcholine, NMT 6% lysophosphatidylcholine in alcohol, safflower oil, glyceryl stearate, coconut oil, and ascorbyl palmitate	Phosal 75 SA/American Lecithin	

However, the fatty acid ester bonds are the most labile (30). Studies of soybean phosphatidylcholine, hydrogenated phosphatidylcholine, partially saturated egg phosphatidylcholine, and phosphatidylglycerol have shown the rate of hydrolysis to be pseudo first order and to depend strongly on pH and temperature. For each of these phospholipids, the rate of hydrolysis reached a nadir at pH 6.5 and accelerated as pH either decreased or increased around this value (30,31). Also, some buffer species showed relatively smaller increases in the rate of hydrolysis related to catalytic effects (30,31). Hydrolytic cleavage of one of the two fatty acids associated with a phospholipid molecule results in the production of one molecule of the corresponding lyso-phospholipid and one molecule of the free fatty acid. Studies have shown that the permeability of liposomes to leakage of calcein was minimal until about 10% of the phosphatidylcholine had hydrolyzed to lysophosphatidylcholine and free fatty acid, after which additional hydrolysis resulted in an increase in the permeability and rate of leakage (30).

To minimize instability due to oxidation, formulators can choose phospholipids comprised only of saturated fatty acids or may consider the addition of antioxidants to formulations containing phospholipids comprised of oxidation-prone unsaturated fatty acids. In addition, maintaining an approximate pH of 6.5 during processing and in the final formulation, as well as avoidance of exposure to excessive heat, will help to minimize oxidation and hydrolysis.

It should also be noted that the use of charged phospholipids, such as the phosphatidylglycerols or phosphatidic acids, may prevent liposome aggregation and fusion. Incorporation of cholesterol into the formulation tends to decrease the fluidity and permeability of the liposomal bilayer membrane and promotes formation of smaller, more stable and more uniformly sized vesicles (31,32).

CONCLUSIONS

Lipids are perhaps one of the most versatile excipient classes currently available, providing the formulator with many potential options for improving and controlling the absorption of poorly water-soluble drugs. These formulation options include lipid suspensions, solutions, emulsions, microemulsions, mixed micelles, SEDDS, SMEDDS, thixotropic vehicles, thermo-softening matrices, and liposomes. The formulator should be aware of the factors that determine the suitability of the various lipids for the intended formulation, such as stability to oxidation, hydrolysis, and polymorphic changes as well as digestibility and stability in the GI environment.

Selected subsets of commercially available lipids and considerations pertinent to their pharmaceutical applications have been summarized in this chapter. The formulator is advised to consult the literature and contact the excipient manufacturers for more detailed information on the properties of any lipid being considered for use in formulations.

REFERENCES

1. Rouldt-Marchaud D, Jannin V. Enhanced bioavailability of Simvistatin in a self-micro emulsifying drug delivery system. Gattefosse Internal publication, 2003.
2. Hauss DJ, Fogal SE, Ficorilli JV, et al. Lipid based delivery systems for improving the bioavailability and lymphatic transport of a poorly water-soluble LTB4 inhibitor. J Pharm Sci 1998; 87(2):164–169.
3. Charman WNA, Stella VJ. Transport of lipophilic molecules by the intestinal lymphatic system. Adv Drug Del Rev 1991; 7:1–14.
4. Ash M, Ash I. Handbook of Pharmaceutical Additives. 2nd ed. Endicott, NY: Synapse Information Resources, 2002:3–777.
5. Morrison R, Boyd R. Carboxylic acids. In: Organic Chemistry. 2nd ed. Boston: Allyn and Bacon, 1969:578–614.
6. O'Keefe S. Nomenclature and classification of lipids. In: Akoh C, Min D, eds. Food Lipids: Chemistry, Nutrition and Biotechnology. 2nd ed. New York and Basel: Marcel Dekker, 2002:1–40.
7. Hauser H, Poupart G. Lipid structure. In: Philip L Yeagle, ed. The Structure of Biological Membranes. CRC-Press, 1992:3–71.
8. http://www.lipid.co.uk/infores/lipids.html (accessed May 2004).
9. O'Neil M, Senior Editor. The Merck Index. 13th ed. Whitehouse Station, NJ: Merck and Co., Inc, 2001.
10. Physical constants of organic compounds. In: Lide D, ed. CRC Handbook of Chemistry and Physics. 82nd ed. Boca Raton, London, New York, Washington, D.C.: CRC Press, 2001:3-1 to 3-330.
11. Dr. James Williams, Principal Scientist, Abitec Corp. Personal Communication.
12. Shinoda K, Kunieda H. Phase properties of emulsions: PIT and HLB. In: Becher P, ed. Encyclopedia of Emulsion Technology, Basic Theory. New York and Basel: Marcel Dekker, 1983, Vol. 1:337–367.
13. http://www.crodausa.com/index.lasso (accessed May 2004).
14. http://www.uniqema.com/ (accessed May 2004).
15. http://www.stepan.com/en/ (accessed May 2004).
16. http://www.abitec.com/ (accessed May 2004).
17. http://www.gattefosse.com/ (accessed May 2004).
18. http://www.sasol.com/sasol_internet/frontend/navigation.jsp?navid=1 (accessed May 2004).
19. The HLB System: A Time-Saving Guide to Emulsifier Selection. Wilmington, Delaware: ICI Surfactants, 1992:1–21.
20. The Croda Product Guide to High Purity Raw Materials for Pharmaceutical and Nutritional Use. Parsippany, NJ: Croda Inc., 2000:22.
21. Min D, Boff J. Lipid oxidation of edible oil. In: Akoh C, Min D, eds. Food Lipids: Chemistry, Nutrition and Biotechnology. 2nd ed. New York and Basel: Marcel Dekker, 2002:335–363.
22. Reische D, Lillard D, Eitenmiller R. Antioxidants. In: Akoh C, Min D, eds. Food Lipids: Chemistry, Nutrition and Biotechnology. 2nd ed. New York and Basel: Marcel Dekker, 2002:489–542.
23. Mead J, Alfin-Slater R, Howton D, Popjak G. Peroxidation of fatty acids. In: Lipids: Chemistry, Biochemistry and Nutrition. New York and London: Plenum Press, 1986:83–99.

24. http://www.sigmaaldrich.com/Area_of_Interest/The_Americas/United_States.html (accessed May 2004).
25. http://www.cognis.de/cognis.html (accessed June 2004).
26. http://www.basf.com/static/index.html (accessed June 2004).
27. Bowtle W. Lipid formulations for oral drug delivery. Pharmaceutical Technology Europe September 2000; 20–30.
28. http://www.avantilipids.com/index.htm (accessed June 2004).
29. http://www.americanlecithin.com/ (accessed June 2004).
30. Crommelin D, Schreier H. Liposomes. In: Kreuter J, ed. Colloidal Drug Delivery Systems. New York, Basel, and Hong Kong: Marcel Dekker, 1994:73–190.
31. Crommelin D, Talsma H, Grit M, Zuidam N. Physical stability on long term storage. In: Cevc G, ed. Phospholipids Handbook. New York, Basel, and Hong Kong: Marcel Dekker, 1993:335–348.
32. Liu R, Cannon J, Li Y. Liposomes in solubilization. In: Liu R, ed. Water-Insoluble Drug Formulation. Denver, CO: Interpharm Press, 2000:355–404.

3

Feasibility Assessment and Considerations for Scaling Initial Prototype Lipid-Based Formulations to Phase I/II Clinical Trial Batches

Paul Sirois

Eli Lilly and Company, Indianapolis, Indiana, U.S.A.

INTRODUCTION

The preferred method for the administration of most drugs is via the oral route as conventional compressed tablet or dry-filled capsule formulations. However, there are a growing number of drugs and candidate drug compounds whose inherent solubility and permeability characteristics result in unacceptably low bioavailability when delivered from conventional oral formulations. Many times, standard manipulations aimed at enhancing bioavailability through improvements in the drug solubility or dissolution rate, such as particle size-reduction, or salt or crystal form selection, are either ineffective or do not enhance absorption sufficiently to make these traditional approaches viable options. In such instances, lipid-based formulations may offer an opportunity to enhance bio-availability through processes that impact physicochemical, and occasionally physiologic, mechanisms controlling drug absorption. Efforts to develop tablet formulations containing sufficient quantities of lipid and surfactant excipients to solubilize a poorly water-soluble drug have met with limited success due to the tendency for these excipients to compromise the physical integrity and mechanical strength of conventional compressed tablets. However, most lipid-based formulations are compatible with either hard gelatin capsule (HGC) or soft gelatin capsule (SGC) shells, which allow the development of commercially viable oral dosage forms. The dynamic nature of fully or partially-solubilized drugs in lipid formulations, however, requires careful control of manufacturing, packaging, and handling conditions to maintain the physical and chemical stability of drug and excipients alike, thereby ensuring consistent product performance.

EXCIPIENT SELECTION: GENERAL CONSIDERATIONS

The relationship between in vitro solubility in aqueous media and in vivo drug absorption is well established (1) and the most common reason that lipid excipients are considered for use in an oral formulation is to enhance drug bioavailability resulting from low aqueous solubility (2,3). However, lipid-based formulations can also improve drug absorption through inhibition of P-glycoprotein-mediated efflux (4,5), enhanced lymphatic drug transport and concomitant reduction of hepatic first pass metabolism (6–8), or through prolongation of gastrointestinal transit time, thereby allowing greater time for drug dissolution and absorption to occur (9). Lipid-based formulations have also proven useful in preparing stable formulations of moisture sensitive drugs (10).

The initial objective in excipient screening is to identify excipients or excipient combinations in which the drug has maximal solubility, with the objective of finding a formulation in which the entire drug dose can be solubilized in the fill volume of a single oral capsule of acceptable size. The selected drug concentration for the final formulation should be somewhat less than the maximum solubility in the chosen excipient mixture over the anticipated range of processing and storage temperatures to safeguard against precipitation of the drug. In instances where the drug dose cannot be fully solubilized in the fill volume of a single capsule, the formulator may choose to deliver the drug as a partially solubilized lipid suspension. In addition to simple lipid solution formulations, emulsions (11), self-emulsifying drug delivery systems (SEDDS) and self microemulsifying drug delivery systems (SMEDDS) (discussed in detail in Chapter 5), are combinations of lipids, surfactants, and cosurfactants, that have found application for enhancing and normalizing drug absorption (12–14).

Developing a viable lipid based oral drug formulation with acceptable performance characteristics requires the formulator to maintain the solubility and stability of the drug in an excipient blend that does not adversely interact with the capsule (15). Unexpected precipitation of the drug in the dosage form may result from a number of factors, including insufficient solubility in the excipient matrix, loss of a volatile solubilizing excipient (e.g., ethanol), changes in storage temperature, or migration of water into the formulation from the capsule shell or the environment. In addition, the potential dehydrating effects of some excipients on HGCs can lead to loss of moisture and brittleness or fracture of the capsule shell, which can sometimes be remedied by using SGC, which contain higher levels of plasticizers (propylene glycol, sorbitol, and glycerol) and water.

Thermo-softening Excipients

The low hygroscopicity of the thermo-softening excipients not only makes them particularly compatible with HGC, but also frequently yields final products that are relatively resistant to moisture-induced drug precipitation (16). These excipients are available within a range of melting points and hydrophile–lipophile balance (HLB) values and provide the formulator with latitude for creating specific drug release characteristics in the final product. Examples of these excipients include the Gelucire® and Capmul® lines of derivatized glyceride excipients from Gattefosse and Abitec respectively, and the Cremophor® or Solutol® lines of polyoxyl castor oil and polyethylene glycol derivatives, respectively, from BASF Corporation. These excipients exist as waxy solids or semisolids at typical ambient temperatures and require melting prior to capsule filling; this limits their use to HGC that tolerate temperatures up to 70°C. In addition to being relatively nonhygroscopic, and therefore compatible with HGC shells, the high viscosity of thermo-softening excipients obviates the need for capsule sealing operations, which are required to prevent leakage when using formulations that are liquid at ambient temperatures. For those compounds intended to remain completely solubilized (in the semi solid matrix) at ambient temperatures it is important to develop a quantitative sense of the potential for in situ precipitation or crystallization upon cooling and storage. Direct determination of drug solubility in the congealed excipient matrix is challenging for obvious reasons; however, a solubility estimate may be obtained by back-extrapolation from drug solubility values determined at a series of temperatures at which the excipient is molten. Alternatively, the physical state of the drug in the congealed matrix can be confirmed by using a combination of analytical techniques, including X-ray diffraction, microscopy (polarized light or hot stage) and thermal analysis [Differential Scanning Calorimetry (DSC) or modulated DSC], which together can identify eutectic mixtures, two phase systems, and glassy states of a drug substance (17). For example, correlating the visual changes in the crystalline form of a formulated drug observed during hot stage microscopy with the quantitative thermal events recorded during DSC analysis can be useful for defining the drug solubility range and physical state in the excipient matrix. In addition to physical characterization, the chemical stability of the drug in the molten excipient matrix should be determined over the time and temperature ranges to which the drug will be exposed during manufacturing operations.

When developing formulations using thermo-softening excipients, it is essential to characterize and control the physical state of the excipient matrix, which can crystallize upon congealing. In order to destroy any preformed crystalline structure and to ensure homogeneous dispersion of the multiple components contained in these excipients (e.g., the lauryl macrogolglycerides), the excipient manufacturers recommend liquefying the entire contents of the bulk container by heating to 10°C above the nominal melting temperature followed by thorough mixing prior to use in formulating. Removal and use of portions of bulk containers prior to the melting and mixing step is not recommended and may produce final products, which vary in physical and performance characteristics. Most manufacturers recommend that a given batch of excipient be exposed to no more than three or four melting/cooling cycles to minimize thermally-induced accumulation of peroxides or free fatty acids, which can catalyze drug degradation. For this reason, it is a good practice for the scientist to divide the melted and mixed bulk excipient material into a number of smaller aliquots to support formulation development activities.

The crystalline forms of these excipients that control drug solubilization and release characteristics, are influenced by the thermal history acquired during the product handling and processing procedures (18,19), which if not adequately controlled, will lead to variation in the product in vitro dissolution profile and possibly, in vivo performance. The crystalline form of the excipient matrix can be controlled through postmanufacturing annealing or by careful and consistent control of the congealing process (20). Annealing that involves holding the final product at a controlled, elevated temperature for a predetermined period of time, is used to accelerate conversion of a thermo-softening excipient to its most stable crystalline form. The annealing time may range from a period of several hours to several days, with the duration inversely related to the annealing temperature. For example, the conversion of Gelucire 50/13 to its stable β' crystalline form, requires several months at 25°C, but can be driven to completion in less than two days by annealing at 40°C (21).

LIPID-BASED HARD GELATIN CAPSULE FORMULATION DEVELOPMENT

As typical fill volumes for HGC fall in the range of 0.2 to 0.9 mL, the formulator may initially target a maximum fill volume of 0.5 to 0.7 mL for estimating the required solubility of the drug in the excipient matrix intended for the prototype formulations (Table 1).

Table 1 Capsule Size and Approximate Volumes (Licaps)

Capsule size	Approximate body volume (cc)
00el	0.89
0el	0.7
00	0.82
0	0.59
1	0.43
2	0.33
3	0.26
4	0.18

HGC are physically incompatible with some of the lower molecular weight solubilizing excipients such as polyethylene glycol (PEG) 400, ethanol, water, and glycerol at concentrations greater than a few percent as higher concentrations of these excipients can result in capsule brittleness or softening (22).

The aqueous dissolution rate of HGC is temperature dependent, requiring a minimum of 35°C to occur at an appreciable rate. The dissolution profile of HGC drug products are also subject to change upon aging, particularly following exposure to a combination of elevated heat and humidity (23), certain chemicals (24), or trace levels of volatile substances contained in various packaging components (25,26). The chemical compatibility of the formulation with the capsule shell may be assessed, by dissolution testing following storage of the encapsulated formulation, placebo, and empty capsule shells for approximately one to two months under conditions of elevated temperature and humidity (50°C, 25°C/60%/RH, and 40°C/75% RH). A formulation that is incompatible with the capsule shell may show evidence of changes in appearance, physical integrity, and in vitro dissolution profile. It is helpful to videotape or photograph the dissolution process and scrutinize the visual appearance of the capsule shell as it dissolves. Careful observation of the difference between a poorly dissolving capsule shell containing formulation versus placepo and empty capsule shell stored under the same environmental conditions, may provide insight into whether the formulation or the storage condition has impaired dissolution.

Decreases in the in vitro dissolution performance are often attributed to "gelatin crosslinking," although physicochemical evidence of crosslinking may be difficult to provide. Despite this deficiency, the terms "internal" and "external" crosslinking are frequently used to describe the subjective visual appearance of an insoluble pellicle. Internal crosslinking describes the situation, where the inner surface of the dissolving capsule shell appears to be less soluble than the outer surface, suggesting incompatibility between gelatin and formulation. Changes in capsule dissolution that appear to originate on the external surface of the capsule shell may suggest that environmental factors (e.g., excessive heat, humidity, or exposure to packaging components) are responsible for the change. Interaction between the formulation and capsule gelatin can be confirmed by replacing the capsule contents with a rapidly dissolving formulation and repeating the dissolution test; an altered dissolution profile is confirmatory of this type of interaction (27). Alternatively, empty capsules that were stored for equivalent time periods under identical conditions of temperature and humidity can be used for this test.

The water content of a HGC is critical for maintaining gelatin plasticity and overall capsule shell integrity, and must be kept within a narrow range (13–16% w/w). Inadequate control of HGC moisture content during processing can result in capsule swelling, shrinkage, turned edges, or accumulation of a static charge, all of which can lead to compromised handling on automated filling and sealing equipment and result in batch failures. These deficiencies may go unnoticed during hand-filling of small test batches and can lead a formulator to incorrectly conclude that problems encountered during scale-up are due to a faulty formulation or improper set-up of processing equipment. Hence, it is wise to confirm that the initial moisture content of the HGC shell is within the limits specified by the manufacturer and is maintained within that range during every step of product manufacture and packaging.

Capsule shell moisture content can be estimated by comparing the average weight of a sample of empty capsules to the acceptance range supplied by the manufacturer or by assessing the weight loss on drying at 105°C for 17 hours (28). A useful, shorter screening test may be developed by correlating the 17-hour "loss on drying" results with those generated at slightly elevated temperatures (29) (between 105°C and 120°C) for shorter time periods (e.g., 5–10 minutes) using a gravimetric analyzer such as the Computrac® 2000 (Arizona Instruments, Phoenix, Arizona, U.S.A.). The relationship between HGC brittleness and moisture content is shown in Figure 1 (30). These data were generated by spreading 100 capsules on a 4-inch diameter circular sample test pan, which was subsequently compressed with a platen and held at 1500 psi for 5 to 15 seconds. The number of capsules broken under these conditions represents the percent brittleness of the sample. Empty capsule shells that have remained outside of controlled environmental conditions (between 68°F and 77°F, and 40% and 60% RH), either in the laboratory or in the manufacturing environment, should be discarded prior to resumption of filling operations. During manufacturing operations, empty capsule shells should not remain in the hopper overnight, during lunch breaks, or over other extended periods of work stoppage.

Since excipients can also significantly influence capsule moisture content and physical integrity, formulations need to be selected with regard to their relative humectant properties. Hygroscopic materials such as glycerol, low molecular weight polyethylene glycols (<1000 molecular weight), and propylene glycol are generally unsuitable for HGC products in appreciable levels since they tend to draw

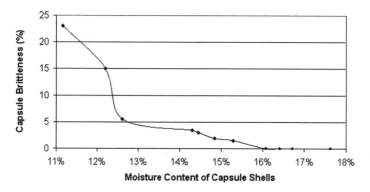

Figure 1   Relationship between hard gelatin capsule shell moisture content and capsule brittleness.

moisture into the capsule shell from humid environments, leading to capsule softening. Conversely, under conditions of low environmental humidity, these excipients can dehydrate the capsule shell leading to brittleness. A variety of simple screening tests can be performed during formulation development to evaluate the moisture affinity profiles of various excipients and their respective compatibilities with the HGC shell (31). One method that requires relatively long periods of time (several weeks), involves evaluating differences in weight gain or loss between small groups or 10 to 20 filled or empty control capsule shells stored under a range of humidity conditions (2.5–65%). Those formulations that maintain their weight within a range of $\pm 2\%$, relative to the empty capsule control, are considered to be hygroscopically compatible with the capsule.

LIPID-BASED SOFT GELATIN CAPSULE FORMULATION DEVELOPMENT

A combination of economic, proprietary, and technical considerations limit the development and manufacture of SGC drug products to a small group of third-party specialist companies. On a relative basis, development and manufacturing costs for SGC products are substantially higher than those for tablets or HGC products, and economic considerations for SGC products usually necessitate round-the-clock manufacturing operations. Consequently, the associated formulations and manufacturing processes must be designed to maintain a continuous supply of capsule fill material that is physically and chemically stable for extended periods of time. SGC that are filled and hermetically sealed in a single operation, find greatest application for low-viscosity (<100 cP), liquid formulation products. A decision to pursue a SGC product is most often driven by a lack of alternative formulation options coupled with a significant commercial opportunity. This decision should also consider the additional costs and potential intellectual property issues associated with any third-party collaboration. Although the average formulator will never be solely responsible for the development of a SGC product, he/she may be required to generate or interpret drug physicochemical, solubility, and excipient compatibility data to facilitate SGC product development by a third-party specialist company.

During the early stages of formulation and drug stability screening, it is possible to obtain strips of SGC gelatin from the capsule manufacturer for use in excipient compatibility screening. This allows the formulator to screen potential incompatibility between the formulation and the gelatin (and its plasticizers and colorants) without committing time and resources to the development of a prototype SGC product. SGC come in a variety of shapes and sizes, but not all can be conveniently delivered by the oral route. The capsule sizes that are acceptable for oral administration are the 20 minim oblong, 16 minim oval, and the 9 minim round shapes, which correspond to volumes of 1.23 mL, 0.99 mL, and 0.55 mL respectively (32). Maximum fill volumes should not exceed 90% of the capsule capacity to guard against rupture or leakage from osmotic or thermally-mediated expansion or from mechanical perturbations of the capsule shell. Filling temperatures must be maintained below 40°C to prevent melting of the capsule shell, which precludes SGC use with most thermo-softening formulations. Compared to HGC, capsule brittleness due to dehydration is less of a problem, since relatively high amounts of plasticizer (40–80% w/w) can be incorporated into the capsule gelatin (32). However, screening of SGC formulations for moisture transfer between the capsule gelatin and formulation nevertheless remains an important criterion during product development.

Immediately after filling, the moisture content of the capsule gelatin is approximately 50% w/w, which necessitates a drying period of several days, during which the formulated drug must be tolerant of the elevated moisture and 21°C to 24°C drying temperature. The potential for drug or excipient to migrate into the shell during the drying period will be dictated by the relative hydrophilicity of these components. Storage or handling of capsules at greater than 60% relative humidity, even for short periods of time, can result in capsule swelling, tackiness, irreversible agglomeration, or cosmetic defects.

While both SGC and HGC possess lower oxygen permeability than conventional film-coated tablets, SGC have higher oxygen permeability than sealed HGC. Achieving a degree of protection from oxygen equivalent to that of a sealed HGC may require inclusion of antioxidants or exclusion of certain oxygen sensitive excipients from the formulation. For example, formulations of oxygen-labile drugs should exclude unsaturated lipid excipients to minimize peroxide formation, which occurs subsequent to fatty acid degradation. In addition, the formulation and excipient screen should consider the use of lipid soluble antioxidants such as butylated hydroxy anisole (BHA) and butylated hydroxy toluene (BHT) (33). The effectiveness of an antioxidant may be assessed by comparing formulations stored in oxygen-enriched atmospheres to those stored under nitrogen or with oxygen-consuming packaging components (34).

The compatible pH range for SGC is between 2.5 and 7.5 (32). Strongly acidic formulations can result in hydrolysis of the capsule gelatin and leakage of the contents. Similarly, basic formulations (including basic salts of weak acid drugs) outside of the compatible pH range can cause gelatin tanning, with subsequent changes in the capsule dissolution profile (32). The ability to buffer basic drugs to an acceptable pH range while maintaining the desired level of solubility should be evaluated by screening pharmaceutically acceptable weak acids, including citric, lactic, and tartaric. Alternatively, consideration of less soluble salts of strongly basic or acidic drug or formulating these drugs as lipid suspensions may provide solutions to SGC incompatibility problems.

Aldehyde impurities that are formed during oxidative degradation of aliphatic alcohols and phenols are frequently present in several excipients including polyethylene glycols, polysorbates, and polyoxyethylenated glycerides. The quantities of these oxidative byproduct impurities generally increase during manufacturing processes involving prolonged exposure to elevated temperatures used during filling of HGC with thermo-softening excipient formulations and have been implicated in capsule shell gelatin crosslinking and changes in the in vitro dissolution rate of the drug product. Although the processing temperatures commonly associated with SGC formulation manufacture are below those typically associated with excipient oxidative degradation, it is still wise to evaluate chemical stability of the pharmaceutical active at temperatures in excess of 30°C for extended periods of time in order to address potential differences in processing times between lab scale and manufacturing batch processing.

When low molecular weight PEG is used for solubility enhancement in a SGC formulation, incorporation of 5% to 10% (w/w) of propylene glycol or glycerin will reduce the migration of these plasticizers from the capsule gelatin into the fill, and decrease the likelihood of capsule brittleness. Inclusion of volatile solubilizing excipients, such as ethanol, should be at concentrations of less than 5% since loss of these excipients may occur during the gelatin drying cycle conducted at 21°C to 24°C and 20% to 30% RH (35).

LIPID SUSPENSION FORMULATIONS

Although fully-solubilized lipid-based formulations generally provide optimal absorption, drugs that cannot be completely solubilized in the lipid excipient matrix may be formulated as partially-solubilized lipid suspensions. Maintaining the physical stability of the dispersed drug in the lipid phase requires control of factors including formulation viscosity, drug particle size, and total solids content, all of which are interdependent with processing times and temperatures.

The physical stability of the dispersion of a solid in a liquid is dependent on the relationship between fluid viscosity and particle diameter, which governs the particle settling rate and in dilute suspensions, and is described by the Stokes Einstein equation:

$$V = [d^2(\rho - \rho_o)g)/18\eta]$$

where, d is the particle diameter, η is fluid viscosity, ρ and ρ_0 are the densities of the particle and fluid respectively, g is the gravity constant, and V is the settling velocity. Although this relationship best applies to dilute suspensions with less than 2% solids content, it illustrates the fundamental concept that settling velocity is proportional to the square of particle diameter and inversely proportional to fluid viscosity. Using this relationship as a guide, the formulator can assess the potential impact of these parameters on a formulation's physical stability or content uniformity and institute controls during development and scale-up of mixing, pumping, and hold time operations.

Predicting the physical and chemical shelf life of suspension formulations from accelerated storage conditions is more challenging than for traditional solid dosage forms, since changes in formulation viscosity and drug solubility induced by elevated testing temperatures may create conditions not reflective of those encountered during product use and storage, thereby leading to erroneous conclusions.

Formulation viscosity, a critical parameter governing the physical stability of suspension formulations, will increase in a nonlinear manner with solids content and will be affected by particle shape and size distribution. The drug particle size, relative crystallinity, and specific crystalline form can all be influenced by changes in the chemical synthetic process, the batch size, or when scaling the milling procedure from bench top to production batches. Since most low solubility drugs will be milled, it is important to understand the impact of different particle size distributions or amorphous content on product performance so that an appropriate control strategy can be established.

From a manufacturing perspective, viscosity has a significant influence on the ease and accuracy of capsule filling and should be closely controlled. Differences in processing temperature, mixing time, shear rate, mixer design and capacity will influence formulation viscosity and can lead to variation in the rate and extent of size attrition of suspended drug particles leading to dosing inaccuracy during filling operations. The mixing rate and shear force required to disperse the solid drug material in the suspending vehicle can be influenced by the formulation batch size, the drug physical properties, the drug loading in the suspending vehicle and the rate of addition of the drug to the vehicle. The formulation scientist should also be aware that the hydrophobic drug particles might aggregate to a greater extent during process scale-up if the rate of addition to the suspending vehicle changes relative to the shear force of the mixer. In this situation, attempting to disrupt the aggregates by mixing at a higher rate of speed may not achieve the intended result if the geometry of the mixing vessel and placement of the mixing blade relative to the surface of the fluid phase are improperly selected. For example, placement of the blade too near the surface could result in incorporation of air into the suspension leading to chemical instability or drug particle aggregation. An increased exposure to heat resulting from longer mixing times with larger batch size, may potentially result in degradation of heat sensitive drug substances. Drug particle size and loading in the suspending vehicle are other factors that can impact required mixing time or shear force necessary to prepare an adequate dispersion. For example, the viscosity of a PEG6000 suspending vehicle at 68°C is typically 300 to 500 centipoise in the absence of suspended drug particles. Introduction of drug particles with a mean diameter of 10 μm at 30% loading may produce a viscosity of approximately 8,000 centipoise, while equivalent loading at an average particle size of 40 microns may increase the viscosity to approximately 10,000 centipoise. Process scale-up of suspensions, particularly from bench scale to first time manufacture, should take into account processing parameter values that are outside of the anticipated manufacturing ranges for time, temperature, and shear rate. This will allow the formulator to compensate for unexpected changes in chemical stability and product performance as the formulation evolves during the development process (36).

ENCAPSULATION OF LIPID-BASED FORMULATIONS

The choice of excipients, the stability of the drug, and the need for heating during the manufacturing process (e.g., to enable filling of thermo-softening formulations) will initially dictate the suitability of a particular capsule format (SGC vs. HGC) for the final product. SGCs and HGCs differ in their excipient compatibility profiles, moisture content, thermal resistance, permeability to oxygen and moisture, and need for special sealing operations.

The potential impact of elevated processing temperatures on formulation stability should be determined over the time intervals corresponding to the typical exposures anticipated during manufacturing. In the case of thermo-softening suspension formulations, the lower viscosities associated with elevated processing temperatures can accelerate the rate of drug particle settling, during cooling of the filled capsules and lead to nonuniform distribution of the drug within the excipient matrix, which can adversely impact in vitro release characteristics (37). It is sometimes possible to compensate for this temperature sensitivity by selecting a drug particle size, small enough to reduce the settling rate to a degree sufficient to maintain a uniform dispersion in the excipient matrix, during the congealing process. Some of the thermal requirements that limit the use of certain excipients with SGC are addressed by the use of HGC, which are less permeable to water and oxygen and tolerate higher filling temperatures than SGC (38). In contrast to SGC, production of liquid-filled HGC products can be routinely handled in most pharmaceutical development organizations with standard processing equipment, provided by manufacturers such as IMA, MG2, Hofliger and Karg, Capsugel, Zanassi, and others. For bench scale preparation of small quantities of prototype capsule formulations, the formulator may choose from the HiBar® Model S0291 (Hibar Systems LTD., Toronto, Canada) or the Liquid Encapsulated Microspray System (LEMS®) CFS 1000 (Capsugel Division of Pfizer, Morris Plains, New Jersey, U.S.A.).

Hard Gelatin Capsule Sealing

The need for postfilling sealing of HGC is determined by the viscosity of the encapsulated formulation. Fluid formulations with viscosities of <100 cP will require sealing, whereas thermo-softening formulations that congeal at ambient temperatures, are inherently leak-proof and, may not require sealing during the prototype assessment stage if kept below 30°C.

Sealing of HGC can be accomplished at bench top scale by either manual or automated means using gelatin banding or solvent fusion. The STI capsule sealer (Schaefer Technologies, Incorporated, Indianapolis, Indiana, U.S.A.) is a typical gelatin banding device useful for sealing small batches of HGC. This device functions by transferring a thin band of molten gelatin to the junction of the capsule body and cap by passing a manually loaded template of 10 capsules across a circular steel plate that gathers gelatin as it rotates through a reservoir of molten gelatin. The model is capable of sealing 100 or 200 capsules per hour and simulates the sealing process of larger production sealing machines (STI S-15 and the Shionogi HICAPSEAL 40/100).

A more recently developed method for sealing HGC is by gelatin fusion, which functions by spraying an aqueous ethanol solution into the junction of the cap and body to fuse the gelatin surfaces together. Following fusion, the capsules are partially dried by momentary application of heated air and subsequently, by overnight tray-drying. This proprietary LEMS technology was developed by the Capsugel Division of Pfizer (Morris Plains, New Jersey, U.S.A.), and requires the use of proprietary, unvented capsules (Licaps®) with a tight cap/body locking ring that prevents liquid seepage into the seal area during the drying process. The Capsugel CFS 1000 is a gelatin fusion sealer, which affords sufficient flexibility of scale and ease of use for both low and high viscosity liquid filling and has a maximum output of 1000 filled and sealed capsules per hour, making it suitable for experimental as well as initial clinical trial batch sizes. The unit is relatively small, weighing approximately 100 kg with physical dimensions of $720 \times 380 \times 520$ mm (L $\times$ W $\times$ H). A 700 mL capacity heated liquid fill reservoir with optional heating suitable for filling thermo-softening formulations is available along with a smaller (30 mL) unheated reservoir, intended for filling small prototype batches of liquid formulations.

SUMMARY

Oral lipid-based formulations provide the formulation scientist with a significant opportunity to address the poor and variable gastrointestinal absorption typically associated with poorly water soluble drugs. In some instances, these formulations may be of benefit for increasing drug exposure resulting from low intestinal permeability or for delivering drugs subject to certain forms of chemical instability. Most lipid-based formulations would preferably deliver the drug in solubilized form. A number of physical and chemical factors including moisture, drug solubility in the excipient matrix, and the crystalline forms of both the excipient and the drug can potentially influence product performance and should be identified and controlled by the formulator. While both HGCs and SGCs can be used to deliver oral lipid-based formulations, a thorough understanding of differences in processing requirements and excipient compatibilities with the capsule shell is required to ensure successful development of a drug product. The mechanical properties and physical integrity of the capsule gelatin are dependent upon establishing a proper balance between water or other plasticizing agents within the gelatin film, controlling the heat and moisture to which the capsule is exposed during processing, and proper selection of the packaging components used to protect the product from the environment. In particular, the equilibrium established between environmental moisture and the pharmaceutical active or excipients contained in the formulation can have a significant impact on the physical and chemical properties of the drug, and the in vitro and in vivo performance of the dosage form. It is important for the formulation scientist to understand, anticipate, and screen for potential differences in equipment performance and processing parameters when scaling from bench top to production size batches. A number of suggestions have been presented in this chapter to enable the formulation scientist to screen for potential changes in drug solubility, physical form, content uniformity, and product performance during the earliest stages of product development. By developing a fundamental understanding of the differences, both subtle and obvious, between bench-top scale and manufacturing equipment and processes, the scientist should be able to develop oral lipid-based drug products that perform effectively and consistently between scales.

REFERENCES

1. Amidon GL, Lennernas VP, Crison JR. A theoretical basis for a biopharmaceutics drug classification: the correlation of in vitro drug product dissolution and in vivo bioavailability. Pharm Res 1995; 12:413–420.
2. Strickley RG. Solubilizing excipients in oral and injectable formulations. Pharm Res 2004; (21)2:210–230.
3. Shah NH, Carvajal MT, Patel CI, Infeld MH, Malick AW. Self emulsifying drug delivery systems (SEDDS) with polyglycolyzed glycerides for improving invitro dissolution and oral absorption of lipophilic drugs. Int J Pharm 1994; 106:15–23.
4. Wasan KM. Formulation and physiologic and biopharmaceutical issues in the development of oral lipid based drug delivery systems. Drug Dev Ind Pharm 2001; 27(4):267–276.
5. Yeh PY. Effect of medium chain glycerides on physiological properties of rabbit intestinal epithelium in vitro. Pharm Res 1994; 11(8):1148–1154.
6. Caliph SM, Charman WN, Porter CJH. Effect of short-, medium-, and long-chain fatty acid-based vehicles on the absolute oral bioavailability and intestinal lymphatic transport of halo tantrine and assessment of mass balance in lymph-cannulated and non-cannulated rats. J Pharm Sci 2000; 89(8):1073–1084.
7. Hauss DJ, Fogal SE, Ficorilli JV, et al. Lipid based delivery systems for improving the bioavailability and lymphatic transport of a poorly water soluble LTB_4 inhibitor. J Pharm Sci 1998; 87(2):164–169.
8. Charman WNA, Stella VJ. Transport of lipophilic molecules by the intestinal lymphatic system. Adv Drug Del Rev 1991; 7:1–14.
9. Welling PG. Influence of food and diet on gastrointestinal drug absorption: a review. J Pharmacokinet Biopharm 1977; 5:292–334.
10. Shah NH, Phuapradit W, Ahmed H. Liquid/semi solid filling in hard gelatin capsules: formulation and processing considerations. Semi-solid formulations and oral absorption enhancement. Bulletin Technique Gattefosse 1996; 27–37.
11. Stegemann S. Liquid and semisolid formulation in hard gelatin capsules. Swiss Pharma 1999; 21(6):21–28.
12. Microemulsions Formulation Guide. Gattefosse technical document MEP 3–18. Pharmaceutical Department Edition, May 1992.
13. Tenjarla S. Microemulsions: an overview and pharmaceutical applications. Crit Rev Ther Drug Carrier Syst 1999; 16:461–521.

14. Charman WN, Porter CJH, Mithani S, Dressman JB. Physicochemical and physio-logical mechanisms for the effects of food on drug absorption: the role of lipids and pH. J Pharm Sci 1997; 86(3):269–282.

15. Serajuddin ATM, Sheen PC, Augustine MA. Water migration from soft gelatin capsule shell to filled material and its effect on drug solubility. J Pharm Sci 1986; 75(1):62–64.

16. Cade D, Madit N. Liquid filling in hard gelatin capsules–preliminary steps. Lecture presented at Gattefosse Symposium, June 1966. Capsugel Library, BAS 1998:191.

17. Craig QM. The physical characterization of Gelucire 50/13. Semi solid formulations and oral absorption enhancement. Bulletin Technique Gattefosse 1996.

18. Duddu SP, Roussin P, Laforet JP, Pad NR. A Gelucire 50/13 theophylline formula-tion. Semi solid formulations and oral absorption enhancement. Bulletin Technique Gattefosse 1996.

19. Sutananta W, Craig DQM, Newton JM. An investigation into the effects of prepara-tion conditions and storage on the rate of drug release from pharmaceutical glyceride bases. J Pharm Pharmacol 1995; 47:355–359.

20. Gelucine® solid product literature. Controlled Release and Increased Bioavailability. PF 96327 page 12, 1st edition, April 1999.

21. Gattefosse internal communication. Controlled Release and Increased Bioavailability. PF 96327 page 12, 1st edition, April 1999.

22. Bowtle WJ. Liquid filling of hard gelatin capsules: a new technology for alternative formulations. Pharm Tech Eur 1998; 10:84–90.

23. Khalil SA, Ali MM, Khalek AMMA. Effects of aging and relative humidity on drug release. Part 1. Chloramphenicol capsules. Pharmazie 1974; 29:36–37.

24. Cade D, Madit N, Cole ET. Development of a test procedure to consistently ross-link hard gelatin capsules with formaldehyde. Pharm Res (New York) 1994; 11(suppl 10):S147.

25. Hartauer KJ, Bucko JH, Cooke GG, Mayer RF, Schwier JR, Sullivan GR. The effect of rayon coiler on the dissolution stability of hard-shell gelatin capsules. Pharm Tech 1993; 17:76–83.

26. Chen GL, Hao WH. Factors affecting zero-order release kinetics of porous gelatin capsules. Drug Dev Ind Pharm 1998; 24(6):557–562.

27. Cade D, Madit N. Liquid filling of hard gelatin—preliminary steps. Capsugel Library Publication 1998.

28. Internal communication with Shionogi Qualicaps.

29. Unpublished internal data.

30. Unpublished internal data generated using Shionogi test method to assess capsule brittleness.

31. Serajuddin ATM, Sheen PC, Augustine MA. Water migration from soft gelatin capsule shell to filled material and its effect on drug solubility. J Pharm Sci 1986; 75:62–64.

32. Stanley JP. Soft gelatin capsules. In: Lachman L, Lieberman HA, Kanig JL. The Theory and Practice of Industrial Pharmacy. 3rd ed. Philadelphia: Lea and Febiger, 1986:398–412.

33. Arthur HK. Handbook of Pharmaceutical Excipients. 3rd ed. Washington, DC: AphA, 2000.

34. Fresh Pax™ oxygen absorbing packet. Multisorb Technologies Inc., Buffalo, New York, U.S.A., 14224–1893.

35. Ebert WR. Soft elastic gelatin capsules: a unique dosage form, Pharm Technol 1977; 1:44–50.
36. AAPS Workshop Committee. Scale-up of liquid and semisolid disperse systems. Pharm Technol 1995; 19(6):52–60.
37. Shah NH, Phuapradit W, Ahmed H. Liquid/semi solid filling in hard gelatin capsules: formulation and processing considerations. Semi-solid formulations and oral absorption enhancement. Bulletin Technique Gattefosse 1996; 27–37.
38. Cole ET. Liquid filled hard gelatin capsules. Pharm Tech 1989; 13(9):124–140.

4

Materials, Process, and Manufacturing Considerations for Lipid-Based Hard-Capsule Formats

William J. Bowtle

*Department of Research and Development,
Encap Drug Delivery, Livingston, U.K.*

INTRODUCTION

The recognition of the potential of lipid-based formulations for improving the gastrointestinal absorption of poorly water-soluble drugs has been a major driver for the development of liquid-filled capsule technology (1–4). Lipid excipients possess a wide range of desirable characteristics, such as broad chemical compatibility, low melting points, surfactant or self-emulsifying properties, and suitability for large-scale manufacture. The increasing application of lipid-based formulations has prompted the production equipment and capsule manufacturers to develop new materials, processing systems, and product formats. Lipid-based capsule formulations are encountered not only in ethical pharmaceutical products but in consumer and "high-end" nutriceutical products as well. The market is therefore diverse and presents numerous technical challenges for the formulation and manufacture of these dosage forms.

This chapter will describe the material-selection and process issues for oral lipid-based formulations with an emphasis on their use in hard-capsule format. It reflects specialist development and manufacturing experience acquired over 15 years and in over 1500 batches of lipid-based capsule products ranging from simple nutriceutical oil formulations to cytotoxics. In order to provide a basis for the successful manufacture of a novel lipid-based oral dosage form, options in

formulation excipients and capsule shell selection will be discussed along with
the main processing routes employed.

THE CONCEPT

The most basic lipid-based formulations are simple fluids (e.g., low-viscosity oils,
<50 cps) or suspensions with drug solids content varying from <0.04% to 40.0%
and with viscosities ranging from 20 to over 25,000 cps. They may be thermo-
softening products or self-emulsifying formulations. Additionally, they may include
multi-phase formats designed to meet more complex and specific technical needs
such as multi-step release-profiles. Certain products, specifically the multi-phase or
thermo-softening formulations with high melting-points, are better suited to the
hard gelatin capsule format as dictated by the processing needs. A limited number
are better suited to soft gelatin capsule encapsulation due to the embrittling or plasticizing effects of the formulation excipients. Lipid-based formulations are well
suited to processing in capsule format, especially as one-piece soft gelatin capsules
or as the more commonly used two-piece hard gelatin capsules. A further type consists of spherical capsules containing an oil/active, which are formed by coextrusion
of the core content and a gelatin/plasticizer solution through submerged nozzles,
forming the so-called "seamless capsule" (5). While the soft gelatin capsule has
been available for liquid-filled products for over 150 years, the liquid-filled, two-
piece hard gelatin capsule has become well established only in the last 5 to 10 years.
This has been due largely to the time required to generate sufficient stability and in
vivo performance data and to gain regulatory approval for these formulations as
well as recent technological developments, which allow for efficient, large-scale
encapsulation of lipid-based products. Figure 1 shows the concept for liquid-filled
two-piece capsules. The active component, as a liquid or as a solid, may be formulated with a liquid, thixotropic, or thermo-softening carrier to form a fluid, which is
filled into hard capsules using capsule filling equipment in which a fluid-filling
pump replaces the powder head. Certain products may require a further process of
capsule sealing, while others require no further processing. Sealing may be required
due to the physical nature of the fill material (e.g., low viscosity liquid), to improve
stability or for regulatory or marketing reasons. The production process therefore is
essentially a mix/fill/seal sequence, which can be simplified for particular products,
for example, by the elimination of the need to seal.

MATERIALS

Capsule Shells

Animal Gelatin

Animal gelatin represents the historical major material for two-piece capsules. Its
properties and most recent issue, transmissible spongiform encephalopathy (TSE),
are well understood (6,7). The major gelatin capsule manufacturers can provide

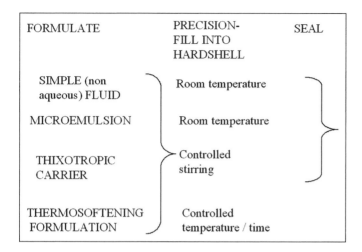

Figure 1   Unit operations involved in the production of liquid filled, two-piece gelatin or HPMC capsules. The active component, as a liquid or as a solid, may be formulated with a liquid, thixotropic, or thermo-softening carrier which is filled into hard capsules using capsule filling equipment in which a fluid-filling pump replaces the powder head. Certain products may require a further process of capsule sealing to ensure against leakage.

variants designed specifically for liquid-filling. While these can offer certain advantages, they are not necessary to all products, according to the nature of the fill material and the processing system being used. Issues of TSE, specific technical properties and consumer preference/religion-based market requirements drive a continuing effort to find substitutes (8). The current alternative material of choice to animal gelatin capsules are those prepared from hydroxypropyl methylcellulose (HPMC). Another recently introduced but less frequently applied alternative to animal gelatin is fish-skin-derived gelatin.

Hydroxypropyl Methylcellulose

Recent advances in capsule sealing technology have improved the commercial attractiveness of HPMC capsules. Many major pharmaceutical companies are proactively including them in their development programs. Their technical properties are compared with those for gelatin in Table 1. HPMC is a mixed-ether of cellulose containing variable proportions of methoxy- and 2-hydroxypropoxy groups. Various grades are suitable for preparing hard capsules and are accepted by the pharmacopoeia in the United States, Europe, and Japan (9). The grades used for capsule manufacture provide shells whose water solubility characteristics compare with those of gelatin. HPMC capsules compare closely in physical size and dimensions to gelatin capsules, allowing them to be processed on standard capsule-filling equipment. However, the various capsule shell manufacturers employ a variety of additives and production techniques, which influence the capsule physical properties and suitability for specific products, particularly

Table 1 Comparison of Gelatin and HPMC Capsule Shells

Selection factor	Gelatin capsule	HPMC capsule
International capsule acceptability	Widespread	Widespread for nutriceuticals; restrictions for ethical pharmaceuticals
Transmissible spongiform encephalopathy certification	Required	Not required
Manufacturer	Capsugel, Qualicaps, Roxlor, and Cardinal Health	Capsugel, Qualicaps, Su Hueng
Liquid-fill variant	Licaps, double ring	None
Moisture content	13–16%	4–6%
Solubility characteristics	Dissolves in acid and neutral condition	Varies according to manufacturer
Working temperature	Up to 75°C	Up to 75°C
Susceptibility to embrittlement	High	Low moisture content confers resistance to embrittlement
Susceptibility to static	High	Low
Susceptibility to Maillard reaction	Yes	No
Permeability to oxygen	Very low	High
Suitability for liquid-filling	Yes	Yes
Suitability for sealing	Yes	Wet-strength of HPMC requires specialized approach
Suitability for coating	Yes	Yes

Abbreviation: HPMC, hydroxypropyl methylcellulose.

liquid-filled products (10). While HPMC capsules are generally suitable for most nutriceutical products, limitations may be encountered in pharmaceutical application due to specific technical issues such as poor solubility at low pH or high oxygen permeability. In addition, costs are much higher than for gelatin capsules. Technical comparisons of gelatin and HPMC capsules are listed in Table 1.

Fish Gelatin

Fish gelatin is derived from the collagen of fish skin and is chemically and structurally similar to mammalian gelatin. Its main commercial attractiveness lies in avoidance of the various health and personal preference issues associated with mammalian gelatin. Commercially available fish gelatin is prepared from species residing in either cold water (CFG) or warm water (WFG), with the two varieties differing in the relative content of the amino acids proline and hydroxyproline. WFG is the only form suitable for the preparation of capsule shells or for band-sealing capsules as the banding process is critically dependent on the occurrence of gelling at temperatures of approximately ≤35°C. The low proportion of proline and hydroxyproline found in CFG requires temperatures of less than 8°C to 10°C for gelling to occur, thus rendering this form of fish gelatin unsuitable for capsule manufacture or as a banding material.

The application of fish gelatin to capsule manufacture is limited primarily by availability, high cost, and lack of inclusion in the various pharmacopoeias, which currently refer to mammalian-derived gelatin exclusively. The safety profile of fish gelatin with regard to persons with fish allergy has not yet been determined. Experience at Encap Drug Delivery in trial manufacturing for nutriceutical oils has shown that these capsules, such as those manufactured by Roxlor (France), are well suited to use in standard manufacture of liquid-filled capsules, although their cost currently precludes their use for commercial liquid-fill products.

Lipid Excipients

Description

Lipid excipients may be used as simple, single-component oily solutions of the drug substance or in more complex systems such as suspensions, microemulsions or self-emulsifying drug delivery systems. For the purposes of this report, they are herewith described as fluids (remaining fluid at or below 25°C) or as thermo-softening materials. Tables 2 and 3 provide summary information, collated from standard texts, manufacturers' literature, and from extensive experience at Encap. A range of related surface-active materials is also described. The simple oil excipients are composed of mono-, di-, or triglycerides or their derivatives, and differ on the content of medium (6 to 12 carbon atoms in chain length) or long-chain (12 or more carbons in chain length) fatty acids. These excipients are water-immiscible and their solvent characteristics for drug substances vary according to the chain length of the fatty acid content. Certain of these excipients, such as the medium chain monoglycerides, have surfactant or self-emulsifying characteristics. Lipid excipients may be selected for some specific purpose, such as product stability improvement or absorption enhancement. Their extensive origination and derivation provide for a wide range of properties suited to liquid-filled formulation and manufacture.

Nomenclature

Nomenclature for the components of fatty oils can be confusing with respect to fatty acid content. When reference is made in the pharmacopoeia to "the fatty-acid fraction of the oil," it pertains to the fatty acid components of the glycerides, as opposed to the free fatty acid content of the oil, which is usually minimal (typical acid values are <1). For example, the European Pharmacopoeia (Ph. Eur.) monograph for "medium-chain triglycerides" includes a listing of five fatty acids under "composition of fatty acids" but makes no reference to "triglyceride" other than in the defining title and description. A parent material, coconut oil, refers to 12 fatty

Table 2 GRAS-Listed and Pharmacopoeial Liquid Excipients for Liquid-Filled Two-Piece Capsules

Material/compliance	Source/chemistry/major fatty acid	Comment	Brand/manufacturer
Liquid excipients (melting point ≤ 25°C), natural or refined			
Arachis oil[a,b]	Oil, vegetable; glyceride (long chain C-18:1; C-18:2)	Refined oil, should not be linked with nut allergy; protect from oxygen and light	Various
Canola oil[a,c]	Oil, vegetable; glyceride (long chain C-18:1; C-18:2; C-18:3)	Rapeseed oil from strains with low erucic acid content	Various
Corn oil (maize oil)[a,b,d]	Oil, vegetable; glyceride (long chain C-18:1; C-18:2)	Protect from oxygen and light	Various
Fractionated coconut oil[a,c]	Oil, vegetable; fractionated; triglycerides (medium chain C-8:0; C-10:0)	Classified as "medium chain triglycerides" in European Pharmacopoeia	Various
Lecithin[b,c]	Oil, vegetable; phosphatidyl esters/triglycerides/fatty acids	E 322[f]; zwitter-ionic; partially soluble in water; emulsifier	Various
Olive oil[b–d]	Oil, vegetable; glyceride (long chain C-18:1)	Protect from oxygen and light	Various
Sesame oil[a,b,d]	Oil, vegetable; glyceride (long chain C-18:1; C-18:2)	Protect from oxygen and light	Various
Soybean oil[a,b]	Oil, vegetable; glyceride (long chain C-18:1; C-18:2; C-18:3)	Protect from oxygen and light	Various
Liquid excipients (M.P. ≤ 25°C), semi- and fully-synthetic			
Caprylic/capric/ succinic triglycerides[c]	Triglyceride (medium chain, C-8:0; C-10:0, succinylated	Carrier	Miglyol 829/ Condea
Caprylic/capric lauric triglycerides[a,c]	Triglyceride (medium chain, C-8:0; C-10:0)	Solubilizer	Captex 355 EP/Abitec Corp

Name	Chemical	Function	Trade name/Supplier
Caprylic/capric triglycerides[a,c,d]	Triglyceride (medium chain, C-8:0; C-10:0)	Solubilizer	Captex 300 EP/Abitec Corp
Caprylic/capric triglycerides[a,c,d]	Triglyceride (medium chain, C-8:0; C-10:0)	Fractionated coconut oil, from *Cocos nucifera*	Miglyol 810/Condea Miglyol 812 N/Condea
Glycerol monolinoleate[a,c]	Mono- and di-glycerides (long chain, C-18:2)	E 471[f]; insoluble in water; very soluble in vegetable oils; self-emulsifying	Maisine 35-1 FCC/Gattefosse
Linoleoyl macrogol-glycerides[a]	Macrogol glyceride (long-chain, C-18:2)	Insoluble but dispersible in water	Labrafil M 2125 CS/Gattefosse
Oleic acid[a-c]	Fatty acids (C-18:1 + others)	Mixture of unsaturated fatty acids; miscible with fixed oils	Various
Propylene glycol dicaprylate/dicaprate[c]	Propylene glycol di-esters of (C-8:0; C-10:0) fatty acids	Carrier	Miglyol 840/Condea

Pharmacopoeial compliance/GRAS status:
[a] European Pharmacopoeia,
[b] United States National Formulary,
[c] GRAS,
[d] Japanese Pharmacopoeia,
[e] United States Pharmacopoeia;
[f] "E abc" etc., is an EEC code, which designates specific food additives.

acids under "fatty acid fraction of the oil" but also makes no reference to "triglyceride." Conversely, the Ph. Eur. monograph for sesame oil does refer to triglyceride content (as determined by fatty acid radicals) in defining limits for particular components (e.g., "a glyceride with two oleic acid and one linoleic acid chains").

Fluid Excipients

Fluid excipients, defined as those that are flowable liquids at ambient room temperature, are comprised of three primary classes based on their derivation: (*i*) natural and fractionated oils, (*ii*) semi-synthetic liquids, and (*iii*) fully synthetic liquids.

Natural and Fractionated Oils

A wide range of natural product oils are available and suitable for use in encapsulated oral formulation products. The majority of these oils are derived from plant sources, which have been subjected to various degrees of refining, including solvent extraction, deodorizing, and bleaching. Chemically, these oils are glyceride esters of a wide range of saturated and unsaturated fatty acids, the exact composition being characteristic of the specific oil itself and subject to variation based on such factors as source and growing season. Certain natural product oils, such as evening primrose oil and the marine oils, find application primarily for their nutritive or health benefits, although they could technically be used as lipid excipients.

Plant Oils

Plant oils are composed primarily of unsaturated fatty acid glycerides containing oleic acid (C-18:1), linoleic acid (C-18:2) and in certain cases, linolenic acid (C-18:3). These oils also contain varying proportions of saturated fatty acid glycerides composed of various medium and long-chain fatty acids, as previously mentioned. The exact mixture of glycerides present in a given plant oil is determined by the particular plant species and can vary with the source or growing season. The particular glyceride mixture dictates the pharmaceutically-important properties of melting point and susceptibility to oxidative degradation. The melting point of a plant oil is controlled by both the glyceride fatty acid chain length and degree of unsaturation, with shorter chain length and higher degree of unsaturation favoring a lower melting point. For instance, soybean oil, a popular pharmaceutical excipient, is fluid at ambient room temperature, whereas its hydrogenated derivative melts at 66°C to 72°C. Fluidity at ambient room temperature is generally considered desirable from a processing standpoint as it obviates the need for capsule filling at elevated temperatures, which can result in varying degrees of degradation of both drug and excipient alike. The relative susceptibility to oxidation is controlled largely by the degree of fatty acid unsaturation, with resistance to oxidation being favored by saturated fatty acid glycerides. The unsaturated glycerides are chemically reactive to oxygen and light, forming peroxides, which can impact the stability of drug substances and affect the integrity of gelatin capsules, necessitating capsule filling in an inert atmosphere (e.g., nitrogen) to prevent in-process oxidation. In addition, the final products may also require protection from oxygen and light during storage and prior to use.

Canola oil (low erucic acid rapeseed oil) is of increasing interest, due to its aggressive marketing and low (<7.1%) level of saturated fatty acids, which is half the level of corn, olive, and soybean oils and one-quarter of the level in cotton seed oil (11). It is derived from rapeseed plant strains, with low levels of erucic acid developed through traditional hybridization and from gene-modification programs. Native rapeseed oil was previously considered unsuitable for use in humans due to its erucic acid content, which has been implicated in muscle wasting. The Ph. Eur. limits the erucic acid content of rapeseed oils to not more than 2% of the total fatty acids present in the oil. Canola oil also contains tocopherol as a natural antioxidant and this contributes to its stability.

Other vegetable oils contain higher levels of saturated fatty acids and glycerides along with varying high levels of (unsaturated) C-18:1 and C-18:2 fatty acids and are vulnerable to oxidation. Various nutriceutical oils (e.g., borage) also contain glycerides of C-18:3 fatty acids and possess similar oxidative lability. However, the (C-18:1 and C-18:2) oils commonly used in pharmaceuticals (Table 2) are regarded as stable, when protected from oxygen and light. Soy bean oil also contains 5% to 10% C-18:3 fatty acid, which makes it somewhat more vulnerable to oxidation. In practice, the pharmacopeias permit inclusion of an antioxidant and these grades are regarded as stable, when protected from atmospheric oxygen.

Fractionated Glycerides

Separation of particular plant oils into their component glyceride fractions, as is carried out commercially for coconut oil and to a lesser extent, palm kernel oil, has been used to prepare excipients that maximize desirable physical and drug absorption-promoting properties, while minimizing such issues as susceptibility to oxidation. Coconut oil, for example, is composed of saturated medium (MCT) (C6:0 to C-12:0) and long-chain (LCT) fatty acid triglycerides (C-12:0 to C-18:0) and is semi-solid at ambient room temperature. Its fluid derivative, fractionated coconut oil (FCO) [e.g., Miglyol 812 (Condea, Witten, Germany) and Captex 300 (Abitec Corporation, Ohio, U.S.A.), which contain ≥95% medium-chain (C-8:0 and C-10:0) saturated fatty acids] finds greater application as a pharmaceutical excipient in soft gelatin encapsulated products such as Advil® (ibuprofen), Robitussin® (guiafenisin), and "Lemsip." MCT have proven particularly suitable as oily excipients for oral drug administration. These products, by virtue of their shorter fatty acid chain length, are liquids at ambient room temperature and, when prepared from natural product oils composed primarily of saturated triglycerides, confer resistance to oxidative degradation. MCT are also more readily hydrolyzed during gastrointestinal lipid digestion than are LCTs (12) and are also less dependent on bile salts for preabsorptive emulsification. For example, lingual lipases continue to hydrolyze di- and triglycerides in the upper small intestine and are unaffected by luminal amphiphiles, including the bile salts (13).

Marine oils: Marine oils are rich in long-chain (≥ 20 carbon atoms in chain length) fatty acids and are distinguished from terrestrial animal oils by their relatively high content of polyvalent unsaturated fatty acids [e.g., C-20:5 omega-3 or eicosapentaenoic acid (EPA), and C-22:6 omega-3 or docosahexaenoic acid (DHA)]. Marine oils are particularly susceptible to oxidation and require protection from oxygen and light, which generally precludes their use as pharmaceutical excipients. Rather, these oils find application primarily for their nutritive benefits due to their content of EPA and DHA as well as various fat-soluble vitamins.

Semi-synthetic Fluids

Several semi-synthetic fluid excipients are currently available as pharmaceutical excipients for oral formulation development. They are derived from plant sources and are comprised primarily of medium-chain (C-8/C-10) saturated fatty acids that have been chemically combined with one or more chemical entities to confer dispersing or self-emulsifying properties on the final product, which may enhance drug absorption (e.g., Labrafil M 2125 CS, Imwitor 780K). These products consist of specific mixtures of propylene glycol esters of mono-, di-, and triglycerides and are generally resistant to oxidative degradation.

In general, the semi-synthetic fluids are well suited for filling into both soft and hard gelatin or HPMC capsules. They are self-emulsifying or dispersible in water and are relatively hydrophilic. Experience in our laboratories has shown that certain materials (e.g., Labrafil M 2125®) may require the addition of a more hydrophobic component, such as a hard fat, to prevent embrittlement of hard gelatin capsules. Such problems, however, may be solved more simply by the use of HPMC capsule shells, since they do not become brittle, even at low moisture content.

Exceptions arise for those excipients containing glycerol, which possesses humectant and gelatin plasticizing properties. Although compatible with soft gelatin capsules that incorporate glycerol as a plasticizing agent, hard gelatin capsules are subject to softening and deformation in the presence of glycerol. Particular proprietary products (e.g., Capmul MCM) may contain glycerol as a secondary component, which thereby precludes use of such excipients for the hard gelatin capsule formats.

Phospholipids: Lecithin is an emulsifying agent derived from soy and consisting of phospholipids, which are similar to triglycerides except that the first hydroxyl of the glycerol molecule has a polar phosphate-containing group in place of a fatty acid. Pharmaceutical grades of lecithin are readily available and this excipient, which is a common ingredient in soft gelatin capsule formulations, is compatible with both hard and soft gelatin capsules. For example, the proprietary products, "capsule filling masses 'SPL' and 'PPL,'"manufactured by Lipoid GMBH (Ludwigshafen, Germany) are viscous fluids that are described as polyunsaturated phospholipids derived from soybean lecithin. The development use of a particular lecithin ("galactolecithin," mixed galactolipids and phospholipids, 70:30) has been described for delivery of insoluble drugs, such as cyclosporin and acyclovir, in soft gelatin capsules (14).

Synthetic Fluids

There are available a number of fully-synthetic monomeric and polymeric liquids that possess sufficient solubilizing power for hydrophobic substances to render them useful as excipients for formulating poorly water-soluble drugs. These excipients, most of which are glycolic in nature, can be used alone or in combination with lipid excipients to improve the overall solubilizing power of the formulation. As they are water-miscible, these excipients can exhibit dose-dependent bioavailability enhancement following dilution in the primarily aqueous contents of the gastrointestinal tract and loss of solubilizing capability, resulting in uncontrolled precipitation of the drug substance.

Propylene glycol: Propylene glycol is a useful solvent for compounds that are either unstable or insoluble in water. Its humectant and plasticizing properties make it a suitable excipient for soft gelatin capsule formulations but prevent its use in hard gelatin capsules, in which it causes softening and deformation.

Poloxamers: Poloxamers are block copolymers consisting of polyoxyethylene-polyoxypropylene glycol. Specific grades are defined in a three-digit format, where the first two digits multiplied by 100, is the approximate average molecular weight of the polyoxypropylene portion, and the third digit, multiplied by 10, is the percentage by weight of the polyoxyethylene portion. For example, the liquid grade "Poloxamer 124" has a polyoxypropylene portion of molecular weight of 1200 and a polyoxyethylene portion comprising 40% of the molecule. This amphiphilic excipient is fluid at room temperature, has wide chemical compatibility, surfactant properties, and may increase the absorption of lipophilic drugs. Formulators should note that the commercial availability development-scale quantities of Poloxamer 124 USNF is very limited in Europe; larger, production-size batches can, however, be obtained. Other technical liquid grades are available but are not suited to use in humans [see section on "Thermo-Softening (Semi-Solid) Excipients" for solid grades and current use].

Macrogols: The macrogols, also known as polyoxyethylene glycols or "PEGs," are available as both liquids and thermo-softening semi-solids, possess molecular weights in the range of 300 to 600 and find wide application as pharmaceutical excipients due to their high solubilizing capacity for many hydrophobic drugs. Similar to propylene glycol, PEGs are widely used in soft gelatin capsule formulations, but find limited use in conjunction with hard gelatin capsules, due to their dehydrating or softening effects, which compromise the capsule physical integrity.

Thermo-softening (Semi-solid) Excipients

Thermo-softening excipients that melt in the range of 26°C to 70°C and exist as waxy semi-solids at ambient room temperatures include both semi-synthetic and fully synthetic products. These excipients are typically filled into capsules in the molten state, with the excipient melting temperature dictating the suitability for hard versus soft gelatin capsules. Hard gelatin capsules can tolerate molten formulations up to 70°C, whereas soft gelatin capsules, which melt at a lower temperature, are only suitable for excipients melting at <40°C.

Semi-synthetic Excipients

The majority of semi-synthetic, thermo-softening excipients are glycerides of saturated fatty acids, and include the hydrogenated oils or hard fats and the macrogolglycerides. A unique semi-solid excipient, d-alpha tocopheryl macrogol 1000 succinate, is a semi-synthetic derivative of vitamin E, which has found limited application in the oral delivery of poorly soluble drugs (see next).

Hard fats: These excipients are hydrogenated glycerides derived from various natural oils and include Gelucire® 30/01 and 43/01 (Gattefosse, Cedex, France) and Sterotex® HM (Abitec Corporation, Ohio, U.S.A.) derived from palm and soybean oils, respectively. They are highly water-insoluble and may be included in formulations primarily to increase viscosity or to increase the hydrophobicity of certain excipients, which may otherwise cause embrittlement in hard gelatin capsules. The relatively low-melting points of many of these excipients (e.g., Type II hydrogenated vegetable oil), which typically fall in the range of 30°C to 45°C, limits their use as single-component formulations in controlled release formulations. "Type 1" hydrogenated vegetable oils have higher melting ranges, typically 57°C to 70°C, and may be more suited to prolonged-release and other specialty applications. For example, experimental work in these laboratories has shown that a formulation containing approximately 50% hard fat, 20% glyceryl monostearate, and 30% of a concentrated sugar syrup provided a chewable base, which had good "mouth feel" and which produced capsules with at least a year's physical stability.

Macrogol glycerides: These excipients that are prepared by chemically combining glycerides with hydrophilic compounds, such as glycol derivatives, comprise a versatile and widely-applied group of excipients suitable for encapsulation. They are prepared by one of three methods: (*i*) partial alcoholysis of a natural product glyceride with PEGs (*ii*) esterification of glycerol and PEG with selected fatty acids, or (*iii*) mixing of glycerol esters and condensates of ethylene oxide with selected fatty acids. The chain length of the selected fatty acid and molecular weight of the corresponding PEG controls the melting point and hydrophile–lipophile balance (HLB) of the final product. Typically, long-chain fatty acids of varying degrees of unsaturation are used in combination with PEG's ranging from 200 to 4000 in molecular weight. Based on the particular combination selected, excipients can be prepared with a wide range of HLB values (2–14) that melt in the range of 33°C to 53°C. The final products may contain low (3–5%) levels of free glycerol and the component PEG as well varying amounts of mono-, di-, and triglycerides and fatty acid mono- and di-esters of the component PEG. These excipients self-emulsify in water, thereby facilitating drug absorption, and their wide range of physical characteristics provide formulators with considerable flexibility for manipulating drug release rates. Care is required in the selection of a particular excipient with regard to the relative levels of free glycerol and PEG and the degree of unsaturation of the component fatty acids. As mentioned previously, the humectant properties of glycerol can lead to deformation or embrittlement of hard gelatin capsules, whereas resistance to oxidative degradation decreases with increasing unsaturation of the fatty acid content. PEGs that commonly form peroxides upon aging, can result in drug degradation and have been implicated in gelatin cross-linking, which prolong capsule shell disintegration and may lead to altered drug release rates. Of special note is that one particular excipient from this class, stearoyl macrogolglyceride, may require TSE certification dependent on the source of the stearic acid, which may be derived from beef tallow.

d-Alpha tocopheryl macrogol 1000 succinate: This self-emulsifying, thermo-softening excipient (vitamin E TPGS, Eastman Chemical, Kingsport, Tennessee, U.S.A.) is a water-soluble form of vitamin E (tocopherol) prepared by chemically attaching PEG1000 to this fat-soluble vitamin via a succinic acid linker. This excipient product has utility not only as a solubilizer for hydrophobic drugs in both liquid and thermo-softening formulations, but also as an absorption enhancer by virtue of its demonstrated inhibition of the p-Glycoprotein efflux transporter (15).

Fully Synthetic Excipients

The high molecular weight PEGs (1350 and greater) and solid-grade poloxamers (e.g., "188 grade") currently dominate the fully-synthetic class of excipients suitable for encapsulation. Of the thermo-softening PEG's, the 4000 and 6000 molecular weight grades are the most widely applied for product formulations. Of the poloxamers, the solid "188" grade (polyoxypropylene portion of molecular weight of 1800 and a polyoxyethylene portion comprising 80% of the molecule) is most widely used in product development. While other grades of these excipients are also available, these particular thermo-softening grades find the widest application due to their desirable solvent and surfactant properties (which are comparable to their fluid grades) and melting ranges, which are well suited for capsule filling operations. In addition, they are well characterized with respect to quality, chemical compatibility, and performance in promoting the absorption of hydrophobic drugs through solubilization or increased wetting of the drug particles. These excipients may also enhance cell membrane permeability and decrease intestinal efflux through inhibition of the p-Glycoprotein transporter (16).

Surfactants

Various nonionic surfactants, such as the polysorbates (e.g., Tween® 80) and polyoxyls (e.g., Cremophor® EL), which cover the HLB range from 2 to 18, may be used in combination with lipid excipients to promote self-emulsification or microemulsification. The acceptable quantities for use of these surfactants in hard and soft gelatin capsules are restricted by their tendency to cause embrittlement, due to their dehydrating effects. Caprylocaproyl macrogolglycerides are related to the thermo-softening macrogolglycerides, differing from the others in the series in being derived from medium-chain saturated triglycerides and from the lowest molecular-weight range of macrogols. These excipients have significant surfactant properties and find application as components of microemulsions. Certain products (e.g., polysorbate 60 and 80) may require TSE certification depending on the source of the long-chain fatty acids (e.g., beef tallow as opposed to plant oils) used in their manufacture.

Regulatory Compliance

As with any substance intended for human use, insufficient data to ensure regulatory compliance has slowed the more wide-spread application of lipid-based oral formulations. This situation is gradually being resolved as these formulations continue to find new applications in the delivery of poorly water-soluble drugs, thereby expanding the body of information required to gain acceptance by the various regulatory agencies.

Tables 2 and 3 refer to generally regarded as safe (GRAS) or pharmacopoeial materials only; excipients intended for the U.S. market are additionally required to meet the relevant regulations described in 21 CFR 210.3 (7). While there are many other examples of lipid-based excipients suited for gelatin encapsulation and appropriate to particular products, their international regulatory status is highly varied and needs to be carefully considered in the development of products intended for global marketing.

Certain of the excipients described here may contain components of animal origin, particularly stearate or oleate derivatives of bovine tallow, which are currently subject to TSE regulation and certification. The Ph. Eur. (7) describes both in general terms and for specific products, the control of materials used in pharmaceuticals that carry TSE risks, which may not always be obvious as is the case for specific polysorbate surfactants ("60" and "80"), which contain an oleate or stearate component that may be derived from beef tallow. The issue of TSE compliance can be addressed in practice by use of (*i*) nonbovine sources (e.g., plant sources) of long chain fatty acids, (*ii*) animal sources from selected geographical areas not associated with high TSE risk, (*iii*) suitably rigorous processes designed to minimize TSE risk by ensuring the destruction of prions, such as the treatment of ossein collagen (used in the preparation of bone-derived gelatin) with 2% to 5% slaked lime for 60 to 120 days ("liming"). Similarly, glycerol and fatty acids derived from beef tallow and subjected to such rigorous processes have been considered unlikely sources of TSE.

Lipid Excipient Properties Affecting Processing and Stability

Oxidation Issues

Lipid excipients vulnerable to oxidation may be protected by inclusion of a selected, lipid-soluble antioxidant in the capsule formulation (e.g., tertiary-butyl

Table 3 GRAS-Listed and Pharmacopoeial Thermo-softening Carriers for Liquid-Filled Two-Piece Capsules

Material/compliance	Source or chemical composition	Melting point (°C)	Comment	Commercial products
Hard Fat [1,4]	Hydrogenated glycerides	34–38	Softisan "138" has lower -OH value/higher melting point and contains beeswax	Softisan 134 [8], Softisan 138 [8], Gelucire 39/01 [9]
Hydrogenated soybean oil [1,4]	Hydrogenated glycerides (long chain, C-16:0;C-18:0)	66–72		Various
Hydrogenated vegetable oil (Type I) [1,2,3,4]	Hydrogenated glycerides	57–70	Multiple sources (e.g., soybean, palm)	Various
Hydrogenated vegetable oil (Type II) [2,4]	Hydrogenated glycerides	20–50		Various
Lauroyl macrogolglycerides [1,5]	Macrogol glyceride (long-chain fatty acids, C-12:0; C-18:0)	33–48	Amphiphilic; self-microemulsifys in water	Gelucire 44/14 [9], Acconon C-44 [6]
Oleoyl macrogolglycerides [1,5]	Macrogol glyceride: (long-chain fatty acids, C-18:1; from apricot kernel oil	40	Amphiphilic; useful for preparing microemulsions	Labrafil M 1944 CS [9]
Poloxamer 188 (and others) [1,4]	Polyethylene-propylene glycol copolymer	52–55	Amphiphilic; may increase absorption of lipophilic substances	Lutrol F 68 [7], Pluronic F 68 [7]
Polyethylene glycol (1000–10000) [1,3a,4]	Macrogol	50–60	Trace levels of peroxides can cause product oxidation; specific incompatibilities	Lutrol E [7], Carbowax [10], Lipoxol [8]
Stearoyl macrogolglycerides [1,5]	Macrogol glyceride (long-chain fatty acids, C-16:0; C-18:0)	50–53	Dispersible in warm water; can self-microemulsify	Gelucire 50/13 [9], Gelucire 53/10 [9]

^aAccording to grade.

Pharmacopoeial compliance/GRAS status: (1) European Pharmacopoeia; (2) GRAS; (3) Japanese Pharmacopoeia; (4) United States National Formulary (5) United States Pharmacopoeia

Manufacturers' addresses: (6) Abitec Corp, Columbus, OH, USA; (7) BASF, Ludwigshafen, Germany; (8) Condea, Witten, Germany; (9) Gattefosse, St Priest Cedex, France; (10) Union Carbide, Danbury, CT, USA.

hydroquinone (TBHQ), 250–500 ppm, or propyl gallate, 25–500 ppm). Inclusion of an antioxidant is particularly important to formulations with a high content of unsaturated fatty acids or derivatives thereof. Alternatively, these formulations may be protected from oxidation by the capsule shell, of which hard gelatin capsules afford the greatest protection due the inherent, low permeability of these capsules to oxygen, which is augmented by the capsule sealing process. Further protection against oxidation can be achieved by gassing of the capsule headspace with nitrogen, which is easily achieved for hard gelatin capsule by incorporation of a nitrogen-feed device at the capsule closing station. The presence of gelatin plasticizers in soft gelatin capsules renders them permeable to oxygen with subsequent, increased liability for product oxidation. HPMC capsules, due to the inherent physicochemical properties of the material used in their manufacture, possess relatively high permeability to oxygen, as well. Protection from oxidation in either soft gelatin capsule or HPMC capsules is therefore limited to the inclusion of an appropriate, lipid-soluble antioxidant in the formulation. For example, evening primrose oil in HPMC capsules can be protected against oxidation by the inclusion of TBHQ at 250 ppm (10).

Polymorphism

Certain of the semi-synthetic thermo-softening lipid excipients, particularly the macrogol glycerides, require specific process controls in their application in order to minimize or control a tendency towards polymorphic changes of the excipient matrix. The vulnerability of these excipients and their formulations to such polymorphic changes, as well as their needs for specific process controls (e.g., controlled-rate capsule cooling), may be assessed by such techniques as modulated differential scanning calorimetry (17). From a processing perspective, such polymorphic changes may lead to prolongation of solidification time, which can adversely impact capsule filling and handling during production. From a performance perspective, polymorphic changes can produce nonuniformity of the solidified formulation matrix with resultant changes in the product release-profile, particularly upon aging. In order to control this phenomenon, these excipients should be fully melted by heating to 20°C above their nominal melting point and thoroughly mixed prior to encapsulation (18). This serves to destroy any preformed crystalline structure and promotes homogeneous dispersion of the multiple components contained in these excipients (e.g., the lauryl macrogolglycerides), which are subject to local separation during storage of commercial bulk packages. The molten material will then behave in a consistent fashion with regard to solidification rate and the final, solidified product will provide a uniform and predictable drug release profile. Removal and use of portions of bulk packages prior to the melting and mixing step is not recommended and may produce final products, which vary in physical and performance characteristics.

MANUFACTURING SYSTEMS

The basic operations involved in the manufacture of liquid-filled capsules include preparation of the bulk mix, followed by capsule filling and, when required, sealing.

Table 4 Major Factors Contributing to Successful Hard-Capsule Processing, by Process Category

Formulation development	Capsule	Filling machine	Sealing machine	Other
Minimize leak potential by increasing viscosity above 100 cps	Select for compatibility with intended sealing process (in-process (Qualicaps Hicap®) or secondary, separate sealing process (Capsugel LEMS®)	Ensure robust system operates for detection of missing capsule parts (including "transparent" formats) and related inhibition of the dosing pump/rejection of unfilled capsules	Control the amount of sealing solution applied to ensure sufficient is applied for seal integrity but avoiding over-wetting of capsule	Control elapsed time between capsule filling and sealing to minimize intra-capsule pressure and formulation seepage between cap and body
Select formulation proportions, which ensure that the fill quantity is not more than 90% of the selected capsule body volume	Select to minimize intracapsule pressurisation, e.g., vented "Qualicaps" or unvented Capsugel "Licaps," according to process equipment	Pay close attention to the need for "clean-running"	Pay close attention to the need for "clean-running"	
	Consider (but do not require) use of speciality "liquid-fill" capsule formats (e.g., LiCaps®)	Avoid "stringing" by nozzle selection and formulation de-gassing	Band-sealing (Qualicaps Hicap®): control sealing-solution viscosity to ensure consistent application of gelatin over entire processing period	

(Continued)

Table 4 Major Factors Contributing to Successful Hard-Capsule Processing, by Process Category (*Continued*)

Formulation development	Capsule	Filling machine	Sealing machine	Other
	Select capsule size to avoid excessive void volume	Select injection nozzle profile to minimize injection speed into capsule body over-drying and embrittlement	Limit drying temperature to that required for removing sealing solvent without causing capsule	
		Control machine speed to avoid intracapsule pressurization	Control sealing machine speed to match filling-machine output and maximize drying time	
		Consider two-stage closing (preclosing and full closing) and the use of "profiled" bottom bushes, which prevent spill seepage into bush bores		

Table 4 details the major technical factors involved in successful processing of liquid-filled hard capsules. Implementation of its main points (formulation design, capsule selection, operation of filling, and sealing machines) has supported full-scale manufacture at Encap Drug Delivery and confirms the robustness of the process.

Bulk Mix Preparation

The equipment utilized for the preparation of bulk fluid or suspension formulations is similar regardless of the excipients comprising the formulation (e.g., lipid vs. traditional excipients). Typically, the bulk formulation vessels have product-relevant facilities for primary agitation, high-shear mixing, vacuum and pressure capability, heating and cooling, and loading and unloading. Homogeneity of the bulk formulation can be maintained by suitable mixer/filler recirculation systems and by local agitation in the filling-machine hopper. Formulations incorporating fluid excipients or those with relatively low-melting points are flexible with respect to process stability and time requirements. However, additional issues arise for formulations based on thermo-softening carriers, which typically require processing at temperatures ranging from 35°C to 70°C. Such temperatures and the maximum associated time limits for holding prior to encapsulation can present product stability issues during manufacturing. In practice, this may require processing in a nitrogen atmosphere to minimize potential oxidation and/or limitation of the batch-size to that, which may be encapsulated within a period dictated by the formulation stability. A product batch with a thermal stability issue will generally be limited to a filling-period not to exceed 24 hours. In practical terms, this will allow for a maximum batch size of approximately 450 k capsules to be prepared in an eight-hour period on a filling machine operating at the typical rate of 60 k capsules per hour. Clearly, selection of excipients requiring minimal processing temperatures provides for flexibility and maximum productivity during manufacturing.

Capsule Filling Systems

Filling Equipment

Commercial-scale machines suited to filling typical lipid-based formulation products are made by such companies as Bosch, MG2 and Qualicaps and derive in design from traditional powder-fill units. Table 5 lists principal features of these capsule filling machines, which offer product flexibility with respect to dose size, temperature control, mixing capability, and fill-material characteristics. Importantly, high-precision dosing is intrinsic in the design of their volumetric liquid pumping mechanisms. Maximum doses of formulated drug substance can be estimated for the various capsule sizes on the basis of a pro-rata quantity of 250 mg to 300 mg total fill (active plus excipients) in a size zero shell, assuming the availability of a pump capable of filling a high-viscosity formulation.

Issues in Operation

The principal operating issues for these capsule filling systems relate to maximum capacity and clean-running. Output rates are much less than those for

Table 5   Features of Capsule Liquid-Filling Machines, by Manufacturer

Feature	Bosch	IMA/ Zanasi	MG2	Qualicaps	Harro-Hofliger	Hibar/ Capsugel
Motion type	Intermittent	Intermittent	Continuous	Intermittent	Intermittent	Bench
Max capacities k/hr[a]	60	55	60	150	10	3 k/day
Special features	Nozzle insertion into capsule	N/A	"Add-ons" for "Futura"	Integrated sealing version available	Use pneumatic pumps	Capsugel unit has integrated sealing
Maximum viscosity range	25,000 cps	N/A	<10,000 cps	<10,000 cps	<10,000 cps	N/A
Missing-capsule detection system	Yes	Yes	Yes	Yes	Yes	N/A

[a]Varies with the particular model.
Abbreviation: N/A, not applicable.

high-speed tablet compression or powder-filling machines for capsules and, at first sight, suggest slow processing for liquid-filled capsule products. However, these filling rates should not be considered in isolation. Although conventional tablet compression-machines can operate at 10 times the speed of these capsule liquid filling systems, the relative complexities of the overall support processes differ significantly. The current disadvantage of relatively low production rate for liquid-filled capsules is offset by the advantage of minimizing other process support activities associated with conventional tablet or capsule dosage forms. For the hard capsule dosage form, a single bulk mix is prepared and can be filled and sealed in one continuous process, whereby formulated drug entering the filling machine is converted into the package-ready final dosage unit in as little as 10 minutes, according to the particular fill-seal system used. There is no need for coating to address product appearance or to provide taste-masking properties, which obviates the need for an otherwise complex series of additional operations. Since the liquid-filling process is essentially dust-free after the initial drug powder dispensing to prepare the bulk formulation, the need for the installation, running, and maintenance of expensive air-filtration facilities is minimized. This is particularly important for such actives as cytotoxics and highly-potent drugs, such as steroids and certain drugs, which act on the central-nervous-system, where support costs in the form of containment and clean-up may not be obvious but are, nevertheless, high.

The design of the liquid handling systems used by these filling machines generally promotes clean-running. However, incidents of empty capsule-feed failure can lead to rapid contamination of machine bushes and external capsule surfaces, resulting in the failure of any subsequent capsule sealing process. The availability and robustness of the filling machine for detecting missing capsule parts in the empty capsule feed system and its ability to subsequently halt the liquid filling pump or machine operation are critical features of these machines. Methods for detecting missing capsule parts may function by mechanical, light or pneumatic methods, or by combinations thereof, depending on the particular machine manufacturer, with each method having its advantages and disadvantages. For example, light-based fault detection systems may not be suitable for use with clear capsules. On the other hand, mechanical fault detection systems may stick whereas pneumatic systems may be vulnerable to the presence of shell fragments. Clean-running is also promoted by degassing of bulk fill material and by appropriate filling-nozzle design. These features are important in avoiding droplets or "pig-tailing" at the filling-nozzle tips, which is a common cause of bush contamination. Maintaining clean nozzle tips is also promoted in certain machines by mechanisms, which make a final, sharp movement between the capsule and nozzle at the end of the filling stroke, giving a "clean break" in the fill material stream at the nozzle tip.

In addition, useful output rates for filling machines need to be matched to those of the corresponding sealing units in order to minimize the time interval between initial capsule filling and final sealing during which leakage of the contents may occur. Currently, practical maximum output rates for single fill/seal machine combinations are around 60 k capsules per hour.

Sealing Systems

The technical need for capsule sealing varies according to the specific product. In practice, sealing is required for products whose melting point is less than 50°C and commonly applies to the lipid excipients considered here.

Sealing Equipment

The two major integrated systems available for capsule sealing include capsule banding and gelatin fusion and they differ in operating principles and in their product flexibility. Table 6 lists principal features of sealing machines. Each may be used in-line with, or separately from, the capsule liquid-filling unit. In the Shionogi capsule banding system, the capsules are passed continuously from a feed system to a conveyor belt, which passes them over a series of rotating disks, which apply the gelatin sealing solution over the cap/body junction. The capsules then pass directly to an inline drying cabinet, after which they are suitable for further processing or packaging. This system was originally developed for hard gelatin capsules, but is suitable for HPMC capsules and accommodates capsules from various manufacturers ranging in size from 0–4. The Qualicaps band sealing machine has an output rate of approximately 60 k capsules per hour, matching the

Table 6   Features of Capsule Sealing Machines, by Manufacturer

Feature	Qualicaps "Hicapseal"	Capsugel "LEMS" (liquid encapsulation microspray sealing)
Basic sealing operation	Gelatin double-banding by rotating-disc application of aqueous gelatin solution	Microspraying of aqueous ethanol
Sealing mechanism	Adhesion of gelatin band to external shell surface	Fusion of cap (inner) and body (outer) surfaces
Primary drying mechanism	Inline drying chamber on moving carriers	Inline drying chamber based on tumbling in warm air
Secondary drying	Not required	Overnight tray drying
Output rate	60 k/hr	30 k/hr
Number of change parts/set	1100	Minimal
Capsule types accommodated	Gelatin or HPMC from the various suppliers	Limited to gelatin "Licaps®"
Leak detection	Immediate	Delayed
Product suitability for subsequent coating	Yes	Can be limited by cap/body "lip" at point of closure

Abbreviation: HPMC, hydroxypropyl methylcellulose.

maximum output of typical high-speed liquid-filling machines and is relatively expensive with respect to the initial capital cost (basic sealing machine plus multiple change-parts to accommodate different capsule size); it also incurs additional operating costs due to the time required for equipment cleaning and part change-over for different capsule sizes. These costs can be significant for operations producing multiple-size products, but will not be an issue for long runs of a single capsule size, as is generally the case with many products. The system is robust in the hands of experienced operators, but remains vulnerable to damage from unskilled operation.

In the alternative continuous sealing system employing gelatin fusion [Liquid Encapsulation Microspray System (LEMS®), Capsugel], which operates at half the capacity (30 k capsules per hour) of the gelatin banding system, an aqueous ethanol solution is microsprayed into junction of the cap and body of the filled capsules. This wets the capsule components and fuses the gelatin surfaces together, after which the capsules are partially dried by tumbling in a rotating heated-air chamber followed by mandatory overnight tray-drying. This sealing system requires the use of special, proprietary, unvented capsules (Licaps®, Capsugel) with a tight cap/body locking ring, which prevents liquid seepage into the seal area during the drying process. One of the drawbacks of the LEMS sealing system is that there is currently no efficient, reliable means for assessing the integrity of the capsule seal immediately prior to final product packaging, which incurs the risk of late postsealing leakage in the capsule product.

Issues in Operation

The major issue involved in capsule sealing is leakage of formulations, which remain fluid to some extent after filling. Leakage may be characterized by its severity (e.g., critical, major, or minor) or by the time of onset relative to filling. While gross leaks are readily detectable at the time of processing, less severe faults may not become evident for some weeks, giving cause for complaint by the consumer. Passive visual examination is insufficient for reliable leak detection for production quality control purposes and in-process inspection methods for detecting leaks, such as fluorescence monitoring, are currently unreliable due to the inherent fluorescence characteristic of gelatin capsule shells. A "stress-test" approach that involves placing the filled capsules under vacuum, has been proven to be a reliable method for leak detection and assessment and can be based on an "acceptable quality level" (AQL) analogous to that used by the capsule shell manufacturers in their product quality systems (19). Finished batches are sampled according to statistical tables, subjected to the vacuum stress test and then visually examined for leaks. These are counted and rated as critical, major or minor, according to a scale defined by the capsule manufacturer, with the numerical results forming the basis for batch "pass/fail" decisions. Leak-producing faults in most capsule types can be shown within an hour of sealing. However, these faults can appear in certain capsule shells (e.g., Licap) at a much later time, and are therefore more difficult to detect during QC inspections.

From the foregoing discussion, it should be apparent that the capsule sealing process is critical to product success and requires skilled operators. Insufficiently controlled, it can lead to the need for labor-intensive sorting to remove potential "leakers." As such, sealing requirements represent a significant disadvantage for liquid-filled capsule dosage forms and emphasize the need for consistently "getting it right the first time." However, a detailed understanding of the causes of leakage can eliminate the need for full-batch monitoring and routine sorting, allowing instead for aliquot testing for batch approval, as has been the case at Encap Drug Delivery for over eight years. Achieving this goal does require detailed attention to product formulation and capsule shell selection, together with appropriate choice of capsule filling and sealing equipment, with adequate operator training being critical to success.

Hydroxypropyl Methylcellulose Capsule Sealing

The requirements for HPMC capsule sealing differ significantly from those for gelatin capsules. Unlike gelatin that is elastic when wet, HPMC shows low wet-strength and can undergo local shell failure during or immediately after sealing and before drying is completed. This may be addressed by various means, such as proper capsule shell selection, manipulation of the sealing solution or design modification of processing equipment, with each factor playing a part in the development of a robust, high-speed process. Encap Drug Delivery has developed and filed patent applications on systems for HPMC capsule processing, which enable liquid-filled HPMC capsules to be manufactured at rates and quality standards comparable to those for gelatin capsule products.

Capsule Coating

Certain capsule products may require coating for various reasons, including cosmetic or functional purposes such as modified release (e.g., enteric coating). Successful coating of liquid-filled capsules, using aqueous or nonaqueous coating systems is critically dependent on freedom from leaks and the resultant egress of the formulation contents onto the capsule surface. Any trace of such surface contamination reduces the adhesion of the coating material to the capsule surface resulting in batch failure. A further factor affecting coating relates to the differing dimensions of the "lip" formed at the cap/body junction, which differ with the particular capsule sealing system employed (e.g., banding vs. gelatin fusion). The seal produced by the banding system provides a continuous, smooth cap/body surface suited to coat deposition, while the seal formed using the microspray system produces a sharply-defined cap/body "step" on which there is more difficulty in assuring complete coat adhesion and integrity.

TECHNICAL DEVELOPMENT FOR MULTI-PHASE PRODUCTS

Currently, oral lipid-based formulations delivered in capsule formats are single-phase products with immediate release delivery profiles. However, there are various cases in which a multi-phase, modified-release product would be appropriate, such as: (*i*) clinical requirements for specific plasma time-course profiles, for the purpose of maximizing therapeutic efficacy or minimizing toxicity, (*ii*) avoidance of site-specific degradation of drug in the gastrointestinal tract, and (*iii*) resolution of chemical incompatibility issues for multi-component products. One method for achieving a modified-release profile takes advantage of the flexibility of liquid-filling machines and the combination of semi-solid and liquid excipients to enable the filling of multiple formulations of the same drug into a single capsule. Technically, the filling operation can be performed in a single or in multiple passes through the filling machine and results in a final product possessing multiple, discrete layers with differing release characteristics (Layercap™, Encap Drug Delivery). Selection of appropriately calculated proportions of the individual formulations would enable the manufacture of a _single capsule with a predetermined, specific release profile. This approach has yet to be marketed on a commercial scale.

The issue of chemical incompatibility between different formulation components has been recently addressed by Encap Drug Delivery through the development of the DuoCap™ multiple capsule system for the delivery of multi-phase lipid formulation products. The concept that has been successfully applied to product manufacture, involves specialist liquid-filling techniques executed on custom-designed filling equipment, which allows the insertion of a prefilled, smaller capsule into a larger, liquid-filled capsule. The smaller, inner capsule may contain either a liquid or semi-solid formulation and, according to the formulation or product requirements, either or both capsules may be of gelatin or HPMC composition and can be coated, if necessary.

The DuoCap™ process is graphically outlined in Figure 2. The inner capsule is first manufactured by using conventional liquid-filling and sealing technology, with the final dosage form being processed on a GKF 1500L liquid-fill machine, which has been re-engineered inhouse by Encap Drug Delivery. This machine utilizes a single, empty-capsule feed station to deliver the outer empty capsule shell to the filling station, where it is then filled to the required volume by "pump 1." A second, specially-designed feed station for the prefilled inner capsule replaces the original "pump 2" mechanism and inserts the inner capsule into the prefilled outer capsule body. The system enables the filling of one capsule (size X) into an outer capsule [size (X + 2) or larger] containing a liquid formulation, (e.g., a #0 capsule containing 0.140 mL of formulation could contain an inner #2 capsule containing 0.325 mL of a second formulation). Capsule total capacities for various combinations are shown in Table 7. The outer capsule is then closed and ejected from the machine by the standard mechanism and is available for subsequent sealing. The machine has various electronic controls to monitor inner capsule and empty outer

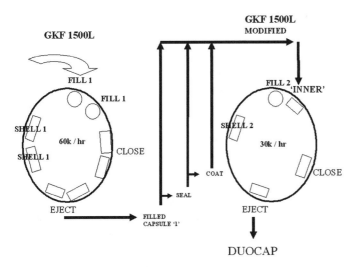

Figure 2 Unit operations involved in the production of the DuoCap™ multiple capsule dosage form. Custom-designed filling equipment is utilized which allows the insertion of a pre-filled, smaller capsule into a larger, liquid-filled capsule The smaller, inner capsule may contain either a liquid or semi-solid formulation Either or both capsules may be of gelatin or HPMC composition and can be coated, if necessary.

Table 7 Capacities of Combination of Inner and Outer Capsules for Duocap™ Format

Capsule size (#)	Maximum capacity (mL)	Capacity (mL), inner/#00 outer	Capacity (mL), inner/#0 outer	Capacity (mL), inner/#1 outer	Capacity (mL), inner/#2 outer
00	0.835	N/A	N/A	N/A	N/A
0	0.600	N/A	N/A	N/A	N/A
1	0.435	0.435/0.235	N/A	N/A	N/A
2	0.325	0.325/0.375	0.325/0.140	N/A	N/A
3	0.250	0.250/0.510	0.250/0.255	0.250/0.110	N/A
4	0.190	0.190/0.585	0.190/0.335	0.190/0.165	0.190/0.076

Abbreviation: N/A, not applicable.

capsule feed and a maximum filling rate of approximately 30 k capsules per hour, which is about half that of the original, single-capsule dual-pump system.

The GKF 1500L capsule filling machine described herein was specifically modified to allow the preparation of dual liquid-filled capsules. However, appropriate modification of the fill-head would readily allow powders or even tablet dosage forms to be combined with a liquid formulation in a single capsule dosage unit. The system is highly versatile, allowing for the preparation of combination dosage forms, with specially-tailored drug-release profiles or for the combination of potentially incompatible components within the same dosage unit, in either coated or uncoated formats.

A practical example of the successful application of the DuoCap™ multiphase, lipid based formulation technology is found in the nutriceutical probiotic product, "Floraguard," launched in 2004 by Biocare U.K., Ltd. and manufactured by Encap Drug Delivery. This product, which is marketed as a dietary supplement, is intended for the restoration of the normal balance of microbial flora within the gut. As such, it finds application in the treatment of diarrhea, which commonly results subsequent to the disturbance of gut flora that frequently follows antibiotic therapy. The main, competing commercial products are simple, freeze-dried granulation formulations of the lactic acid bacteria, *Lactobacillus acidophilus, Lactobacillus casei, Enterococcus faecium*, and *Bifidobacterium bifidum*, which must be protected from excessive heat and moisture. Exposure to moisture during manufacture or storage results in early activation of the organisms, which in the absence of nutrients typically encountered in the gut following ingestion, results in the devitalization of the organisms and loss of product potency. In addition, since the beneficial activity of these organisms is targeted to the colon, early activation during passage through the stomach can reduce the viability of those organisms reaching the colon. Finally, the organisms in the granulation formulations are mechanically fragile and relatively unprotected against the effects of heat, thereby necessitating refrigerated storage.

The DuoCap™ probiotic formulation described here addresses all of the deficiencies of the simple granulation formulations by incorporating live, freeze-dried *Lactobacillus acidophilus* and *Bifidobacterium bifidum* organisms into a multi-component, oil-filled, and enteric coated capsule formulation. The issue of early activation by environmental moisture is addressed by suspending the freeze-dried organisms in a protective oily vehicle, which is filled into a low-moisture content HPMC inner capsule (4–6% moisture content as opposed to the 13–16% moisture content of hard gelatin capsules). The greater resistance of HPMC capsules to embrittlement and cracking subsequent to extraction of moisture by the hydrophilic freeze-dried fill further adds to the attractiveness of HPMC capsule shells for this product. From a physiological standpoint, early activation of the organisms in the stomach prior to arrival in the colon was addressed by coating the inner capsule with a new, pH-dependent food-grade aqueous–coat system based on shellac (patent pending, Encap Drug Delivery), which met standard pharmacopoeial requirements for enteric-coat performance. The product also required coadministration of a second oily formulation, which was incompatible with the probiotic since it possessed native antimicrobial activity. The final product consisted of a sealed, liquid-filled ("Formulation 2") outer size 00 HPMC capsule into which had been inserted a sealed, enteric-coated, size 1 HPMC capsule containing an oily suspension of the freeze-dried microorganisms ("Formulation 1"). Critical requirements for meeting the label claim pertaining to the viability of the organisms (4×10^9 cfu's/capsule, information provided by courtesy of BioCare Ltd., U.K.) were met using the DuoCap™ drug delivery system, as demonstrated by microbiological monitoring based on plate-counts of lactic acid bacteria (20). Thus, by addressing multiple and complex product stability issues in a single dosage unit, the DuoCap™ technology allowed maintenance of the product label claim over a shelf-life that was both competitive and commercially-attractive. This example clearly demonstrates the versatility of multi-component lipid-based formulations as well as their suitability for large-scale manufacture.

CONCLUSIONS

Liquid-fill technology for hard gelatin or HPMC capsules is well suited to the manufacture of lipid-based products. It allows considerable flexibility for addressing issues relating to poor drug bioavailability or product stability as well as providing a unique and flexible option for achieving a modified drug-release profile. Application of this technology is readily achieved through the services of specialist drug delivery companies. Ongoing technical development is being actively pursued by these companies as well as by the major capsule and excipient manufacturers and promises future expansion in the versatility of these drug delivery systems.

REFERENCES

1. Bach AC, Babayan VK. Medium chain triglycerides: an update. Am J Clin Nutr 1982; 36:950–962.

2. Charman WN. Lipids, lipophilic drugs and oral delivery. Some emerging concepts. J Pharm Sci 2000; 9:967–978.
3. Chen M. Lipid-based oral dosage forms—regulatory perspective. Am Pharm Review 2002; Fall:30–35.
4. Hauss D. Lipid-based systems for oral drug delivery: enhancing the bioavailability of poorly soluble drugs. Am Pharm Review 2002; Winter:1–6.
5. Wojcik M, Ellis M, Patel K. Production of seamless hard shell and soft firm mini-capsules. In: Hardshell and Softgel Capsule Technology, Atlantic City. Ann Arbor, Michigan: Pharmaceutical Production TechSource Inc., 2004:452–515.
6. Jones RT. Gelatin: manufacture and physico-chemical properties. In: Podczeck, Fridrun; Jones, Brian E, eds. Pharmaceutical Capsules. 2nd ed. London: The Pharmaceutical Press, 2004:23–60.
7. Minimising the risk of transmitting animal spongiform encephalopathy agents via human and veterinary medicinal products. European Pharmacopoeia, Edition 5.0 (1), Council of Europe, Strasbourg, France, 2004, 463–471.
8. Jones BE, Nagata S. Gelatin alternatives. In: Podczeck, Fridrun, Jones BE, eds. Pharmaceutical Capsules. 2nd ed. London: The Pharmaceutical Press, 2004.
9. Ogura T, Furuya Y, Matsuura S. HPMC capsules—an alternative to gelatin. Pharm Tech Europe 1998; 10:32–42.
10. Young V, Bowtle W. Suitability of two-piece HPMC capsules for oxidation-sensitive liquids. AAPS Pharm Sci Supp 1999; 1(4):2310.
11. Scarth R, McVetty PBE. Designer oil canola—a review of new food-grade Brassica oils with focus on high oleic, low linolenic types. In: Proceedings of the 10th International Rapeseed Congress, Canberra, Australia, 1999. http://www.regional.org.au/au/gcirc/4/57.htm.
12. Greenberger NJ, Rodgers JB, Isselbacher KJ. Absorption of medium and long chain triglycerides: factors influencing their hydrolysis and transport. J Clin Invest 1966; 45:217–227.
13. Carey MC, Small DM, Bliss CM. Lipid digestion and absorption. Ann Rev Physiol 1983; 45:651–677.
14. Gren T, Hutchison K, Kaufmann P. Galacticles™ oral lipid matrix in liquid-filled softgel capsule drug delivery system for improved oral bioavailability. Drug Delivery Technology 2002; 2(7). http://www.drugdeliverytech.com/scgi–bin/articles.cgi?idArticle=83.
15. Wu SHW. Vitamin E TPGS as a vehicle for drug delivery systems. In: Formulating with Lipids, AAPS Short Course, Parsippany, NJ, June 1998; American Association of Pharmaceutical Scientists, Alexandria, U.S.A., 1998. http://www.aapspharmaceutica.com/meetings/distance/cdroms/lipcd/index.asp.
16. Aungst B. Intestinal permeation enhancers. J Pharm Sci 2000; 89:429–442.
17. Taylor KMG, Craig DQM. Physical methods of study: differential scanning calorimetry. In: Torchilin VP, Weissig V, eds. Liposomes A Practical Approach. 2nd ed. Oxford, U.K.: Oxford University Press, 2003:79–104.
18. Formulation and processing. In: Gelucire Technical Dossier. 1st ed. Saint Priest Cedex, France: Gattefosse, 1996:9.
19. Visual quality. In: The Two-Piece Gelatin Capsule Handbook. Shionogi Qualicaps: Whitsett, U.S.A., 2002:34–37.
20. Miles AA, Misra SS. The estimation of the bactericidal power of the blood. J Hyg 1938; 38:732–749.

5

Liquid Self-Microemulsifying Drug Delivery Systems

Mette Grove

LEO Pharma A/S, Ballerup, Denmark

Anette Müllertz

Department of Pharmaceutics and Analytical Chemistry, The Danish University of Pharmaceutical Sciences, Copenhagen, Denmark

INTRODUCTION

The utility of solubilizing lipid-based formulations for improving the gastrointestinal (GI) absorption of poorly water-soluble, hydrophobic drugs is well documented in the literature (1–6). While the primary mechanism by which these formulations are thought to improve drug absorption is through elimination of the need for preabsorptive drug solubilization by the gastrointestinal tract (GIT), other mechanisms may include protection from chemical and enzymatic degradation localized in the aqueous environment and promotion of lymphatic drug transport, which circumvents hepatic first-pass metabolism (Fig. 1) (7,8).

The physicochemical characteristics of the drug substance, the lipid excipients themselves, and the dispersibility of the formulation in vivo will determine both the uptake of the drug in the GIT as well as the degree of participation of the portal venous and mesenteric lymphatic pathways in overall drug absorption. This chapter will focus on the use of lipid-based, self-emulsifying drug delivery system (SEDDS) and self-microemulsifying drug delivery system (SMEDDS) as alternative formulations for improving and normalizing the GI absorption of poorly water-soluble, hydrophobic drugs (hereafter referred to as "poorly soluble" drugs).

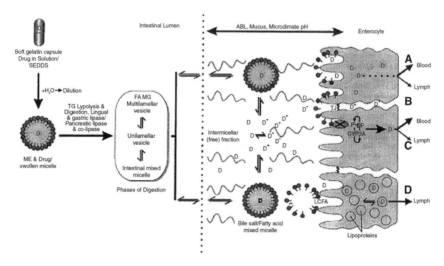

Figure 1 Schematic diagram of intestinal drug transport from lipid-based formulations via the portal and the mesenteric lymphatic routes. (**A**) Increased membrane fluidity facilitating transcellular absorption, (**B**) opening of tight junctions to allow paracellular transport, (**C**) inhibition of P-gp and/or CYP450 to increase intracellular concentration and residence time, and (**D**) stimulation of lipoprotein/chylomicron production. *Abbreviations*: ABL, aqueous boundary layer; D, drug; D-, ionized drug substance; FA, fatty acid; LCFA, long chain fatty acid; ME, microemulsion; MG, monoglyceride; SEDDS, self-emulsifying drug delivery system; TG, triglyceride; TJ, tight junction. *Source*: From Ref. 62.

SELF-EMULSIFYING DRUG DELIVERY SYSTEMS

SEDDSs and SMEDDSs are easily manufactured and physically stable isotropic mixtures of oil, surfactant, cosurfactant and solubilized drug substance that are suitable for oral delivery in soft and hard gelatin [(or hard hydroxypropyl methylcellulose (HPMC)] capsules. These formulations that rapidly and spontaneously form fine oil in water emulsions or microemulsions upon dilution in water (8), owe their self-emulsifying properties to a negative or low free energy requirement for emulsion formation (9). Thus, self-emulsifying formulations are readily dispersed in the GI tract, where the motility of the stomach and small intestine provides the agitation necessary for emulsification (10). Self-emulsifying properties are conferred upon a formulation by proper selection of the lipid/surfactant pair as well as the optimum ratio concentrations of lipid and surfactant (10–13). In addition, the use of surfactant blends to achieve the hydrophilic–lipophilic balance (HLB) value required for emulsification has often been proven to provide superior self-emulsifying properties relative to the use of a single surfactant possessing the desired HLB (9,14).

One or more cosolvents are often added to the formulation to assist in solubilizing high concentrations of the drug (5). SEDDS produce opaque, white emulsions with lipid droplet sizes of approximately 100 nm, while SMEDDS form transparent microemulsions with a droplet size of less than 50 nm (8).

The small lipid droplet size and associated greater lipid surface area produced by SEDDS and particularly, SMEDDS formulations facilitates lipid digestion, resulting in more rapid incorporation of the drug into bile salt mixed micelles. The end result is an increase in the degree and uniformity of drug absorption relative to that associated with simple lipid solutions of drug (3). In addition, there is evidence suggesting that the lipid droplets formed by self-emulsifying formulations may facilitate drug absorption directly, independent of the bile salt mixed micelle transport system (15). The improved drug absorption provided by self-emulsifying formulations is contingent upon the maintenance of the drug in the solubilized state until it can be absorbed from the GIT (4). In instances where the lipid vehicle hydrolysis rate exceeds that of drug absorption, lumenal precipitation can occur resulting in suboptimal and more variable drug absorption. This situation was encountered with tributyrin formulations of the poorly soluble antineoplastic drug, penclomedine, which resulted in substantially lower drug absorption as compared to solution formulations of the drug in long chain fatty acids (16). In this instance, the facile GI dispersion and rapid hydrolysis of the more polar tributyrin led to precipitation of penclomedine in the intestinal lumen before it could be absorbed.

SELECTION OF EXCIPIENTS IN SELF-EMULSIFYING FORMULATIONS

The primary consideration in selecting appropriate excipients for any lipid-based formulation lies in identifying an excipient or excipient combination that will solubilize the entire drug dose in a volume acceptable for unit oral administration. But equally, if not more important, the drug must be physically and chemically stable in the formulation and the drug release characteristics must remain constant as the formulation ages. This latter requirement is dependent on the physical and chemical stability of the excipients, which like the drug substance, must be carefully monitored during formulation development.

Excipient toxicity has assumed greater importance to regulatory agencies and guidelines are now available describing the safety evaluation of new pharmaceutical excipients (17). The United States Food and Drug Administration (FDA) has published a list of "generally recognized as safe" (GRAS) excipients, which are considered nontoxic to humans and animals and thus, do not require additional toxicity testing when used in formulations. In addition, the agency has published another list of acceptable inactive ingredients currently utilized in previously approved products that most likely will not require additional safety evaluations prior to clinical application (18). However, as formulations often consist of more than one excipient, the possibility of an additive toxicological effect should always be considered.

Lipid Component

Lipid excipients are comprised of a large group of physically and chemically diverse substances, which provide the formulator with considerable latitude in formulation design. These excipients can readily be used to orally deliver drugs as solutions (liquid and semi-solid), suspensions, emulsions, microemulsions, SEDDS, or SMEDDS. In general, lipid based formulations have been found to yield greater and more uniform bioavailability than polyethylene glycol (PEG) solutions of the drug, which are water miscible and can precipitate upon aqueous dilution in the GIT. Two examples of this include Ro 15-0778 and seocalcitol, for which lipid based formulations provided superior bioavailability relative to simple water miscible solutions of the drug (Table 1). In other studies, Charman et al. (13) and Lin et al. (19) reported similar improvements in bioavailability, relative to conventional solid formulations, of the drugs WIN 54954 and L-365,260, respectively, when administered to dogs as either PEG 600 solutions or as SEDDS formulations. While both the SEDDS and PEG 600 solution formulations provided similar drug exposure, the SEDDS formulations provided more uniform plasma concentration profiles, suggesting more consistent solubilization of drug in the GIT.

Despite the considerable potential that lipid excipients offer, very few lipid-based formulations have reached the pharmaceutical marketplace. We believe this to be largely due to insufficient information regarding the relatively complex physical chemistry of lipids and concerns about formulated drug chemical and physical stability. In addition to these concerns, the interaction of a lipid-based formulation with the GI environment and its impact on drug absorption need to be considered. For instance, digestible lipids have been shown to be considerably more efficient enhancers of poorly soluble drug absorption, as compared to nondigestible lipids (e.g., liquid paraffin) and fatty acid chain length of the lipid can influence drug absorption, as well (1,20–23).

Influence of the Lipid Dose

The amount of lipid contained in a formulation will influence drug absorption primarily via solubilization in the GIT and potentially, through activation of GI lipid digestion resulting in increased secretion of pancreatic juice and bile. Although the minimum lipid quantity required to activate lipid digestion has not been fully elucidated, oral administration of the poorly soluble antimalarial drug, halofantrine, to dogs in a small, pharmaceutically relevant lipid volume [0.3 g of long chain triglycerides (LCT) or mixed long chain mono- and diacylglycerols], triggered the processes of GI lipid digestion and lymphatic drug transport (24). In another study in which conscious, restrained rats received single oral doses of benzo(a)pyrene administered as a solution in 50 or 500 μmol olive oil, the lipid volume had no effect on benzo(a)pyrene bioavailability (25).

These findings are far from conclusive but suggest that the formulator should consider the impact of any lipid-based formulation on the lipid digestion processes, particularly when multiple dosage units of a lipid-based formulation are administered as a single dose, which is common for many anti-HIV drugs.

Choice of Surfactants

The self-emulsifying or self-microemulsifying properties of SEDDS and SMEDDS formulations, respectively, require the incorporation of relatively large amounts of

(Text continues on page 114.)

Table 1 In Vivo Studies with Drug Substances Dissolved in SEDDS and SMEDDS[a]

Drug substance	SMEDDS/SEDDS	In vivo observation	Reference
Coenzyme Q$_{10}$	SEDDS 6% CoQ$_{10}$ 38% Myvacet 9-45 50% Labrasol 9% Lauroglycol	Relative bioavailability in dogs: SEDDS (2-fold) > powder	(60)
Cyclosporine A	Neoral® 100 mg Cyclosporine A 75 mg Propylene glycol 150 mg Ethanol 345 mg Partial glycerides 405 mg Cremophor RH40	Sandimmune® 100 mg Cyclosporine A 100 mg Ethanol 416 mg Maize oil 300 mg Labrafil M2126 Neoral > Sandimmune: reduced inter- and intrapatient variability, dose linearity and reduced food effect	(38,39,61)
Danazol	MC-SMEDDS 5% Danazol 36% Captex 355 18% Capmul MCM 36% Cremophor EL 10% Ethanol	LC-SMEDDS 5% Danazol 29% Soybean oil 29% Maisine 35-1 30% Cremophor EL 7% Ethanol Relative bioavailability in dogs: Soybean oil solution~LC-SMEDDS (5-fold) > MC-SMEDDS > powder	(43)
Halofantrine	MC-SEDDS 5% Halofantrine 46.5% Captex 355 23.3% Capmul MCM 15% Cremophor EL 10% Etanol	LC-SMEDDS 5% Halofantrine 29% Soybean oil 29% Mansine 35-1 30% Cremophor EL 7% Ethanol Absolute bioavailability in dogs: LC-SMEDDS (67.3%)~MC-SMEDDS (52.7%)~MC- SEDDS (51.6%) > tablet	(32)

(Continued)

Table 1 In Vivo Studies with Drug Substances Dissolved in SEDDS and SMEDDS[a] (*Continued*)

Drug substance	SMEDDS/SEDDS		In vivo observation	Reference
Halofantrine (*Continued*)	MC-SMEDDS 5% Halofantrine 33.3% Captex 355 16.7% Capmul MCM 35% Cremophor EL 10% Ethanol			
	MC-SMEDDS 5% Halofantrine 29% Captex 355 29% Capmul MCM 30% Cremophor EL 7% Ethanol	LC-SMEDDS 5% Halofantrine 29% Soybean oil 29% Mansine 35-1 30% Cremophor EL 7% Ethanol	Lymphatic transport in dogs: LC-SMEDDS (28.3% of dose) >MC-SMEDDS (5.0% of dose) Relative plasma availability in dogs: MC-SMEDDS~LC-SMEDDS	(24)
	MLM-SMEDDS 5% Halofantrine 29% MLM lipid 29% Maisine 35-1 30% Cremophor EL 7% Ethanol	LML-SMEDDS 5% Halofantrine 29% LML lipid 29% Mansine 35-1 30% Cremophor EL 7% Ethanol	Lymphatic transport in dogs: LML-SMEDDS (27.4% of dose) >MLM SMEDDS (17.9% of dose) Plasma availability in dogs: MLM-SMEDDS (56.9%) >LML-SMEDDS (37.2%)	(50)
L-365,260	SEDDS 56% Labrafil M2125 30% Tween 80 14% L-365,260		Absolute bioavailability in dogs: SEDDS (60%) ~PEG600 (60%) >suspension (9%)~tablet	(19)
Ontazolast	SEDDS(50/50) 50% Gelucire 44/14 50% Peceol	SEDDS(80/20) 80% Gelucire 44/14 20% Peceol	Absolute bioavailability in rats: Emulsion (8.4%) ~SEDDS (80/20) (7.3%) ~SEDDS (50/50) (6.3%) >suspension	(42)

Drug	Formulation / Composition	Bioavailability	Ref.
Ro 15-0778	SEDDS Comp. not described	Relative bioavailability in dogs: SEDDS (3-fold) > PEG400 > capsule with milled powder > tablet	(10)
Seocalcitol	MC-SMEDDS 25% Fr. Coconut oil 27% Akoline MCM 45% Cremophor RH40	Absolute bioavailability in mini-pigs: MC-SMEDDS (32%)~MCT (22%) ~propylene glycol (17%)	(44)
	MC-SMEDDS 25% Fr. coconut oil 27% Akoline MCM 45% Cremophor RH40 LC-SMEDDS 25% Sesame oil 27% Peceol 45% Cremophor RH40	Absolute bioavailability in rats: MCT (24%)~LCT (22%)~MC-SMEDDS (18%) ~LC-SMEDDS (18%)	(31)
Simvastatin	SMEDDS 37% Carpryol 90 28% Cremophor EL 28% Carbitol 7% Simvastatin	Relative bioavailability in dogs: SMEDDS (1.5-fold) > tablet	(40)
WIN 54954	SEDDS 40% Neobee M5 25% Tagat TO 35% WIN 54954	Absolute bioavailability in dogs: SEDDS~PEG600	(13)
Vitamin E	SEDDS 40% Tween 80 20% Span 80 40% Palm oil	Relative bioavailability in humans: SEDDS (2-fold) > oil solution	(41)

[a]The composition of the SEDDS/SMEDDS is described in the table as well as in vivo observation and in vivo model used.

Abbreviations: Cremophor EL, polyoxyl 35 castor oil; LC-SMEDDS, LCT containing SMEDDS; LCT, long chain triglycerides; LML-SMEDDS, SMEDDS with structured triglycerides containing long, medium, long chain fatty acid; MC, medium chain; MCM, medium chain monoglycerides; MCT, medium chain triglycerides; MC-SMEDDS, SMEDDS containing medium chain triglycerides; MLM-SMEDDS, SMEDDS containing structured triglycerides with medium, long, medium chain fatty acids; SEDDS, self-emulsifying drug delivery system; SMEDDS; self-microemulsifying drug delivery system, PEG, polyethylene glycol.

surfactant in the formulation in addition to the oily drug carrier vehicle. The surfactants used in these self-emulsifying formulations should possess relatively high HLB values to enable rapid and facile dispersion in the GIT as a very fine oil-in-water emulsion and also to reduce the risk of drug precipitation following dilution in the GI fluids (4,9). While surfactants of natural origin [e.g., lecithin, Akoline® medium chain monoglycerides (MCM), and Peceol®] are preferred over synthetic surfactants for safety reasons, natural surfactants often provide less efficient self-emulsification compared to the synthetics (8). Attempts have been made to evaluate the toxicity of pharmaceutical excipients and SEDDS or SMEDDS formulations in vitro in Caco-2 cell monolayers (26–28). While this in vitro model cannot reproduce the dynamic environment of the GIT, it may be of value in early screening for excipient toxicity. Regardless, in vivo excipient toxicity studies are mandated by the regulatory agencies and close collaboration between pharmaceutical formulators and toxicologists to assess excipient toxicity, independent of the drug substance, is crucial.

For preparing self-emulsifying formulations, nonionic surfactants are normally preferred over their ionic counterparts due to more favorable safety profiles and greater emulsion stability over a wider range of pH and ionic strength (29). In addition, nonionic surfactants can produce reversible changes in intestinal mucosal permeability, further facilitating absorption of the coadministered drug (8). Surfactant concentrations employed in SMEDDS formulations typically range from 30% to 60% of the total formulation volume, which can potentially result in GI mucosal irritation (8). However, the extremely small lipid droplet size produced by SMEDDS formulations promotes rapid stomach emptying and wide dispersion throughout the GIT, minimizing exposure to high local surfactant concentrations and thus reducing the irritation potential (13). The anticipated frequency and duration of dosing are other factors that should be taken into account in assessing the potential for local and systemic toxicity resulting from these formulations.

Examples of excipients that have found application in self-emulsifying formulations include medium chain (MC) glycerides derived from coconut oil, which are GRAS-listed and are known to act as absorption promoters (29) and Cremophors, which are semi-synthetic, pegylated forms of castor oil containing complex mixtures of hydrophobic and hydrophilic molecules that are highly effective solubilizing and self-emulsifying excipients for hydrophobic drugs (30). An SMEDDS containing long chain triglycerides (MC-SMEDDS) formulation of seocalcitol containing Cremophor® RH40 and the cosurfactant, Akoline MCM (mono-, di-, and triglycerides) was described by Grove, et al. (31).

In Vitro Characterization of SEDDS/SMEDDS

Pouton (4) classified lipid-based formulations into three categories based on the polarity of the excipient blends (Table 2). Due to their relative simplicity Type I formulations, which are simple solutions of the drug in triglycerides and/or mixed glycerides, are a reasonable starting point in the search for a lipid-based formulation. Type II formulations that add a lipophilic surfactant (HLB <12), are employed when

Table 2 Typical Properties of Type I, II, IIIA, and IIIB Lipid Formulations

	Increasing hydrophilic content			
	Type I	Type II	Type IIIA	Type IIIB
Composition (%)				
Triglycerides or mixed glycerides	100	40–80	40–80	<20
Surfactants	—	20–60 (HLB <12)	20–40 (HLB >11)	20–50 (HLB >11)
Hydrophilic cosolvents	—	—	0–40	20–50
In vivo performance				
Particle size of dispersion (nm)	Coarse	100–250	100–250	50–100
Significance of aqueous dilution	Limited importance	Solvent capacity unaffected	Some loss of solvent capacity	Significant phase changes and potential loss of solvent capacity
Significance of digestibility	Crucial requirement	Not crucial but likely to occur	Not crucial but may be inhibited	Not required and not likely to occur

Abbreviation: HLB, hydrophilic–lipophilic balance.
Source: From Ref. 4.

SEDDS and greater drug solubilizing capacity is desired in a formulation. Type III formulations include the further addition of hydrophilic surfactants (HLB <12) and cosolvents to further improve the self-emulsification process in the GIT, thereby yielding a SMEDDS formulation. Type III formulations are further subdivided into Types IIIA and IIIB, where Type IIIB contains a greater ratio of hydrophilic to lipophilic components than the former. While Type IIIB formulations are associated with more facile self-emulsification and smaller lipid droplet size than Type IIIA, they carry a greater risk of drug precipitation as the hydrophilic components may separate from the oil phase during dispersion in the GIT leading to a loss of drug-solubilizing capacity.

Excipient combinations yielding SEDDS/SMEDDS formulations are identified by construction of ternary phase diagrams (Fig. 2). Each point in the phase diagram represents a given combination of oil, surfactant, and cosurfactant. In instances where combinations of more than three excipients must be tested, a fixed ratio between two of the excipients (e.g., the surfactant and cosurfactant) is selected and treated as a single component. As a practical example, mixtures consisting of different amounts of the selected excipients are evaluated for their self-emulsifying properties by the addition of pharmaceutically-relevant amounts of the formulation to 250 mL of water or a biorelevant, simulated physiological

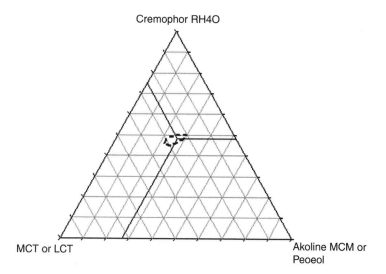

Figure 2 The area in the phase diagram represents microemulsions with either medium chain triglycerides or long chain triglycerides as lipid phase, Cremophor RH40 as surfactant and Akoline MCM or Peceol as cosurfactant obtained after addition of 250 mL water to 1 g of SMEDDS giving a droplet size of less than 100 nm. The SMEDDS in the area are mono-phasic at room temperature. *Abbreviations*: LCT, long chain triglycerides; Akoline MCM, pharmaceutical surfactant containing medium chain monoglycerides; MCT, medium chain triglycerides; SMEDDS, self-microemulsifying drug delivery system.

fluid. The resulting dispersion is examined by direct visualization and by dynamic light scattering to accurately determine the lipid droplet size, thereby allowing classification of the formulation as a SEDDS or SMEDDS. The number of combinations of drug and excipients resulting in a microemulsion, which is typically small, defines the microemulsion existence field on the ternary phase diagram: the area enclosed in the broken line in Figure 2 represents the microemulsion existence field for various combinations of medium chain triglycerides (MCT) or LCT, Cremophor RH40 and Akoline MCM or Peceol.

At the molecular level, the structures formed between water and the lipid and surfactant components of the formulation change with the excipient to water ratio (Fig. 3). During the initial stages of dilution in water, the surfactant molecules form inverse micelles that trap water molecules in their hydrophilic interior (A); continued addition of water will form a w/o microemulsion in which water droplets are surrounded by surfactant and cosurfactant molecules; as dilution progresses further, a viscous liquid-crystalline state results, which is comprised of cylindrical formations of surfactant molecules with their polar headgroups oriented towards a hydrophilic interior (B). Still further dilution with water results in the reorientation of the surfactant molecules into lamellar structures in which planar sheets of water molecules are sandwiched between surfactant bi-layers (C).

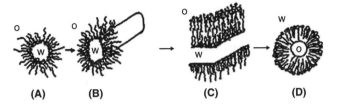

(A)   **(B)**   **(C)**   **(D)**

Figure 3 Schematic presentation of the mechanism happening during titration of a mixture containing oil and surfactants with water. (**A**) Water droplets in continuous oil phase; (**B**) water cylinders in oil; (**C**) lamellar structures; (**D**) oil droplets in continuous phase. *Source*: From Ref. 63.

In the final stages of dilution, the lamellar structure disintegrates giving rise to a continuous phase in which oil droplets, trapped within the hydrophobic interiors of spherical micellar structures formed by surfactant and cosurfactant molecules, are dispersed in water thus forming the emulsion (D).

Gross visual evaluation of the resulting emulsions has proven to be a reliable means of estimating the oil droplet size (8,14,32). Transparent to slightly bluish, opalescent dispersions possess oil droplet sizes between 20 nm and 40 nm and are thus classified as microemulsions, which are defined as dispersions containing oil droplets of less than 50 nm in size. (8,14,32,33). Opaque, milk-white dispersions result as the size of the dispersed oil droplets increases to and exceeds 100 nm (14).

The effect of aqueous dilution on the drug-solubilizing capacity of a self-emulsifying formulation is determined by the relative amount and physicochemical and biopharmaceutical properties of the drug substance as well as the specific types and amounts of incorporated excipients. The incorporation of HPMC into traditional SEDDS formulations as a means for delaying the postdilutional precipitation of paclitaxel from SEDDS formulations was recently described by Gao et al. (34) and was correlated with improved drug absorption in rats relative to a standard SEDDS formulation.

The influence of lipid fatty acid chain length on the ease of self-emulsification has been described by Deckelbaum et al. (23) who attributed the more facile self-emulsifying properties of medium chain triglycerides (MCT), relative to LCT, to the greater water solubility and smaller molecular size of the former. These properties are associated with greater mobility in the lipid/water interface and more rapid lipid hydrolysis in vivo and can lead to improved drug absorption (35). Grove et al. (14) described Type III SMEDDS formulations of seocalcitol, a Biopharmaceutics Classification System Class II drug, comprised of similar fractions (25%) of either LCT or MCT oil emulsified with Cremophor RH40 (48%) and either Akoline MCM or Peceol (27%). In comparison to the MCT-containing SMEDDS, the LCT-containing SMEDDS was relatively difficult to emulsify and required an increased concentration of Cremophor RH40 in order to yield a SMEDDS with the performance characteristics comparable to the MCT-SMEDDS (14).

Influence of Emulsion Droplet Size on Drug Absorption

Although improved drug absorption is generally assumed to be associated with smaller lipid droplet size, many examples exist in which drug absorption is not influenced by droplet size. Khoo et al. (32) evaluated the bioavailability of the poorly soluble antimalarial drug, halofantrine, in dogs following administration of either MC-SEDDS (mean lipid droplet size of 119 nm) or MC-SMEDDS (mean lipid droplet size of 52 nm) formulations; both yielded comparable bioavailability. These findings are in contrast to the findings of Tarr and Yalkowsky (36) who reported an increase in cyclosporine bioavailability from emulsions, when the lipid droplet size was reduced from 4 to 2 μm. However, these experiments were obtained in a rat in situ perfusion model, which lacks the lipid processing capabilities and hydrodynamic characteristics of the GIT in an intact animal. More recently, Odeberg et al. (37) demonstrated comparable bioavailability of cyclosporine in humans administered emulsion formulations possessing lipid droplet sizes of 0.2 μm or 16 to 20 μm.

In another study, de Smidt et al. (15) demonstrated comparable bioavailability of penclomedine in rats administered the drug as a solution in MCT oil or as microemulsions with lipid droplet sizes of either 160 nm or 710 nm. However, administration of the lipolysis inhibitor, tetrahydrolipstatin (THL), resulted in a substantial drop in penclomedine bioavailability when administered in MCT oil relative to the microemulsion formulations, from which biovailability was similar and unaffected in the present of THL.

Studies conducted in humans comparing the Sandimmune® formulation of cyclosporine, which forms a crude emulsion in the GIT, to that of the self-microemulsifying Neoral® formulation demonstrated improved performance of the latter with regard to the rate, extent, uniformity, and linearity of cyclosporine exposure as a function of dose. In addition, absorption of cyclosporine from the Neoral formulation was relatively unaffected by food as compared to the Sandimmune formulation (38,39).

From the foregoing discussion, it is difficult to determine the impact of lipid droplet size on drug absorption. It should be noted, however, that the cited studies utilized different lipid and surfactant systems, which can also influence drug absorption and confound the experimental results, thus making it difficult to draw conclusions. However, these findings collectively suggest that lipid droplet size may be less likely to impact formulation performance unless the normal lipid digestion process, which inherently produces a fine emulsion from ingested lipid, is compromised.

In Vivo Studies with SEDDS/SMEDDS

Several published studies describing modest to substantial increases in drug bioavailability from SEDDS and SMEDDS formulations, relative to conventional solid dosage forms, water-miscible glycol solutions [e.g., PEG and propylene glycol (PG)] or simple oil solutions are summarized in Table 1. Relative to conventional solid dosage forms, increases in drug bioavailability from self-emulsifying formulations ranged from 1.5-fold for simvastatin (40) to approximately seven-fold for L-365,260 (cholecystokinin antagonist) (19). The results of these studies suggest that the physicochemical properties of the drug substance, as well as the excipients selected for the formulation, appear to determine the bioavailability enhancing potential of a particular formulation for a given drug substance.

EFFECT OF DISPERSION ON BIOAVAILABILITY

Compared to simple oil solutions of the drug, only modest improvements in drug bioavailability were generally observed from self-emulsifying formulations (Table 1). However, it is important to note that these studies were conducted in different species, with different formulations and with different lipid and surfactant doses, which sometimes differed within an individual study. It should also be noted that only healthy test subjects, with fully functioning GI lipid handling pathways, were studied. As noted earlier in this chapter, self-emulsifying formulations appear to provide better absorption enhancement, when the normal physiological processes enabling lipid digestion and dispersion are compromised (15).

Julianto et al. (41) reported a two-fold increase in vitamin E bioavailability, when dosed to humans as a SMEDDS as compared to a marketed lipid solution formulation (Natopherol®). However, since a greater amount of lipid was dosed in the SMEDDS than in the Natopherol formulation, it is not possible to determine if the superior bioavailability provided by the SMEDDS formulation was a result of better dispersion or a greater amount of administered lipid, relative to the Natopherol formulation.

Hauss et al. (42) compared the bioavailability of the poorly soluble leokotriene B_4 (LTB$_4$) biosynthesis inhibitor, ontazolast, when administered to rats as four lipid-based formulations [soybean oil emulsion, two SEDDS, and a Peceol (Gattefosse, S.A.)] solution or a reference aqueous suspension formulation. The soybean oil emulsion and the SEDDS formulations all significantly increased ontazolast bioavailability to a similar degree relative to the suspension formulation. While the SEDDS formulations did not provide greater drug exposure than the crude soybean oil emulsion or Peceol solution, significant differences were noted in the absorption profiles, with the SEDDS providing more rapid and less variable absorption.

Studies conducted by Porter et al. (43) demonstrated a significant increase in the bioavailability of danazol, administered as either a LCT solution or a LC-SMEDDS formulation, relative to either a conventional solid dosage form or a MC-SEDDS formulation. The presence of a high concentration of surfactant in the SMEDDS containing long chain triglycerides (LC-SMEDDS) formulation did not improve danazol absorption over that seen from the simple LCT solution, which supported the findings of Grove et al. (31) who demonstrated similar bioavailability of seocalcitol, when administered to rats as simple MCT or LCT solutions or following addition of high concentrations of surfactant to yield MC-SMEDDS or LC-SMEDDS formulations, respectively. It should be noted that the

SMEDDS formulations of danazol described by Porter et al. (43) were not controlled for the ratio amounts of oil, surfactant, or cosurfactant, which makes it difficult to accurately assess the impact of dispersion on drug absorption.

Grove, et al. (31) reported similar bioavailability for seocalcitol, when administered to rats as either a solution in MCT oil or as a MCT-containing SMEDDS (MC-SMEDDS). In this study, similar volumes of the lipid were dosed in each formulation, which provided unequivocal evidence that the presumed, superior dispersion or resistance to precipitation provided by the MC-SMEDDS formulation was not contributing to seocalcitol absorption above and beyond that, which was due to solubilization in the lipid vehicle. However, when the study was repeated in minipigs, a tendency towards higher bioavailability was seen for the MC-SMEDDS formulation relative to the MCT oil solution formulation (44).

In the study by Porter et al. (43), danazol was administered to dogs as either a solution in LCT oil or as a LCT-containing SMEDDS (LC-SMEDDS). While greater bioavailability was seen with the LCT solution, a total of 3 g of LCT oil was administered in each dose as compared to the 1.8 g of LCT oil administered in the LC-SMEDDS formulation. Again, since the administered lipid volume was not controlled, it is not possible to assess the contribution of the presumed, superior dispersion or resistance to precipitation provided by the SMEDDS formulation on the absorption of danazol.

In Vivo Studies of Lymphatic Transport with Dispersed Formulations

Lymphatic drug transport, which is dependent on concomitant GI lipid absorption, can contribute significantly to the overall uptake of lipophilic drugs from the GIT. Since the efficient absorption of lipids and cosolubilized hydrophobic xenobiotics from the GIT is dependent on the initial formation of a fine oil-in-water dispersion in the intestinal lumen, the influence of dispersion on lymphatic transport has been investigated. Porter et al. (45) found similar contributions of lymphatic transport to the overall uptake of the antimalarial drug, halofantrine, following oral administration of a micellar solution, an emulsion and a lipid solution to conscious, mesenteric lymph cannulated rats. However, when the study was repeated with anesthetised rats in which the GI motility and the ability to disperse the administered lipid was compromised, the relative contribution of lymphatic uptake of halofantrine to overall drug absorption was directly related to the degree of lipid dispersion associated with the administered formulation (46). Conflicting findings were reported by Karpf et al. (47) who studied the lymphatic transport of halofantrine in conscious, mesenteric lymph fistula rats administered halofantrine as either a triglyceride (TG) solution or following oil-in-water emulsification with either Cremphor RH40 or lecithin. Compared to a TG solution, the emulsion formulations showed similar and significantly increased lymphatic drug transport. This finding was attributed to increased drug absorption in the proximal regions of the small intestine resulting from more facile lipid digestion and absorption associated with the emulsion formulations.

The lymphotropic potential of SEDDS/SMEDDS formulations of the LTB_4 biosynthesis inhibitor, ontazolast, was studied in conscious, mesenteric lymph fistula rats by Hauss et al. (42). Formulations containing 50:50 or 80:20 ratio concentrations of Gelucire® 44/14 (Gattefosse, S.A.) and Peceol (Gattefosse, S.A.), a solution in Peceol, and a LCT emulsion all provided similar increases in ontazolast bioavailability relative to an aqueous reference suspension. However, the SEDDS formulations promoted the most rapid ontazolast absorption and produced the highest concentrations of ontazolast in the lymph whereas the LCT emulsion resulted in the greatest fractional uptake of ontazolast in the mesenteric lymph. These findings suggested that while SEDDS may have potential as lymphotropic delivery systems, a balance between the concentrations of surfactant and lipid components should be found, which maintains the drug substance in solution in the GIT during absorption while simultaneously providing adequate lipid substrate for the optimal production of drug-carrying chylomicrons.

The results of the foregoing studies can be explained by the work of Ichihashi et al. (48) who determined that mesenteric lymphatic transport of mepitiostane occurred predominantly from the proximal region of the small intestine and Clark et al. (49), who demonstrated that lipoprotein secretory activity is greater in the proximal regions of the small intestine and is limited primarily by the rate of lipid absorption.

Influence of Lipid Components on Lymphatic Transport

The mesenteric lymphatic transport of halofantrine, administered in SMEDDS containing either MCT or LCT as the lipid component, has been studied in conscious dogs (24). The fraction of the administered dose of halofantrine transported in the lymph after administration of the LC-SMEDDS was 28.3% compared with only 5.0% after administration of the MC-SMEDDS. The marginal lymphatic transport of halofantrine associated with the MC-SMEDDS formulation is explained by its content of mono- and diglycerides of MCTs, which unlike long chain fatty acid (LCFA), are not lymphotropic. The foregoing study was repeated by Holm et al. (50) using SMEDDS formulations in which the MCT and LCT lipid components were replaced with "structured triglycerides" [medium long medium chain fatty acid (MLM) $[C_{8:0}-C_{18:2}-C_{8:0}]$ and long medium long chain fatty acid (LML) $[C_{18:2}-C_{8:0}-C_{18:2}]$, respectively]. Structured triglycerides are prepared by selectively esterifying medium and long chain fatty acids to specific positions on the glycerol backbone of the TG molecule. The fraction of the administered dose of halofantrine transported in the lymph from the MLM-SMEDDS increased to 17.9% (compared to the MC-SMEDDS), but for the LML-SMEDDS, was similar to that of the LC-SMEDDS (27.4% vs. 28.3%, respectively). The apparent, greater extent of halofantrine transport observed for the structured lipid, MLM-SMEDDS relative to that seen with the MC-SMEDDS formulation, however, may be an artifact resulting from the relatively high LCFA content of the surfactant, Maisine 35-1 (Gattefosse S.A.), used in the MLM-SMEDDS to promote microemulsification.

The foregoing investigations demonstrate the potential utility that SEDDS or SMEDDS formulations have as lymphotropic drug delivery systems. These effects appear to be mediated by incorporation of excipients containing LCT, which favors chylomicron synthesis, and by the increased dispersion of these formulations in the GIT, which appears to promote lymphatic drug transport by facilitating lipid digestion and absorption.

INFLUENCE OF SELF-EMULSIFYING LIPID-BASED FORMULATIONS ON FOOD EFFECT

Increased drug exposure, relative to the fasted state, following postprandial administration of poorly water-soluble drugs in conventional solid formulations is well documented in the literature [e.g., isotretinoin (51); danazol (43,52,53); L-683,453 (54); DPC 961 (55); halofantrine (56). It has been postulated that the magnitude of the exposure increase may indicate the maximum extent of absorption possible when the drug is administered in a lipid-based formulation (43). The effect of food on the bioavailability of poorly water-soluble, hydrophobic drugs is determined by multiple factors, including the physicochemical properties of the drug substance, the dose, the nature of the formulation and the amount and composition of the ingested food (57). Postprandial changes in the GIT that can increase drug absorption, relative to the fasted state, include: (*i*) increased drug solubilization by bile salt mixed micelles, and (*ii*) increased intestinal membrane permeability secondary to the presence of bile and lipid digestion products. Since food effect can lead to exaggerated pharmacologic responses or unexpected toxicity (57), clinical trial guidelines routinely require studies comparing drug exposure in fed and fasted subjects.

Although limited in number, studies showing the efficacy of self-emulsifying lipid-based formulations for mitigating food effect have been described in the literature. Grove et al. (44) studied the influence of food on the bioavailability of seocalcitol in minipigs following administration as either a solution in MCT, a MC-SMEDDS, or a solution in propylene glycol (PG). The fasted state bioavailability of seocalcitol was 15%, 21%, and 28% for the PG, MCT, and MC-SMEDDS formulations, respectively. In the postprandial state, the seocalcitol bioavailability from the PG solution nearly doubled to 29%, but was unchanged, relative to the fasted state, for both the MCT and MC-SMEDDS formulations. These results suggest a common mechanism by which food and lipid-based formulations improve the absorption of poorly soluble drugs. Other poorly soluble drugs for which lipid-based formulations have reduced the effect of food on drug absorption include danazol (52) and L-683,453 (54) and cyclosporine (38).

CHEMICAL AND PHYSICAL STABILITY

Optimal performance of lipid-based formulations relies on maintaining the drug in the fully-solubilized state within the excipient matrix, which can lead to potential physical and chemical stability issues during storage. A commercially-viable formulation must show <5% degradation during two years of storage under ambient conditions (25°C/60% RH), which translates into no more than 7% degradation within three months under accelerated conditions (40°C/75% RH) (58). Grove et al. (31) described 10% degradation of seocalcitol, when formulated as either a LCT or MCT SMEDDS; in comparison, less than 3% degradation was observed when the drug was formulated as simple MCT or LCT solutions. Although the exact degradation mechanism was not identified, these findings suggest the surfactant (Cremophor RH40) or the cosurfactants (Akoline MCM and Peceol) to be responsible for the poorer drug stability observed in the SMEDDS formulations. Another, similar example of poor drug chemical stability was observed for a SEDDS formulation of paclitaxel [containing varying amounts of Triton WR-1339 (tyloxapol), D-alpha-tocopheryl PEG 1000 succinate and sodium deoxycholate], which underwent approximately 20% degradation when stored for 24 hours at 37°C (59). These findings highlight the need for additional work aimed at providing a greater understanding of the physical and chemical mechanisms governing drug stability in lipid-based formulations.

The physical stability of a lipid-based formulation is also crucial to its performance, which can be adversely affected by precipitation of the drug in the excipient matrix. In addition, poor formulation physical stability can lead to phase separation of the excipients, affecting not only formulation performance, but visual appearance as well. In addition, incompatibilities between the formulation and the gelatin capsule shell can lead to brittleness or deformation, delayed disintegration, or incomplete release of drug. Recently introduced alternatives to gelatin capsules that may be more appropriate for encapsulation of SEDDS/SMEDDS and other lipid-based formulations include HPMC or polyvinylalcohol hard capsules (30) and are discussed in greater detail elsewhere in this book.

CONCLUSION

Properly designed SEDDS and SMEDDS formulations provide the formulator with an opportunity to manipulate the drug absorption profile as well as a means for improving overall absorption relative to non-self-dispersing lipid-based formulations. Formulation performance that can include resistance to food effect, relies on identifying the correct combinations of lipid carrier vehicles and surfactants to ensure facile self-emulsification, while providing resistance to lumenal drug precipitation prior to absorption. Potential limitations to the application of self-emulsifying formulations include poor chemical stability of the drug substance due to excipient catalyzed degradation or precipitation of the drug substance in the excipient matrix. A greater understanding of the chemical and physical mechanisms surrounding these incompatibilities is needed to resolve these issues and unlock the full potential of self-emulsifying formulations.

REFERENCES

1. Yamahira Y, Noguchi T, Takenaka H, Maeda T. Biopharmaceutical studies of lipid-containing oral dosage forms: relationship between drug absorption rate and digestibility of vehicles. Int J Pharm 1979; 3:23–31.

2. Fouad FM, Farrell PG, Marshall WD, van de Voort FR. In vitro model for lipase-catalysed lipophile release from fats. J Agric Food Chem 1991; 39(1):150–153.

3. Humberstone AJ, Charman WN. Lipid-based vehicles for the oral delivery of poorly water-soluble drugs. Adv Drug Deliv Rev 1997; 25(1):103–128.

4. Pouton CW. Lipid formulations for oral administration of drugs: non-emulsifying, self-emulsifying and "self-microemulsifying" drug delivery systems. Eur J Pharm Sci 2000; 11(suppl 2):S93–S98.

5. Gershanik T, Benita S. Self-dispersing lipid formulations for improving oral absorption of lipophilic drugs. Eur J Pharm Biopharm 2000; 50(1):179–188.

6. Stuchlik M, Zak S. Lipid-based vehicle for oral drug delivery. Biomed Pap Med Fac Univ Palacky Olomouc Czech Repub 2001; 145(2):17–26.

7. Porter CJ, Charman WN. Uptake of drugs into the intestinal lymphatics after oral administration. Adv Drug Deliv Rev 1997; 25(1):71–89.

8. Gursoy RN, Benita S. Self-emulsifying drug delivery systems (SEDDS) for improved oral delivery of lipophilic drugs. Biomed Pharmacother 2004; 58(3):173–182.

9. Constantinides PP. Lipid microemulsions for improving drug dissolution and oral absorption: physical and biopharmaceutical aspects. Pharm Res 1995; 12(11):1561–1572.

10. Shah NH, Carvajal MT, Patel CI, Infeld MH, Malick AW. Self-emulsifying drug delivery systems (SEDDS) with polyglycolyzed glycerides for improving in vitro dissolution and oral absorption of lipophilic drugs. Int J Pharm 1994; 106(1):15–23.

11. Pouton CW. Self-emulsifying drug delivery systems:assessment of the efficiency of emulsification. Int J Pharm 1985; 27(2–3):335–348.

12. Wakerly MG, Pouton-CW, Meakin BJ. Evaluation of the self-emulsifying preformance of a non-ionic surfactant-vegetable oil mixture. J Pharm Pharmacol 1987; 39:6P.

13. Charman SA, Charman WN, Rogge MC, Wilson TD, Dutko FJ, Pouton CW. Self-emulsifying drug delivery systems: formulation and biopharmaceutic evaluation of an investigational lipophilic compound. Pharm Res 1992; 9(1):87–93.

14. Grove M, Pedersen GP, Nielsen JL, Mullertz A. Bioavailability of seocalcitol I: relating solubility in biorelevant media with oral bioavailability in rats-effect of medium and long chain triglycerides. J Pharm Sci 2005; 94(8):1830–1838.

15. de Smidt PC, Campanero MA, Troconiz IF. Intestinal absorption of penclomedine from lipid vehicles in the conscious rat: contribution of emulsification versus digestibility. Int J Pharm 2004; 270(1–2):109–118.

16. Myers RA, Stella VJ. Systemic bioavailability of penclomedine (NSC-338720) from oil-in-water emulsions administered intraduodenally to rats. Int J Pharm 1992; 78(1–3):217–226.

17. FDA 2005. Guidance for Industry Nonclinical Studies for the Safety Evaluation of Pharmaceutical Excipients. U.S. Department of Health and Human Services.

18. FDA 2006. www.accessdata.fda.gov/scripts/cder/lig/index.cfm. U.S. Food and Drug Administration.

19. Lin JH, Chen IW, Lievens H. The effect of dosage form on oral absorption of L-365260, a potent CCKB receptor antagonist, in beagle dogs. Pharm Res 1991; 8:S-272.

20. Gallo-Torres H, Ludorf J, Brin M. The effect of medium-chain triglycerides on the bioavailability of vitamin E. Int J Vit Nutr Res 1978; 48(3):240–249.

21. Palin KJ, Wilson CG, Davis SS, Phillips AJ. The effect of oils on the lymphatic absorption of DDT. J Pharm Pharmacol 1982; 34(11):707–710.

22. Palin KJ, Winson CG. The effect of different oils on the absorption of probucol in the rat. J Pharm Pharmacol 1984; 36(9):641–643.

23. Deckelbaum RJ, Hamilton JA, Moser A, et al. Medium-chain versus long-chain triacylglycerol emulsion hydrolysis by lipoprotein lipase and hepatic lipase: implications for the mechanisms of lipase action. Biochemistry 1990; 29(5):1136–1142.

24. Khoo SM, Shackleford DM, Porter CJ, Edwards GA, Charman WN. Intestinal lymphatic transport of halofantrine occurs after oral administration of a unit-dose lipid-based formulation to fasted dogs. Pharm Res 2003; 20(9):1460–1465.

25. Laher JM, Rigler MW, Vetter RD, Barrowman JA, Patton JS. Similar bioavailability and lymphatic transport of benzo(a)pyrene when administered to rats in different amounts of dietary fat. J Lipid Res 1984; 25(12):1337–1342.

26. Gershanik T, Haltner E, Lehr CM, Benita S. Charge-dependent interaction of self-emulsifying oil formulations with Caco-2 cells monolayers: binding, effects on barrier function and cytotoxicity. Int J Pharm 2000; 211(1–2):29–36.

27. Gursoy N, Garrigue JS, Razafindratsita A, Lambert G, Benita S. Excipient effects on in vitro cytotoxicity of a novel paclitaxel self-emulsifying drug delivery system. J Pharm Sci 2003; 92(12):2411–2418.

28. Palamakula A, Khan MA. Evaluation of cytotoxicity of oils used in coenzyme Q10 self-emulsifying drug delivery systems (SEDDS). Int J Pharm 2004; 273(1–2):63–73.

29. Tenjarla S. Microemulsions: an overview and pharmaceutical applications. Crit Rev Ther Drug Carrier Syst 1999; 16(5):461–521.

30. Strickley RG. Solubilizing excipients in oral and injectable formulations. Pharm Res 2004; 21(2):201–230.

31. Grove M, Mullertz A, Nielsen JL, Pedersen GP. Bioavailability of seocalcitol II: development and characterisation of self microemulsifying drug delivery systems (SMEDDS) for oral administration containing medium and long chain triglycerides. Eur J Pharm Sci 2006; 28(3):233–242.

32. Khoo SM, Humberstone AJ, Porter CJ, Edwards GA, Charman WN. Formulation design and bioavailability assessment of lipidic self-emulsifying formulations of halofantrine. Int J Pharm 1998; 167(12):155–164.

33. Christensen JØ. Evaluation of an in vitro lipid digestion model—testing poorly soluble drug substances and lipid-based formulations. Ph.D. Thesis Ed., Department of Pharmaceutics, The Danish University of Pharmaceutical Science, Copenhagen, Denmark, 2004.

34. Gao P, Rush BD, Pfund WP, et al. Development of a supersaturable SEDDS (S-SEDDS) formulation of paclitaxel with improved oral bioavailability. J Pharm Sci 2003; 92(12):2386–2398.

35. Alander J, Wärnheim T. Model microemulsions containing vegetable oils part 1: nonionic surfactant systems. J Am Oil Chem Soc 1989; 66:1656–1660.

36. Tarr BD, Yalkowsky SH. Enhanced intestinal absorption of cyclosporine in rats through the reduction of emulsion droplet size. Pharm Res 1989; 6(1):40–43.

37. Odeberg JM, Kaufmann P, Kroon KG, Hoglund P. Lipid drug delivery and rational formulation design for lipophilic drugs with low oral bioavailability, applied to cyclosporine. Eur J Pharm Sci 2003; 20(4–5):375–382.

38. Mueller EA, Kovarik JM, van Bree JB, Grevel J, Lucker PW, Kutz K. Influence of a fat-rich meal on the pharmacokinetics of a new oral formulation of cyclosporine in a crossover comparison with the market formulation. Pharm Res 1994; 11(1):151–155.

39. Mueller EA, Kovarik JM, van Bree JB, Tetzloff W, Grevel J, Kutz K. Improved dose linearity of cyclosporine pharmacokinetics from a microemulsion formulation. Pharm Res 1994; 11(2):301–304.

40. Kang BK, Lee JS, Chon SK, et al. Development of self-microemulsifying drug delivery systems (SMEDDS) for oral bioavailability enhancement of simvastatin in beagle dogs. Int J Pharm 2004; 274(1–2):65–73.

41. Julianto T, Yuen KH, Noor AM. Improved bioavailability of vitamin E with a self emulsifying formulation. Int J Pharm 2000; 200(1):53–57.

42. Hauss DJ, Fogal SE, Ficorilli JV, et al. Lipid-based delivery systems for improving the bioavailability and lymphatic transport of a poorly water-soluble LTB4 inhibitor. J Pharm Sci 1998; 87(2):164–169.

43. Porter CJ, Kaukonen AM, Boyd BJ, Edwards GA, Charman WN. Susceptibility to lipase-mediated digestion reduces the oral bioavailability of danazol after administration as a medium-chain lipid-based microemulsion formulation. Pharm Res 2004; 21(8):1405–1412.

44. Grove M, Mullertz A, Pedersen GP, Nielsen JL. Bioavailability of seocalcitol III: administration of lipid-based formulations to mini-pigs in the fasted and the fed state. Eur J Pharm Sci 2007; in press.

45. Porter CJ, Charman SA, Charman WN. Lymphatic transport of halofantrine in the triple-cannulated anesthetized rat model: effect of lipid vehicle dispersion. J Pharm Sci 1996; 85(4):351–356.

46. Porter CJ, Charman SA, Humberstone AJ, Charman WN. Lymphatic transport of halofantrine in the conscious rat when administered as either the free base or the hydrochloride salt: effect of lipid class and lipid vehicle dispersion. J Pharm Sci 1996; 85(4):357–361.

47. Karpf DM, Holm R, Kristensen HG, Mullertz A. Influence of the type of surfactant and the degree of dispersion on the lymphatic transport of halofantrine in conscious rats. Pharm Res 2004; 21(8):1413–1418.

48. Ichihashi T, Kinoshita H, Takagishi Y, Yamada H. Effect of oily vehicles on absorption of mepitiostane by the lymphatic system in rats. J Pharm Pharmacol 1992; 44(7):560–564.

49. Clark SB, Lawergren B, Martin JV. Regional intestinal absorptive capacities for triolein: an alternative to markers. Am J Physiol 1973; 225(3):574–585.

50. Holm R, Porter CJ, Edwards GA, Mullertz A, Kristensen HG, Charman WN. Examination of oral absorption and lymphatic transport of halofantrine in a triple-cannulated canine model after administration in self-microemulsifying drug delivery systems (SMEDDS) containing structured triglycerides. Eur J Pharm Sci 2003; 20(1):91–97.

51. Colburn WA, Gibson DM, Wiens RE, Hanigan JJ. Food increases the bioavailability of isotretinoin. J Clin Pharmacol 1983; 23(11–12):534–539.

52. Charman WN, Rogge MC, Boddy AW, Berger BM. Effect of food and a monoglyceride emulsion formulation on danazol bioavailability. J Clin Pharmacol 1993; 33(4):381–386.

53. Sunesen VH, Vedelsdal R, Kristensen HG, Christrup L, Mullertz A. Effect of liquid volume and food intake on the absolute bioavailability of danazol, a poorly soluble drug. Eur J Pharm Sci 2005; 24(4):297–303.

54. Matuszewska B, Hettrick L, Bondi JV, Storey DE. Comparative bioavailability of L-683,453, a 5a-reductase inhibitor, from a self-emulsifying drug delivery system in Beagle dogs. Int J Pharm 1996; 136(1–2):147–154.

55. Aungst BJ, Nguyen NH, Taylor NJ, Bindra DS. Formulation and food effects on the oral absorption of a poorly water-soluble, highly permeable antiretroviral agent. J Pharm Sci 2002; 91(6):1390–1395.

56. Humberstone AJ, Porter CJ, Charman WN. A physicochemical basis for the effect of food on the absolute oral bioavailability of halofantrine. J Pharm Sci 1996; 85(5):525–529.

57. Charman WN, Porter CJ, Mithani S, Dressman JB. Physiochemical and physiological mechanisms for the effects of food on drug absorption: the role of lipids and pH. J Pharm Sci 1997; 86(3):269–282.

58. Pope DG. Accelrated stability testing for prediction of drug product stability. Drug Cosmetic Industry 1980; 1276:48–116.

59. Gursoy N, Garrigue JS, Razafindratsita A, Lambert G, Benita S. Excipient effects on in vitro cytotoxicity of a novel paclitaxel self-emulsifying drug delivery system. J Pharm Sci 2003; 92(12):2411–2418.

60. Kommuru TR, Gurley B, Khan MA, Reddy IK. Self-emulsifying drug delivery systems (SEDDS) of coenzyme Q10: formulation development and bioavailability assessment. Int J Pharm 2001; 212(2):233–246.

61. Kovarik JM, Mueller EA, van Bree JB, Tetzloff W, Kutz K. Reduced inter- and intraindividual variability in cyclosporine pharmacokinetics from a microemulsion formulation. J Pharm Sci 1994; 83(3):444–446.

62. O'Driscoll CM. Lipid-based formulations for intestinal lymphatic delivery. Eur J Pharm Sci 2002; 15(5):405–415.

63. Attwood D. Microemulsions. In: Kreutted J, ed, Colloid Drug Delivery Systems, 1st ed. New York: Marcel Dekker Inc., 1994:31–71.

64. Wu AL, Clark SB, Holt PR. Transmucosal triglyceride transport rates in proximal and distal rat intestine in vivo. J Lipid Res 1975; 16(4):251–257.

65. Charman WN, Stella VJ. Effect of lipid class and lipid vehicle volume on the intestinal lymphatic transport of DDT. Int J Pharm 1986; 33(1–3):165–172.

6

Lipid-Based Isotropic Solutions: Design Considerations

Navnit H. Shah, Wantanee Phuapradit, Yu-E Zhang, Hashim Ahmed, and A. Waseem Malick

Pharmaceutical and Analytical Research and Development, Roche, Nutley, New Jersey, U.S.A.

INTRODUCTION

The advent of combinatorial chemistry and high throughput screening as the primary technologies for drug discovery has resulted in the generation of a preponderance of potential drug candidates, which do not possess favorable "drug-like" biopharmaceutical properties. Specifically, these candidate compounds are highly lipophilic (Log P > 5) and possess very poor solubility (<10 mg/mL) in physiological fluids, resulting in poor and highly variable absorption, after oral administration, that is often strongly influenced by the presence of food in the gastrointestinal (GI) tract (1). In many instances, the GI absorption of these challenging compounds can be significantly improved through the use of lipid-based formulations (2,3).

In addition to improving and normalizing the absorption of poorly water-soluble drugs, lipid based formulations can be used to address other formulation issues, including stabilization of oxygen and moisture sensitive compounds (4), improving content uniformity of the dosage form (5) and allowing for controlled drug release (6,7). Despite the promise that lipid formulation technology holds for addressing challenging formulation issues, research and development activities in this area have been limited and only a few marketed products employ lipids as primary excipients.

Physiological factors that can influence the rate and extent of drug absorption from a lipid-based formulation include GI lipid digestion (8–10) and the emulsion droplet size formed upon mixing with the GI fluids (2,11,12). From a manufacturing perspective, the solubility of the drug substance in the lipid vehicle controls the drug loading of the formulation, whereas the stability of the drug can be influenced by the excipient peroxide and acid values and the degree of lipid fatty acid saturation and hygroscopicity. During manufacturing of semi-solid lipid dispersion formulations, the rate of shear applied during mixing should be carefully evaluated and monitored (4) and the rate of cooling of the formulation must be controlled as it can influence the formulation final viscosity, content uniformity, dissolution rate, and efficiency of the encapsulation process.

CLASSIFICATION OF LIPID-BASED FORMULATIONS

The various categories of lipid formulations have been previously classified with respect to composition, content of hydrophilic cosolvents, dispersion droplet size, impact of aqueous dilution, and digestibility in vivo (13).

In this chapter, we will classify lipid formulations based on the miscibility of the system components (e.g., single phase or isotropic lipid solutions or two-phase systems, such as lipid suspensions or lipid semi-solid dispersions). Case-studies of lipid formulations used to address issues pertaining to poor bioavailability will be presented.

Isotropic Solutions

An isotropic solution is a single-phase system and includes lipid solutions, self-emulsifying drug delivery systems (SEDDS) and self-microemulsifying drug delivery systems (SMEDDS). Isotropic solutions find application primarily for oral delivery of lipophilic drugs for which a unit dose can be solubilized in an acceptable volume of the lipid vehicle. This type of lipid formulation is effective for improving the bioavailability of lipophilic drugs as well as for stabilizing oxygen and moisture sensitive drugs. Commonly used lipophilic vehicles that are the solubilizing excipients that form the basis of isotropic solution formulations, are presented in Table 1. SEDDS and SMEDDS formulations incorporate, in addition to a lipophilic vehicle, an emulsifier and often, a coemulsifier. Commonly used emulsifiers that typically possess hydrophilic–lipophilic balance (HLB) values greater than 10, are shown in Table 2 and commonly used coemulsifiers, which typically possess HLB values in the range of four to six, are shown in Table 3.

Lipid Solutions

Lipid solution formulations are simple solutions of the drug in a single lipid vehicle. Following administration, the preabsorptive emulsification of these formulations relies on the presence of surfactants that are present in normal intestinal fluids (e.g., bile acids). Due to the critical importance of lipid emulsification on drug

Table 1 Commonly Used Lipophilic Vehicles

Classification	Lipophilic vehicles
Fatty acids	Oleic acid, myristic acid, caprylic acid, and capric acid
Ethanol ester	Ethyl oleate
Triglycerides of long-chain fatty acids	Soybean oil, peanut oil, arachis oil, and corn oil
Triglycerides of medium-chain fatty acids	Miglyol 812, Captex 355, and Labrafac

Table 2 Emulsifiers that Are Commonly Used in Isotropic Lipid-Based Solutions

Classifications	Emulsifiers
Polyglycolyzed glycerides	PEG-8 glyceryl caprylate/caprate (Labrasol)
	PEG-32 glyceryl laurate (Gelucire 44/14)
	PEG-32 glyceryl palmito stearate (Gelucire 50/13)
Polyoxyethylene sorbitan fatty acid esters	Polyoxyethylene 20 sorbitan monolaurate (Tween 20)
	Polyoxyethylene 20 sorbitan monostearate (Tween 60)
	Polyoxyethylene 20 sorbitan monooleate (Tween 80)
Sorbitan fatty acid esters	Sorbitan monolaurate (Span 20)
	Sorbitan monostearate (Span 60)
	Sorbitan monooleate (Span 80)
Polyoxyethylene castor oil derivatives	Polyoxyl 35 castor oil (Cremophor EL)
	Polyoxyl 40 hydrogenated castor oil (Cremophor RH 40)
Polyethylene glycol based derivatives of vitamin E	d-Alpha-tocopheryl polyethylene glycol-1000 succinate
Phospholipids and PEG based phospholipids	Lecithin and modified lecithin

Abbreviations: EL, ethoxylated; PEG, polyethylene glycol.

absorption, selection of the lipid vehicle can significantly impact formulation performance in vivo (8,14,15). Lipid solution formulations comprised of "predigested" lipids of medium chain fatty acids, such as monoglycerides of caprylic/capric acids [Capmul® medium chain monoglyceride (MCM)], or the semi-synthetic propylene glycol monoesters of medium chain fatty acids, readily form emulsions in the gut in the presence of bile salts and have been successfully applied in formulations of poorly water-soluble drugs.

As an example, a medium-chain monoglyceride lipid solution formulation of a poorly water-soluble HIV protease inhibitor improved drug absorption in humans three-fold relative to a conventional capsule formulation administered in

Table 3 Coemulsifiers that Are Commonly Used in Isotropic Lipid-Based Solutions

Classifications	Coemulsifiers
Polyglycolyzed glycerides	Polyethylene glycol-6 glyceryl monooleate (Labrafil M1944 CS)
Monoglycerides of long-chain fatty acids	Glycerol monooleate, and glycerol monostearate
Monoglycerides of medium-chain fatty acids	Glyceryl caprylate/caprate (Capmul MCM)
Mono and diglycerides of medium-chain fatty acids	Imwittor 972 and Imwittor 988
Propylene glycol monoester of medium-chain fatty acids	Propylene glycol monocaprylate (Capmul PG-8; Capryol 90)
Propylene glycol diester of medium-chain fatty acids	Propylene glycol dicaprylate/dicaprate (Captex 200)
Poly-glycerol esters	Glyceryl tri-oleate and decaglycerol mono-oleate

Abbreviations: MCM, medium chain monoglyceride; PG, propylene glycol.

Table 4 Bioavailability of an HIV Protease Inhibitor in Human Under Fed Conditions from Powder Filled in Hard Gelatin Capsules vs. Lipid Solution Filled in Soft Gelatin Capsules

Formulation	C_{max} (ng/mL)	T_{max} (h)	AUC (ng.h/mL)
Powder (filled in hard gelatin capsules)	61.85 (62.3)	4.5	194.9 (59.3)
Lipid solution (filled in soft gelatin capsules)	334.6 (70.9)	1.5	701 (80.9)

Note: Data represent the mean (CV in parentheses).
Abbreviation: AUC, area under the curve.

the fed state (Table 4). The compound had poor solubility in simulated gastric fluid (0.08 mg/mL), which was pH-dependent, resulting in the compound being practically insoluble in simulated intestinal fluid. The poor bioavailability of the compound, when administered in conventional dosage forms, was attributed to its low aqueous solubility, which resulted in incomplete absorption.

Self-Emulsifying Drug Delivery Systems

In the absence of water, properly formulated mixtures of lipid vehicles and non-ionic surfactants exist as transparent isotropic solutions (SEDDS), which upon dilution in aqueous media and with mild agitation, form fine oil-in-water emulsions with mean lipid droplet diameters ranging from 1 to 10 microns, depending on the degree of dilution. Following oral administration, normal GI motility provides sufficient energy for the emulsification of these formulations (16). The application of SEDDS for improving the GI absorption of poorly water-soluble drugs is the subject of several excellent publications (11,13,17).

The absorption of the retinoid compound, Ro 15-0778, a naphthalene derivative with poor water solubility (<0.01 mg/mL) and relatively high peanut oil solubility (95 mg/mL), was evaluated in unfasted dogs following administration of a 200 mg dose as a proprietary SEDDS formulation or as three other formulations: (*i*) a 1.2% drug solution in polyethylene glycol 400 (PEG400); (*ii*) a tablet containing micronized drug; (*iii*) a capsule containing 55% wet-milled spray dried powder (11). The exposure (C_{max} and AUC) of Ro 15-0778 from the SEDDS was at least three-fold greater than that of the other dosage forms (Table 5). The in vitro release of Ro 15-0778 from each formulation was determined in a United States Pharmacopeia (USP) XXII dissolution Apparatus 2 in 900 mL of water containing 5% of the nonionic surfactant, Alkamuls EL-719 (HLB = 16) that was added to achieve sink conditions. The superior in vitro drug release observed for the PEG400 solution (Fig. 1), which was not reflected in the in vivo results, may be the result of drug precipitation in vivo, which was not observed in vitro due to the presence of the solubilizing surfactant in the dissolution medium.

Self-Microemulsifying Drug Delivery Systems

SMEDDS are isotropic solutions of a drug in a mixture of a lipid vehicle, a surfactant and a cosurfactant. These formulations emulsify spontaneously upon contact with the GI fluids, forming finely dispersed lipid droplets with a typical mean diameter of less than 50 nm, the size of which is relatively independent of the dilution factor and degree of agitation. The resulting microemulsion is a thermodynamically stable, clear isotropic dispersion of two immiscible liquids (e.g., the lipid vehicle and water) stabilized by an interfacial film of surfactant molecules (18). SMEDDS formulations, by virtue of their smaller lipid droplet size, may provide improved and less variable drug absorption relative to lipid solution or SEDDS formulations, and due to the typically higher surfactant content, may provide additional absorption enhancement resulting from surfactant-induced membrane permeability increases as well as inhibition or reduction of transporter-mediated drug efflux (19).

Table 5 Pharmacokinetics Parameters of Ro 15-0778 from Different Formulations in Dogs Under Fed Conditions

Formulation	C_{max} (μg/mL)	T_{max} (h)	AUC (μg.h/mL)	% Relative bioavailability
Self-emulsifying drug delivery systems	5.57	2.5	29.77	389.0
Drug solution in PEG 400 as control	1.44	2.0	7.64	100.0
Capsule formulation from wet-milled spray dried powder	0.78	3.0	2.69	35.3
Tablet formulation with micronized drug	0.58	2.0	1.32	17.2

Abbreviation: AUC, area under the curve.

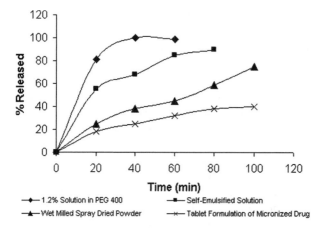

Figure 1   In vitro release profiles of Ro 15-0778 from different formulations. *Abbreviation*: PEG, polyethylene glycol.

Sandimmune Neoral® (20), a SMEDDS preconcentrate formulation of cyclosporine that upon dilution in aqueous media, forms a mean lipid droplet diameter of 30 nm, has been shown to reduce the inter- and intrapatient variability and the effect of food on drug absorption and other key pharmacokinetic parameters (e.g., C_{max}, C_{min}, T_{max}) relative to the previous Sandimmune® formulation, a crude emulsion, which yielded a mean lipid droplet diameter of 2 to 5 µm (21).

Lipid Suspensions and Lipid Semi-solid Dispersions

Lipid suspensions and lipid semi-solid dispersions, covered in greater detail elsewhere in this book, are two-phase formulations in which the finely divided drug substance is dispersed in the lipid excipient matrix. These formulations that do not fully solubilize the drug, find application in addressing drug delivery, stability, or manufacturing issues in the following ways:

1. Reduced drug degradation by protection from oxygen and moisture.
2. Improved content uniformity by eliminating electrostatic charges and facilitating de-agglomeration of the drug by dispersion in the lipid excipient matrix.
3. May provide sustained drug release capability.

CONSIDERATIONS IN DESIGN ISOTROPIC SOLUTIONS

When selecting among the various isotropic solution options available for a poorly soluble drug (e.g., lipid solutions, SEDDS, and SMEDDS), careful considerations of the drug physicochemical properties and the choice of lipid excipients is essential. Drug physico-chemical parameters that influence the design of isotropic solutions include solubility, HLB, partition coefficient, dielectric constant, and molecular weight (MW). Critical excipient properties to consider include surface tension and degree of lipid fatty acid saturation. Ternary phase diagrams (discussed in section "Optimal Drug:Surfactant Ratio") are very useful in determining the optimal ratios of drug, lipid, surfactant, and cosurfactant to use when developing a SEDDS or SMEDDS formulation.

Physical–Chemical Considerations

Solubility

Solubility of the drug in the formulation is one of the most critical parameters controlling the absorption-enhancing performance of a lipid-based formulation. As a general rule of thumb, the total capsule fill weight (drug dose plus excipients) should not exceed 1 g.

Insufficient solubility of the drug in the excipient matrix requires administration of multiple dosage units for a single dose and is generally viewed as unacceptable. This situation is most frequently encountered in dealing with moderate potency compounds requiring doses in the range of 100 to 200 mg.

During initial excipient screening activities, drug solubility is routinely determined in various oils, surfactants, and cosurfactants. A typical screening protocol involves combining an excess of the drug (approximately 500 mg) with 1 to 2 mL of the excipient in a screw-capped glass vial followed by heating to 60°C in a water-bath, brief agitation with a vortex mixer, holding for 48 hours at 25°C to 30°C, and centrifugation at 2000 to 3000 g to separate the undissolved drug. The supernatant containing the solubilized drug should be a clear, monophasic liquid at ambient room temperature, and should be of sufficiently low viscosity to allow for facile dispersion upon dilution in aqueous media. Drug solubility determinations are made with high-pressure liquid chromatography (HPLC) following dilution of aliquots of the supernatant with a suitable organic solvent.

In silico prediction of drug solubility in a lipid vehicle remains a challenging task. However, the work of Dumanli et al. (22) has identified several factors that could be useful in predicting drug solubility in a particular excipient. These factors include the solubility parameter (δ), HLB value, partition coefficient, MW, dielectric constant (ε), excipient fatty acid chain length, saponification value, surface tension, and viscosity. These parameters will now be discussed in the following sections.

Solubility parameters (δ): The solubility parameter of a substance is defined as the square root of its cohesive energy density, expressed as the energy of vaporization. When the solubility parameters of two materials are similar, one would expect them to be miscible, and thus provide some guidance in selecting an appropriate lipid vehicle for maximum solubilization of a drug. There are a number of direct and indirect methods available that are used for determining the solubility parameter of a substance. These include vapor pressure or boiling point determinations, miscibility in liquids with known cohesive energy, solution calorimetry, surface energetic measurements, and calculations using the group contribution method (23,24).

The solubility parameter (δ) of a drug or excipient can be determined by the following relationship described by Fedors (23):

$$\delta = [\Delta\Sigma e/\Delta\Sigma v]^{1/2} \tag{1}$$

where Δe is the additive atomic group contributions for the energy of vaporization and Δv is the additive atomic group contributions for the molar volume.

The magnitude of the solubility parameter that reflects the relative degree of polar and other intermolecular interactions occurring with a particular substance, rises in direct proportion to the relative substance hydrophilicity. In general, substances within two to three solubility parameter units of one another can be considered molecularly similar, and therefore are soluble or miscible (e.g., "like dissolves in like").

An alternative measurement, the Hildebrand solubility parameter (HSP), is also useful for estimating the solubility of hydrophobic drugs in lipid excipients. The HSP is derived from several fundamental molecular properties, including boiling point (expressed in °K), MW, and specific gravity (SG).

$$HSP(d) = \frac{[(23.7 \cdot BP + 0.02 \cdot BP^2 - 2950) - 1.98 \cdot T]^{1/2}}{(MW/SG)} \tag{2}$$

As the difference between the HSP values for two substances increases, their miscibility decreases.

Hydrophilic–Lipophilic Balance

The drug release rate from a SEDDS or SMEDDS has been shown to be dependent on the HLB of the surfactant (11). The HLB value is empirically determined from the following relationship:

$$HLB = 20 (1 - S/A)$$

where S is the saponification number of the ester and A is the acid number of the fatty acid (16,25,26). The HLB value of a surfactant quantifies its relative polar character, with greater HLB values reflecting greater relative polarity. Shah et al. investigated the impact of fatty acid chain length and PEG MW of polyglycolyzed glyceride (PGG) surfactants on self-emulsification of a triglyceride and the rate of drug release from SEDDS formulations prepared from these excipients and found that adequate drug release was dependent on the degree of polarity conferred on the dispersed oil droplets by the surfactant (11). The effect of HLB on the in vitro release rate of the lipophilic drug, Ro 15-0778 from a SEDDS formulation at 60% surfactant content is shown in Figure 2. Drug release was optimal from a SEDDS formulation prepared with the surfactant, Labrafac CM10 BM 287 (HLB approximately 10); drug release declined as the surfactant HLB either increased or decreased from this optimal value. For the surfactant, Labrasol® (HLB 14), immiscibility of the low HLB oil vehicle with

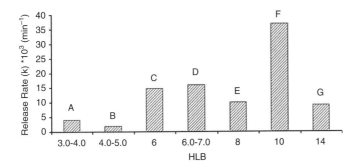

Figure 2 Effect of hydrophilic–lipophilic balance on the release rate of Ro 15-0778 from peanut oil based solution containing 60% of emulsifier (Paddles, 50rpm, 900mL of 5% Cremophor EL aqueous solution). *Key*: A, Labrafil M2125; B, Labrafac Hydro; C, Labrafac CM6 BM290; D, Labrafil WL2609; E, Labrafac CM8Bm 284; F, Labrafac CM 10 BM 287; G, Labrasol. *Abbreviation*: HLB, hydrophilic–lipophilic balance.

the surfactant resulted in the formation of a nonisotropic (two-phase) solution, which presumably retarded drug release due to poor dispersability in the test media. For surfactants with HLB values of less than 10, the surfactant fatty acid chain length and degree of saturation appeared to be responsible for influencing drug release from the SEDDS. The SEDDS formulation prepared with Labrafac CM 10 (C_8-C_{10} fatty acid chain length) was found to result in more rapid drug release than either Labrafil M 10 or Labrafil NA 10 surfactants, both of which are composed of long chain fatty acids (Fig. 3). In comparing the drug release rate from SEDDS prepared from the latter two surfactants, it was observed that drug release was slightly faster with Labrafil M 10 than with Labrafil NA 10, which is thought to be due to the greater degree of nonsaturated fatty acid present in Labrafil M 10 ($C_{18:2}$) as compared to Labrafil NA 10 ($C_{18:1}$). In another study, Bachynsky et al. (27) showed that the HLB of the emulsifier, as well as the fatty acid chain length of the monoglycerides, can have a significant effect on the dispersability of a SEDDS formulation. The results demonstrated that surfactants with a HLB in the range of 10 to 15 and medium-chain monoglycerides were the most effective, there are specific concentrations of emulsifier and oil, which maximize the dispersion efficiency.

Partition Coefficient

The lipophilicity of a molecule can be quantified by its Log P value, which describes (as the common logarithm) its degree of partitioning between an aqueous and a lipophilic phase (usually water and n-1-octanol, respectively) (28). In many instances, the partition coefficient of a drug and its melting point have been shown to be key factors in determining solubility in lipids. While drugs with Log P > 4 tend to possess greater solubility in lipid vehicles than those of lower lipophilicty, there are several exceptions to this rule (29).

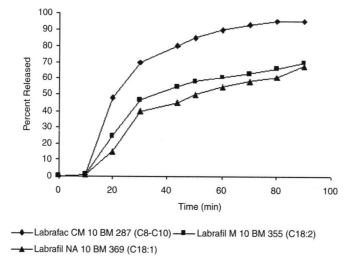

Figure 3 Effect of chain length and saturation of fatty acid present in the glyceride on drug release of Ro 15-0778 from peanut oil based solution containing 60% of emulsifier with hydrophilic–lipophilic balance of 10 (Paddles, 50 rpm, 900 mL of 5% Cremophor EL aqueous solution).

The effect of the surfactant (Labrafac CM10) concentration on the drug oil–water partition coefficient, lipid droplet size, and drug release rate from a SEDDS formulation was investigated by Shah et al. (Fig. 4) (11). Increased surfactant concentrations were correlated with both a smaller lipid droplet size and a reduced oil–water partition coefficient for the drug, which in turn, were associated with more rapid drug release, as determined in 900 mL of 5% aqueous solution of Alkamuls EL-719, in a USP XXII, Dissolution Apparatus 2.

Dielectric Constant (ε)

The dielectric constant that increases in proportion to the relative polarity of a molecule, is determined by oscillometry and is defined as the ratio of the capacity of a condenser (made with the test substance as the dielectric material) to the capacity of the same condenser with air as the dielectric, as determined at a frequency of 1 MHz (30). Given the general assumption that "like dissolves in like," substances with similar dielectric constants are typically miscible with one another.

Formulation Considerations

In Vivo Performance of Lipids

An understanding of the GI processing of lipid excipients (covered elsewhere in this book) is critical in that this phenomenon can exert a considerable influence on drug absorption from lipid-based formulations. This processing involves lipid digestion, in which lipids are degraded into component fatty acids and monoglycerides

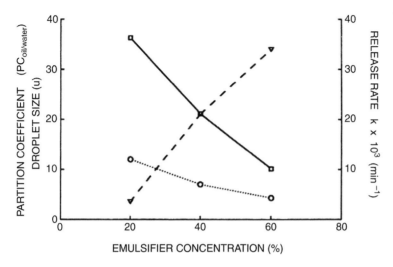

Figure 4 Effect of concentrations of emulsifier, Labrafac CM 10 BM 287, on partition coefficient (□) droplet size (o), and the release rate (▽) of Ro 15-0778 from peanut oil based solution.

followed by emulsification by endogenous bile acids, leading to the creation of complex micellar species, which are intimately related to drug absorption. In general, lipids that are nondigestible, should be avoided due to the poor drug absorption typically associated with these excipients. In addition, the fatty acid chain length of glyceride excipients controls the rate of lipolysis and consequently, drug absorption. Glyceride excipients comprised of long chain fatty acids are lipolysed relatively slowly, whereas lipolysis of medium chain glycerides occurs more readily, which can be associated with more rapid and complete drug absorption (31). In addition, the surfactant component of a formulation can adversely affect the digestion process by sterically hindering the attachment of lipase enzymes at the oil–water interface, resulting in sub-optimal drug release (9,31). Given these limitation, lipid excipients that don't rely on preabsorptive lipolysis as a prerequisite to drug release (e.g., medium chain monoglycerides, fatty acids, and monoesters of fatty acids) are often preferred for lipid-based oral formulations.

Drug Loading

Drug loading can influence both the physical characteristics and long-term physical stability of a lipid-based formulation. Thus, it is important to determine the saturation solubility of the drug in the chosen formulation. A plot of formulation viscosity as a function of drug concentration (Fig. 5) can be used to establish the approximate saturation solubility, which occurs in the region above the inflection point of the plotted data (32). Excessive drug loading in a lipid solution can result in gelling or drug crystallization under shear conditions or during storage, as well as drastic changes in the formulation dispersibility, which is associated with an

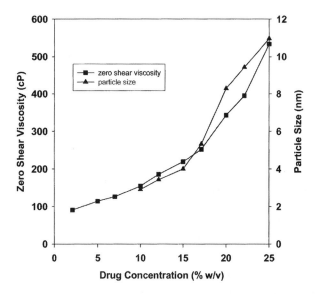

Figure 5   Effect of drug loading on zero shear viscosity and particle size of lipid solutions.

increase in the mean emulsion droplet diameter (MEDD) due to droplet coalescence and or aggregation.

Optimal Drug: Surfactant Ratio (Phase Diagram Construction)

The stability, maximum drug loading, and self-emulsifying behavior of a binary nonionic surfactant–oil mixture is dependent on both temperature and surfactant. Pseudo-ternary phase diagrams are useful for identifying the optimum concentrations, or concentration ranges, of oil, surfactant and cosurfactant necessary to form an efficient self-emulsifying formulation. In the absence of water, mixtures of oils, surfactants, and cosurfactants can exist as either clear isotropic solutions or as oily dispersions depending on the characteristics of the individual excipients and the formulation oil-to-surfactant ratio. The self-emulsifying properties of any SEDDS formulation will be influenced by the physicochemical properties of the incorporated drug (e.g., polarity and surface activity) and its concentration. Hence, in the search for a formulation with optimal self-emulsifying properties (as determined by the size of the dispersed lipid droplets), the SEDDS phase diagram should be constructed by varying not only the concentrations of the excipients but also that of the drug. In addition to oil droplet size, an acceptable SEDDS will exhibit the following characteristics:

- Facile formation of a fine emulsion with a lipid droplet size of less than 5 μm upon dilution with aqueous media and following mild agitation (11,33).
- Dispersed oil droplets possess sufficient polarity to promote rapid transfer of drug into the aqueous phase.

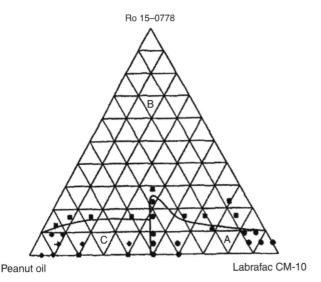

Ro 15–0778

Peanut oil   Labrafac CM-10

Figure 6 Phase diagram for peanut oil/emulsifier, Labrafac CM-10 BM 287/Ro 15-0778 system. (●) region A: good and efficient self-emulsifying system; (■) region B: poor self-emulsifying system; (♦) region C: intermediate self-emulsifying system.

For illustrative purposes, a pseudo-ternary phase diagram for a SEDDS formulation prepared from peanut oil, Labrafac CM-10 (surfactant) and a model drug is presented in Figure 6. Regions describing combinations of drug, surfactant, and oil that produce good, intermediate and poor SEDDS formulations, as defined by the above characteristics, are clearly delineated.

Phase diagrams can be constructed with relatively small quantities of drug and excipients. The test formulations, containing varying concentrations of the drug and excipients are sequentially diluted with water and allowed to equilibrate. The resulting dispersions are next examined with optical microscopy under crossed polar filters to determine lipid droplet size, check for drug precipitation, verify the emulsion isotropic behavior and detect liquid crystalline behavior, which will be indicated by birefringence. The information so gathered is used to construct the phase diagram, which allows determination of the optimal ratios of drug, lipid, surfactant, and cosurfactant to use when developing a SEDDS or SMEDDS formulation.

Hygroscopicity of the Lipid

Hygroscopicity of a lipid excipient may dehydrate hard or soft gelatin capsules resulting in brittleness and fracture of the capsule shell. Moisture sorption isotherms of various excipients that are typically used in lipid based formulations are presented in Figure 7. From the opposite perspective, it is critical to ensure that the formulation can withstand influx of water, when soft gelatin encapsulation is employed, a process, which involves exposure to relatively large amounts of

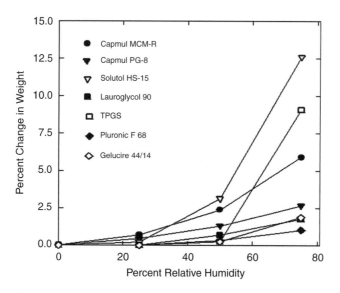

Figure 7   Moisture isotherms of typically used lipid excipients. *Abbreviations*: HS, hydroxystearate; MCM, medium chain monoglyceride; PG, propylene glycol; TPGS, tocopherol polyethylene glycol succinate.

moisture as compared to hard gelatin encapsulation. These dynamic changes must be thoroughly investigated in the early stages of development.

Formulation Evaluation

Mean Emulsion Droplet Diameter

Upon dilution in aqueous media, the MEDD that is inversely proportional to the amount of surfactant in the formulation, is a critical parameter controlling drug release from a SEDDS formulation. In addition, the specific choice of surfactant can influence the lipid droplet size, as well. Smaller oil droplets, with their associated greater surface area, favor more rapid drug release, either by faciliation of partitioning into the aqueous phase or by promoting digestion by lipase enzymes, a process, which is critical to drug absorption from a lipid vehicle (Fig. 4); a reduced drug oil:water partition coefficient has also been shown to favor drug release, as well (11,33–35). The MEDD of a SEDDS is typically assessed by diluting 125 μL of the formulation to 250 mL in a volumetric flask followed by gentle mixing by repeated inversion. The droplet size distribution upon aqueous dilution, which is influenced by the specific composition of the SEDDS (17), is then determined initially and after equilibration for 24 hours by one of the following two techniques, depending on the anticipated lipid droplet size:

- Low-angle laser light diffraction (MEDD of >1 μ)
- Quasi-elastic light scattering (MEDD of <1 μ)

The influence of the MEDD on formulation performance was clearly demonstrated for the Neoral and Sandimmune formulations of cyclosporine. Neoral that forms a microemulsion with a MEDD of approximately 30 nm, has improved and less variable bioavailability compared to the earlier Sandimmune formulation, which formed a coarse emulsion with a MEDD of 2 to 5 μm.

The lipid droplet size distributions of two different SEDDS formulations containing varying amounts of the self-emulsifying lipid excipient, Labrafil M2125 CS, and a poorly water-soluble benzodiazepine drug were compared (17). A control SEDDS that contained no drug, was prepared as a reference. The formulations were prepared by first combining all of the excipients (except the water) and dissolving the drug in the resulting mixture followed by addition of the water. The percentage proportions of the different components in the three formulations are shown next:

Components	Formulation 1	Formulation 2	Formulation 3
Labrafil M2125 CS	62	60	56
PG	3	3	3
Tween 80	30	30	30
Distilled water	5	5	5
Model drug	0	2	6

As shown in Figure 8, the droplet size distributions for Formulations 1 and 2 were found to be bimodal, while the distribution for Formulation 3 was unimodal, which is preferred as it ensures more reproducible drug bioavailability.

Drug Release

As discussed previously, drug release and absorption from a SEDDS formulation is dependent on the physicochemical characteristics of both the drug and excipients, as well as their interaction with the GI milieu, all of which determine the MEDD (36). The amount of drug that diffuses from an oil droplet to a surrounding aqueous phase is a function of the oil droplet radius and the oil:aqueous phase partition coefficient ratio of the drug and can be described from the following relationship:

$$Q(t) = f(1/r \times K)$$

where $Q(t)$ is the amount of drug transferred to the aqueous phase at time t, r is the oil droplet radius, and K is the oil:aqueous phase partition coefficient of the drug. Thus, increased concentrations of surfactant, which typically result in smaller lipid droplet size, tend to promote more rapid release of drug from a SEDDS formulation (Fig. 4).

In addition, drug release is directly correlated with aqueous solubility and inversely correlated with affinity for the lipid phase. Assuming that membrane permeability is not an absorption rate-determining step, the fraction of the drug dose absorbed (Fa) is proportional to aqueous solubility (S) and the volume of the GI fluids (Vg), and is inversely proportional to the dose (D) (37).

$$Fa \propto S \cdot Vg/D$$

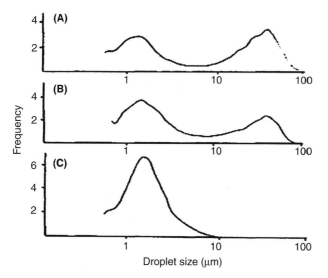

Figure 8 Droplet size of emulsions prepared from (**A**) Formulation 1, (**B**) Formulation 2, and (**C**) Formulation 3.

When evaluating the effect of an oily vehicle on drug release, the following equation should also be considered.

$$Mw = Mo/(K\phi)$$

where Mw is the quantity of drug in the aqueous solution, Mo is the quantity of drug in the lipid phase, K is the partition coefficient (o/w), ϕ is the volume ratio of lipid to aqueous phase.

As can be seen from this relationship, as the volume ratio, ϕ, decreases the rate and quantity of drug released from lipid to aqueous phase increases.

As with conventional formulations, identification of a biorelevant in vitro test method for evaluating drug release from SEDDS formulations is highly desirable for guiding formulation development and for ensuring batch-to-batch consistency of the manufactured product. However, compared to conventional formulations, development of in vitro tests for lipid-based formulations is considerably more complex due to the poor solubility of lipid excipients in conventional aqueous dissolution test media and the need to faithfully reproduce the complex process of GI lipid digestion. One such method, the dynamic in vitro lipolysis model described by Zangenberg et al. (38) (covered in Chapter 11 in this book) has sought to reproduce GI lipolysis in a dissolution test format that allows evaluation of drug release from a lipid-based formulation in vitro. Although the model has shown promise, it is not routinely applied due to its complexity. Conventional dissolution testing methods for lipid-based formulations, which employ aqueous media have relied on the use of surfactants or hydro-alcoholic media to promote drug release from the lipid matrix. Exposure of gelatin capsule shells to such media, however, may result in

Table 6 Summary of In Vitro and In Vivo Results for Nifidepine Lipid Solution

Formulation	Solubility (mg/g)	% Dissolution at 60 min.	Partition coefficient (o/w)	Mean particle size (nm)	AUC_{0-24} mean ± SD (ng.h/mL)[a]	C_{max} mean ± SD (ng/mL)[a]
Miglyol 812	3.36 ± 0.03	50.19 ± 1.44	5.6 ± 0.45	Coarse	173 ± 115[b]	56 ± 31[c]
Miglyol 810/ Cremophor EL	4.86 ± 0.04	97.23 ± 2.52	1.1 ± 0.02	10.0 ± 1.0	231 ± 106[b]	105 ± 36[c]

[a]Fasted beagle dogs (N = 6) using a single dose (2.5 mg nifidepine) crossover design.
[b]Not significant different (p value is 0.27, t-test for paired value for means).
[c]Significant different (p value is 0.036, t-test for paired value for means).
Abbreviations: AUC, area under the curve; EL, ethoxylated.

gelatin cross-linking, which slows dissolution of the capsule shell and retards drug release. For example, the popular anionic surfactant, sodium lauryl sulfate (SLS) has been shown to promote gelatin cross-linking, either through direct hydrophobic interactions with gelatin, or at pH < 5 through interaction with ionized basic amino acids contained in gelatin (39,40). In addition, SLS promotes drug release in aqueous systems primarily through micellar solubilization, a process much different from emulsification, which is thought to be responsible for in vivo drug release and absorption from lipid-based dosage forms, and in which the type of lipid and its digestibility, formed oil droplet size and subsequently mixing with bile salts all play significant roles in drug absorption. Another popular cationic surfactant, cetyl trimethyl ammonium bromide (CTAB), may alter drug release from lipid-based dosage forms by interacting with anionic lipid excipients (e.g., fatty acids). Due to the potential interactions of ionic surfactants with both lipid excipients and gelatin capsule shells, it is recommended that in vitro release testing of hydrophobic drugs in lipid-based formulations rely on the use of nonionic surfactants, such as Tween 20, Tween 80, and Cremophor EL-15.

In a study in which nifedipine was administered to dogs as a coarse emulsion (Miglyol 812) or as a nanoemulsion (Miglyol 810/Cremophor EL) formulation, the C_{max} was significantly (P = 0.036) higher for the nanoemulsion (Table 6). Although not statistically significant, the extent of nifedipine absorption (AUC 0–24 h) was also higher for the nanoemulsion formulation. In addition, the improved absorption seen with the nanoemulsion was correlated with more rapid and complete in vitro release as well as a lower oil-water partition coefficient for the drug (Table 6) (22).

CONCLUSION

The design of self-emulsifying lipid formulations of poorly water-soluble drugs has been described and examples, where these formulations approaches were successfully applied to challenging drug molecules associated with poor bioavailability. The bioavailability of a poorly soluble drug administered in a lipid solution, SEDDS or SMEDDS formulation is dependent upon several factors including:

- digestability of the lipid and the type of lipid vehicle used in which the drug is solubilized,
- droplet size of the formed emulsion that is produced following exposure to GI fluids,
- release rate of the drug from the emulsified oil droplets, which is determined by the relative droplet polarity and surface area.

REFERENCES

1. Lipinski C, Lombardo F, Dominy B, et al. Experimental and computational approaches to estimate solubility and permeability in drug discovery and development settings. Adv Drug Deliv Rev 1997; 23(1–3):3–25.
2. Muranishi S. Modification of intestinal absorption of drugs by lipoidal adjuvants. Pharm Res 1985; 1:108–117.
3. Charman W. Lipids, lipophilic drugs and oral drug delivery-some emerging concepts. J Pharm Sci 2000; 89(8):967–978.
4. Phuapradit W, Shah NH, Lou Y, et al. Critical processing factors affecting rheological behavior of a wax based formulation. Eur J Pharm Biopharm 2002; 53(2):175–179.
5. Shah NH, Phuapradit W, Ahmed H. Liquid filling in hard gelatin capsules: formulation and processing considerations. American Pharmaceutical Review 2003; 6(1):14–21.
6. Craig D. Lipid matrices an academic overview. Bulletin Technique Gattefosse 2004; 97:9–19.
7. Vadas E. Sustained release formulations with lipid derived excipients: big pharma perspectives- why and when. Bulletin Technique Gattefosse 2004; 97:21–27.
8. Yamahira Y, Noguchi T, Takenaka H, et al. Biopharmaceutical studies of lipid-containing oral dosage forms: relationship between drug absorption rate and digestibility of vehicles. Int J Pharm 1979; 3(1):23–31.
9. MacGregor K, Embleton J, Lacy J, et al. Influence of lipolysis on drug absorption from the gastro-intestinal tract. Adv Drug Deliv Rev 1997; 25(1):33–46.
10. Charman WN, Porter CJH, Mithani S, et al. Physicochemical and physiological mechanisms for the effects of food on drug absorption: the role of lipids and pH. J Pharma Sci 1997; 86(3):269–282.
11. Shah NH, Carvajal MT, Patel CI, et al. Self-emulsifying drug delivery systems (SEDDS) with polyglycolyzed glycerides for improving in vitro dissolution and oral absorption of lipophilic drugs. Int J Pharm 1994; 106(1):15–23.
12. Shah NH. Self emulsifying delivery system of improving oral absorption of poorly soluble drugs. Bulletin Technique Gattefosse 1993; 86:45–54.
13. Pouton CW. Lipid formulations for oral administration of drugs: non-emulsifying, self-emulsifying and "self-microemulsifying" drug delivery systems. Eur J Pharm Sci 2000; 11(suppl 2):S93–S98.
14. Embleton JK, Pouton CW. Structure and function of gastrointestinal lipases. Adv Drug Deliv Rev 1997; 25(1):15–32.
15. Bloedow D, Hayton W. Effect of lipids on bioavailability of sulfisoxazole acetyl, dicumarol, and griseofulvin in rats. J Pharm Sci 1976; 65:328–334.

16. Groves MJ, De Galindez DA. The self-emulsifying action of mixed surfactants in oil. Acta Pharm Suec 1976; 13:361–372.
17. Craig D. The use of self emulsifying systems as a means of improving drug delivery. Bulletin Technique Gattefosse 1993; 86:21–31.
18. Eccleston GM. Microemulsions. In: Swarbrick J, Boylan JC, eds. Encyclopedia of pharmaceutical technology. New York: Marcel Dekker, 1992; 9:375–421.
19. Swenson ES, Curatolo WJ. Intestinal permeability enhancement for proteins, peptides and other polar drugs: mechanisms and potential toxicity. Adv Drug Del Rev 1992; 8(1):39–92.
20. Holt DW, Mueller EA, Kovarik JM, et al. The pharmacokinetics of sandimmune neoral: a new oral formulation of cyclosporine. Transplant Proc 1994; 26: 2935–2939.
21. Kovarik JM, Mueller EA, van Bree JB, et al. Reduced inter- and intraindividual variability in cyclosporine pharmacokinetics from a microemulsion formulation. J Pharm Sci 1994; 83:444–446.
22. Dumanli I, Lipid Delivery System. Ph.D. Dissertation, University of Rhode Island, 2002.
23. Fedors RF. A method for estimating both the solubility parameters and molar volumes of liquids. Polymer Engineering and Science 1974; 14(2):147–154.
24. Hancock BC, York P, Rowe RC. The use of solubility parameters in pharmaceutical dosage form design. Int J Pharm 1997; 148(1):1–21.
25. Attwood D. Microemulsions. In: Kreuter J, ed. Colloidal drug delivery systems. New York: Marcel Dekker, 1994:31–71.
26. Osborne DW, Middleton CA, Rogers RL. Alcohol-free microemulsions. J Dispersion Sci Technol 1988; 9:415–423.
27. Bachynsky MO, Shah NH, Patel C, et al. Factors affecting the efficiency of a self-emulsifying oral delivery system. Drug Dev Ind Pharm 1997; 23(8):809–816.
28. Szuts EZ, Harosi FI. Solubility of retinoids in water. Arch Biochem Biophys 1991; 287:297–304.
29. Charman WN, Stella VJ. Estimating the maximal potential for intestinal lymphatic transport of lipophilic drug molecules. Int J Pharm 1986; 34(1):175–178.
30. Klein AE. physical properties of drug molecules. In: Martin A, Bustamante P, Chun AHC, eds. Physical pharmacy. 4th ed. Philadelphia: Lea & Febiger, 1993:77–100.
31. Hutchison K. Digestible emulsions and microemulsions for optimum oral delivery of hydrophobic drug. Bulletin Technique Gattefosse 1994; 87:67–74.
32. Dumanli I. Characterization of gelling phenomenon of a lipid-based formulation. master thesis, University of Rhode Island, 1998.
33. Charman SA, Charman WN, Rogge MC, et al. Self-emulsifying drug delivery systems: formulation, and biopharmaceutical evaluation of an investigational lipophilic compound. Pharm Res 1992; 9(1):87–93.
34. Pouton CW. Self-emulsifying drug delivery systems: assessment of the efficiency of emulsification. Int J Pharm 1985; 27(2–3):335–348.
35. Tarr BD, Yalkowsky SH. Enhanced intestinal absorption of cyclosporine in rats through the reduction of emulsion droplet size. Pharm Res 1989; 6(1):40–43.
36. Armstrong NA, James KC. Drug release from lipid-based dosage forms. II. Int J Pharm 1980; 6(3–4):195–204.
37. Dressman JB, Amidon GL, Fleisher D. Absorption potential: estimating the fraction absorbed for orally administered compounds. J Pharm Sci 1985; 74:588–589.

38. Zangenberg NH, Mullertz A, Kristensen HG, et al. A dynamic in vitro lipolysis
     model, I. Controlling the rate of lipolysis by continuous addition of calcium. Eur J
     Pharm Sci 2001; 14(2):115–122.
39. Pillay V, Fassihi R. A new method for dissolution studies of lipid-filled capsules
     employing nifedipine as a model drug. Pharm Res 1999; 16(2):333–337.
40. Zhao F, Malayev V, Rao V, et al. Effect of sodium lauryl sulfate in dissolution
     medium on dissolution of hard gelatin capsule shells. Pharm Res 2004; 21(1):
     144–148.

7

Lipid-Based Self-Emulsifying Solid Dispersions

Madhav Vasanthavada and Abu T. M. Serajuddin

Novartis Pharmaceuticals Corporation, East Hanover, New Jersey, U.S.A.

INTRODUCTION

The widespread application of combinatorial chemistry and high-throughput screening in drug discovery that began in the early 1990s favors the selection of poorly water-soluble new chemical entities (NCEs), often making oral drug product development very challenging (1). A poorly water-soluble drug is defined as one for which the dissolution time of a single dose in the gastrointestinal (GI) fluids exceeds the normal transit time through the absorptive regions of the gastrointestinal tract (GIT) (2). The absorption of these compounds is dose-dependent and controlled by the dissolution rate in the GIT (3). Particle size reduction and salt formation, which are common strategies for improving dissolution rate, are not always successful at achieving the desired extent of absorption enhancement. There are practical limitations to the degree of particle size reduction achievable by conventional means, which limits the usefulness of this technique. Salt formation that requires an ionizable functional group on the pharmacophore, may not be feasible for very weakly acidic or basic compounds. Even when a salt is formed, it may prove ineffective to achieve the desired absorption enhancement due to pH-mediated precipitation of the drug in the GIT following initial dissolution. Attempts have been made to improve the absorption of poorly water-soluble compounds by solubilizing them in formulations. Such formulations that are typically liquid in nature, rely on micellar or solvent/cosolvent solubilization techniques, oil-in-water emulsions, pH-adjusted solutions, or the use of complexing agents. However, the usefulness of these formulations can be limited by their inability to solubilize the entire drug dose in the volume of a single gelatin capsule suitable for oral administration. Solid dispersion formulations that may not require full solubilization of the drug in the excipient matrix can provide highly effective oral formulations of poorly water-soluble drugs, when the above-mentioned options fail.

Solid Dispersion

A solid dispersion has traditionally been defined as "the dispersion of one or more active ingredients in an inert excipient or matrix" (4), where the active ingredients could exist in finely crystalline, solubilized or amorphous states. Pharmaceutical solid dispersions have been studied for close to half a century as a means for increasing the dissolution rate and oral bioavailability of poorly water-soluble drugs (5,6).

A schematic diagram illustrating the advantages of a solid dispersion as compared to a conventional capsule or tablet formulation is shown in Figure 1 (7). The drug dissolution rate from conventional tablet and capsule formulations is controlled by the size of the primary drug particles, which are limited to a minimum size of around 2 to 5 μm. In most cases, however, powders with particle sizes larger than the minimum 2 to 5 μm ranges are preferred in capsules and tablets for ease of handling, formulation, and manufacturing. In comparison, a portion of the drug contained in a solid dispersion dissolves immediately upon contact with the GI fluid, resulting in a saturated or supersaturated solution for rapid absorption, and the excess drug precipitates in the GI fluid, forming amorphous or crystalline particles in the sub-micron size range with high surface area and a correspondingly high dissolution and absorption rate. These characteristics often result in substantially improved drug absorption from a solid dispersion as compared to a conventional tablet or capsule formulation. Despite

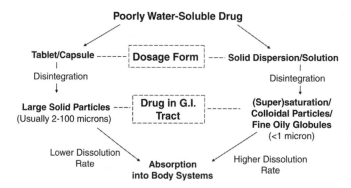

Figure 1 Advantages of a solid dispersion formulation, as compared to conventional capsule or tablet formulations, for enhancing dissolution rate and consequent bioavailability of poorly water-soluble drugs. *Source*: From Ref. 7.

these potential advantages, the commercial application of solid dispersion formulations has been limited (7).

Serajuddin (7) reviewed various issues that formerly impeded the commercial development of solid dispersions, which include: (*i*) inability to scale bench-top formulations to manufacturing-sized batches, (*ii*) difficulty to control physicochemical properties, (*iii*) difficulty in delivering solid dispersion formulations as tablet or capsule dosage forms, and (*iv*) physical and chemical instability of the drug and/or the formulation itself. However, the author further discussed how the relatively recent introduction of surface-active and self-emulsifying excipients, that are solid at room temperature, has greatly renewed the interest in commercial development of solid dispersions. Formulations incorporating these new excipients may not only increase dissolution rates of poorly water-soluble drugs, but they may also be filled directly into hard gelatin capsules in the molten state, thus obviating the need for prior milling, blending, and so on. More recently, hot-melt extrusion technology has shown much promise in resolving some of the manufacturing issues generally associated with solid dispersions (8).

Lipid-Based Solid Dispersion

Many investigators have described the utility of lipid-based formulations for enhancing the bioavailability of poorly water-soluble drugs (9–12). These formulations range from simple solutions of drugs in dietary triglycerides (oil) to the use of complex mixtures of triglycerides, partial glycerides, surfactants, cosurfactants, and cosolvents to solubilize drugs. Depending on the formulation composition, they are described as nonemulsifying drug delivery systems, self-emulsifying drug delivery systems (SEDDS) or self-microemulsifying drug delivery systems (SMEDDS). Pouton attempted to provide a scientific basis of classifying various self-emulsifying lipid-based formulations based on the lipid droplet sizes formed upon mixing with aqueous media, which may range from $>100\,\mu$m (Type I) to 50 to 100 nm (Type IIIB) (11). Despite the potential for the use of lipid-based systems to formulate many poorly water-soluble drugs, Gursoy and Benita (12) reported that there were only four lipid-based commercially marketed products available in 2004, of which two were for cyclosporine A and the other two for ritonavir and sequinavir; all of these products were encapsulated liquids. The primary limitation of lipid-based dosage forms is the requirement that the drug possess sufficient solubility in the formulation to allow delivery of a single dose in a standard oral capsule dosage form. In instances where insufficient solubility in the formulation precludes the development of a fully-solubilized lipid-based formulation, preparation of a solid dispersion of the drug in a semi-solid, lipid-based formulation could provide a viable path forward.

Most surface active and self-emulsifying excipients used in solid dispersions may be categorized as lipids or lipid-like because they are either glycerides or chemically related to the glycerides. In the present article, lipid-based solid dispersions will be discussed in broad terms by including various surface active carriers in the lipid category. Mixtures of surface active carriers with nonsurface active vehicles [e.g., polyethylene glycols (PEGs), different polymers, etc.] will also be discussed. Particular consideration will be given to the physicochemical advantages and limitations of these formulations as viable drug delivery systems as well as the different methodologies applicable to commercial product development.

The performance of nonself-emulsifying solid dispersions (e.g., those prepared using PEGs) is often limited by the relatively rapid dissolution rate of the water-soluble excipient matrix as compared to that of the dispersed drug substance. This results in the formation of a highly concentrated solution of drug, which precipitates on the surface of the dissolving excipient plug, forming a poorly soluble coating that prevents further dissolution of dispersed drug contained within the excipient matrix. For this reason, solid dispersions must be pulverized and sifted to increase their surface area in order to facilitate drug release. This is a difficult task as solid dispersions prepared with such common excipients as PEGs are usually soft and tacky and may not be readily milled. Moreover, the powders thus produced often have poor flow and mixing properties and are difficult to fill into capsules or compress into tablets.

In comparison, solid dispersion formulations prepared from surface-active lipid or lipid-like excipients prevent the formation of a poorly water-soluble drug surface layer on the excipient plug during dissolution. While a portion of the released drug may still precipitate in the dissolution medium once its dissolved concentration exceeds the saturation solubility, it would typically be present in a finely divided state due to the surface active properties of the excipient. The associated high surface area of the finely divided drug substance would facilitate its rapid dissolution in the GI fluid. This is shown schematically in Figure 2 for solid dispersions filled into hard gelatin capsules.

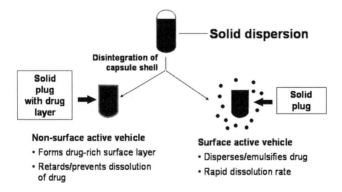

Figure 2   Incorporation of surface active or lipid carriers promotes dissolution of poorly water-soluble drugs administered in solid dispersions by preventing precipitation of a water insoluble, drug-rich layer on the surface of the dissolving formulation plug.

Another major advantage of solid dispersion formulations prepared from lipid or surface active excipients is realized in the relative ease with which they are manufactured. Solid dispersions prepared from these excipients may be directly filled into hard gelatin capsules in the molten state, which subsequently solidify upon cooling to ambient room temperature, thus eliminating the need for grinding, sifting, and mixing. The melting temperature of the molten excipient, however, must not exceed ~70°C, which is the maximum acceptable fill temperature for hard gelatin capsules (13).

EVALUATION OF NEED FOR SOLID DISPERSION

As discussed previously, solid dispersions typically enhance the dissolution rate, and hence the bioavailability of poorly water-soluble drugs and can provide a viable path forward in the development of dosage forms for challenging NCEs. However, it must be borne in mind that compared to conventional tablet and capsule dosage forms, solid dispersion formulations are relatively complex drug delivery systems, requiring a substantially greater commitment of time, effort, and resources for development. Initial formulation development strategies for NCEs should seek to conserve precious time and resources; therefore, less complex approaches, such as particle size reduction or salt formation should first be considered prior to embarking on the development of a solid dispersion formulation. These initial formulation development strategies should be guided by careful in vitro assessment of the NCE biopharmaceutical properties and the relevance of these findings to the projected in vivo formulation performance (3).

Johnson and Swindell (14) described a simple method for assessing the likelihood that a NCE might be subject to poor absorption following oral administration. This determination is made by estimating the maximum absorbable dose (MAD) of an NCE using the following relationship:

$$MAD = S \times K_a \times SIWV \times SITT$$

where S is aqueous solubility (mg/mL) at pH 6.5, K_a is intestinal absorption rate constant (min^{-1}) obtained from a rat intestinal perfusion study (which is considered to provide data similar to that in humans) (15), SIWV is small intestinal water volume in mL (which is considered to be 250 mL), and SITT is the small intestinal residence time (which is generally assumed to be three hours). The MAD concept serves as an initial guide to whether potential absorption issues are present for a compound. If the value is higher than the anticipated human dose, it is usually assumed that there will be no bioavailability issues encountered with conventional formulations. On the other hand, if it is lower, one should be concerned about potential absorption issues and alternative formulation strategies, such as solid dispersion, may be explored to assure satisfactory oral bioavailability. It should, however, be noted that the foregoing MAD estimation does not consider the surface area of the drug, nor is consideration given to in vivo drug solubilization that could be a function of lipids, surfactants, and mixed micelles present in the GI fluids. Therefore, one should carefully consider these factors in any dosage form decisions based on MAD values.

Most poorly water-soluble drugs with good intestinal permeability (Biopharmaceutical Classification System or BCS Class II compounds) require a more rigorous analysis of potential drug absorption issues, which includes both dose and drug particle size, to determine whether an absorption-enhancing formulation will be required and if so, which approach is likely to provide the desired result with the minimum effort. When drug absorption is limited by dissolution in the GI fluids, the fraction of the dose absorbed will decrease with an increase in the dose size if the drug particle size or surface area is held constant (Fig. 3). On the other hand, if the dose size is held constant, the fraction of the dose absorbed will increase with a reduction in particle size or an increase in the particle surface area. If it is determined that complete absorption of the dose might be obtained by reducing the particle size to approximately 2 to 5 μm (within the range of standard manufacturing capability), a conventional tablet or capsule dosage form may still be feasible. However, if it is determined that particle size reduction to the sub-micron range is necessary, a solid dispersion may provide a viable alternative. In silico absorption modeling with software packages, such as GastroPlus® (SimulationsPlus, Lancaster, California, U.S.A.), have demonstrated utility in determining the impact of particle size reduction on drug absorption (16). For the hypothetical example presented in Figure 3, the drug particle size must be below 1 μm for a dose of 1 mg to be completely absorbed. For the 25-mg and 500-mg doses, particle size reduction is not likely to be effective in enabling complete absorption of the dose and alternative dosage form development strategies would most likely be required.

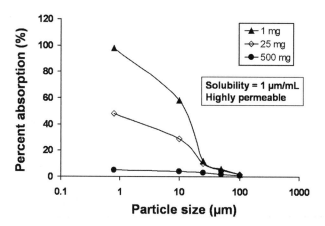

Figure 3   Simulation of the effect of dose and particle size on the extent of absorption of a poorly water-soluble drug with a water solubility of 1 μg/mL. A solubility-enhancing formulation should be considered to ensure complete absorption of the 25 mg and 500 mg doses if particle size reduction to the sub-micron range cannot be readily achieved.

STRUCTURE OF SOLID DISPERSION

Solid dispersions are complex mixtures of a drug and one or more carrier. The molecular structures of solid dispersions are critical as they determine the physicochemical stability, release characteristics and ultimately, the therapeutic efficacy of the formulated drug. While it is frequently impossible to determine the exact physical state of a drug in a solid dispersion formulation, it is generally agreed that the drug exists in one or more of the following forms:

- Reduced particle size, relative to the bulk drug substance used in preparation of the formulation.
- Metastable crystalline form.
- Partial or complete conversion of the drug into an amorphous form.
- Full or partial solubilization of the drug in the carrier matrix.

This section will focus on the preparation and characterization of solid dispersion formulations prepared by combining the drug with the molten carrier a technique that is frequently used for preparation of solid dispersions. The concepts discussed here may as well be applicable to solid dispersion formulations prepared by melt extrusion or solvent evaporation techniques. When a melt technique is used, the structure of a solid dispersion would depend on whether the drug is miscible or immiscible with the molten carrier. If the drug is poorly soluble in the molten carrier, one would not expect a significant change in the crystalline morphology of the drug upon congealing. On the other hand, if the drug is solubilized in the molten carrier, then upon cooling the drug could either remain fully solubilized in the congealed formulation, precipitate in a crystalline or semi-crystalline state, or remain entrapped within the carrier matrix in an amorphous state. Factors that would determine the final state of the drug in the formulation include intrinsic drug crystallization tendency, drug loading, drug-carrier interaction, crystallinity of the carrier, and cooling rate of the molten formulation.

Eutectic Solid Dispersions

A eutectic mixture is a two-phase system of a specific composition in which the drug and the carrier(s) exhibit complete miscibility in the molten state, but are immiscible in the solid state and form an intimate mixture of the finely divided crystalline drug and carrier. When solid A (drug) and solid B (carrier) are combined at the "eutectic composition" defined by point Y (Fig. 4), the melting point of the mixture is lower than the melting point of either drug or carrier alone (X and Z, respectively). While some researchers claim eutectics to be an intimate but inert physical mixture of components, others claim that the reduction in the melting point of eutectic mixtures is a direct evidence of a molecular interaction between the drug and the carrier (17–19). Eutectics find application in pharmaceutical dosage forms because of their ability to increase dissolution rate and absorption of poorly soluble drugs mostly via particle size reduction.

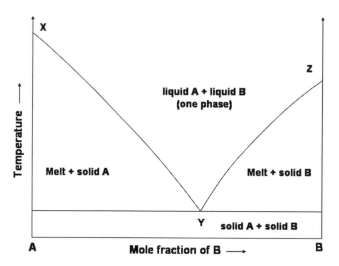

Figure 4 Phase diagram of a simple eutectic system. At temperatures below curve XY or YZ, either drug (A) or carrier (B) solidify first from the molten mixture, respectively. At eutectic composition Y, both drug and carrier solidify simultaneously as a mixture of finely divided crystalline components.

The eutectic composition for a drug and a carrier is usually identified by constructing phase diagrams using differential scanning calorimetry (DSC) scans of their physical mixtures with various drug-carrier ratios. The melting temperature for each mixture is recorded and plotted against the drug-carrier ratio to yield the eutectic composition. A significant limitation to the use of eutectics as pharmaceutical dosage forms is the amount of drug loading that can be achieved at the eutectic composition.

Amorphous Solid Dispersions

Amorphous solid dispersions result when the drug and carrier are miscible in the molten state, but upon cooling, the drug loses miscibility in the carrier and solidifies in its amorphous state. While the amorphous form of a drug typically possesses a higher rate of dissolution, and correspondingly higher bioavailability than its stable crystalline form (20), a major limitation of amorphous dosage forms has been an inconsistent and unpredictable tendency to spontaneously crystallize upon aging and under various storage conditions (e.g., elevated temperature and humidity), thereby leading to a drop in dissolution rate and bioavailability (21,22).

Solid Solutions

Solid solutions are homogeneous, single-phase systems in which the components are completely miscible with one another, on a molecular scale, in the solid state. In Figure 5, if a molten mixture of A (drug) and B (carrier) is cooled from point

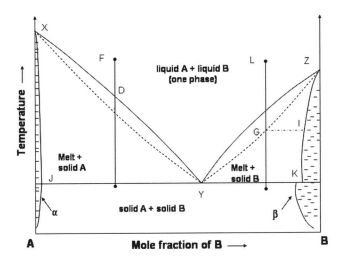

Figure 5 Phase diagram illustrating the formation of a solid solution when a molten mixture of drug (A) and carrier (B) is cooled; a certain fraction of carrier could remain dissolved in drug (region defined by α) and certain fraction of drug could remain dissolved in carrier (region defined by β). The dotted line represents solidus curve when the liquid completely converts into solid form.

F to below its liquidus curve (defined by point D on line XY), the drug will begin to precipitate in the molten carrier as either a crystalline or amorphous solid. During such precipitation, it is possible for a fraction of carrier to remain molecularly dispersed with the precipitating drug. Similarly, solid solution of drug in carrier can result if mixture at point L is cooled below its solidus curve (point G). The fraction of drug that remains dissolved at G is given by point I. When the two-phase mixture of solid solution (segmented zone) and liquid solution of drug-in-carrier is cooled further, the concentration of drug in solid solution increases. Upon further cooling below the line JK, the two solid phases begin to separate out as the α-phase, which is the saturated solid solution of carrier-in-drug and the β-phase, which is the saturated solid solution of drug-in-carrier.

Unlike metallic alloys, pharmaceutical melts typically do not form crystalline solid solutions. In the case of polymers such as PEG and polyethylene oxide (PEO), which are semi-crystalline, solid solution formation is rare but the possibility cannot be ruled out, since the semi-crystalline nature of such polymers can permit drug to remain entrapped as a solid solution in the polymer amorphous regions. Amorphous solid solutions have been described in the pharmaceutical literature using polymers such as polyvinylpyrrolidone (PVP), hydroxypropylmethyl cellulose (HPMC), hydroxypropyl cellulose (HPC), and alike (23). A solid solution is believed to exist in the amorphous mixture if there is a composition-dependent change in the glass transition temperature (T_g) of the drug-excipient mixture (24).

Although drug-carrier miscibility in the solid state can help to enhance the drug dissolution rate and possibly, the bioavailability, the physical stability of the solid dispersion under conditions of elevated temperature and humidity is of concern. Drug-carrier phase separation and drug crystallization can result in a reduction in the drug release rate. One obvious approach to minimize such drug crystallization is to experimentally identify a drug concentration, which would not result in crystallization upon storage. This drug concentration is referred to as the "apparent solid-solubility" and has been determined using thermal analysis and X-ray diffraction (25–27).

EXAMPLES OF LIPID-BASED AND SELF-EMULSIFYING SOLID DISPERSIONS

Gelucires®

One excipient that has stimulated interest in lipid-based solid dispersion formulations is Gelucire 44/14 (Gattefossé Corp., St. Priest, France). This self-emulsifying excipient that exists as a waxy semi-solid at ambient room temperature is a mixture of glyceryl and PEG 1500 esters of long-chain fatty acids and is listed in the European Pharmacopoeia as laurylmacrogolglycerides and in the United States Pharmacopoeia as lauroylpolyoxyglycerides. The suffixes, 44 and 14, in the excipient trade name refer to its melting point and hydrophilic–lipophilic balance (HLB), respectively. Serajuddin et al. (28) compared properties of different formulations of the poorly water-soluble drug, REV5901, which were prepared by dissolving the drug in molten PEG1000, PEG1450, PEG8000, or Gelucire 44/14; the molten formulations were filled into size 0 hard gelatin capsules in amounts that contained 100 mg of REV5901 and 550 mg of the excipient. Upon congealing of the formulations at ambient room temperature, the incorporated drug existed as either a molecular dispersion (solution) or in the amorphous state within the excipient matrix. REV5901 is a weakly basic drug with a pK_a value of 3.6 and a maximum solubility of 0.95 mg/mL at pH 1 and 37°C; the aqueous solubility at pH 6.8 was less than 2 μg/mL (29). Although sink conditions existed in the 900 mL volume of simulated gastric fluid USP (without enzyme) used for dissolution testing of the drug capsules, dissolution from all of the PEG-based solid dispersions was incomplete, whereas Gelucire 44/14 provided complete dissolution (Fig. 6). The results of this study demonstrate the potential value of surface active excipients for enhancing dissolution of poorly water-soluble drugs. When the dissolution study was repeated in water (pH ~6) in which the drug was practically insoluble, the Gelucire 44/14-based solid dispersion completely released the drug in the dissolution medium, forming a milky dispersion of the free drug as fine, metastable oily globules. In contrast, no such release of drug in water by any of the PEG formulations was observed. From this study, it was concluded that, relative to a simple PEG dispersion, a poorly water-soluble drug formulated in a surface-active excipient (e.g., Gelucire 44/14) would either dissolve completely in aqueous media or be

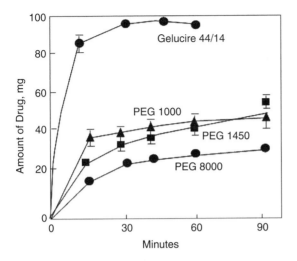

Figure 6 Relative dissolution rates of REV5901 from solid dispersion formulations of various polyethylene glycols and Gelucire 44/14 in 0.1 M HCl. Each capsule contained 100 mg of drug in a total fill weight of 550 mg. Capsules were prepared by filling with the molten formulations. *Abbreviation*: PEG, polyethylene glycol. *Source*: From Ref. 28.

released in a finely divided particulate state, thus increasing its dissolution rate and bioavailability. Clinical testing of a Gelucire 44/14 solid dispersion formulation of REV5901 in normal fasted volunteers revealed substantially improved bioavailability relative to a conventional tablet formulation prepared from micronized drug and containing a wetting agent (30).

Aungst et al. (31) observed that the bioavailability in dogs of a PEG-based formulation of the poorly water-soluble HIV protease inhibitor, DMP323, decreased 10-fold when the dose was increased from 100 to 350 mg. In contrast, bioavailability from a Gelucire 44/14 solid dispersion was relatively unaffected by the delivered dose of DMP323 (69% and 50% after doses of 85 mg and 350 mg, respectively). The bioavailability of another HIV protease inhibitor, ritonavir, was also substantially enhanced, relative to a conventional formulation, by using a solid dispersion formulation prepared from a mixture of Gelucire 50/13, polysorbate 80 and polyoxyl 35 castor oil (32).

Barker et al. (33) reported an increase in α-tocopherol (vitamin E) bioavailability from a Gelucire 44/14 solid dispersion formulation, which was attributed to the formation of fine emulsion droplets containing the vitamin following dispersion of the formulation in the aqueous contents of the GIT (Fig. 7).

Gelucire 44/14 has also been extensively used in combination with other surfactants and solubilizing agents to enhance the performance of solid dispersions. For example, Vippagunta et al. (34) observed higher dissolution rate of crystalline nifedipine from solid dispersion in a mixture of Gelucire 44/14 and Pluronic F68 as compared to the neat crystalline drug substance milled to the same particle size.

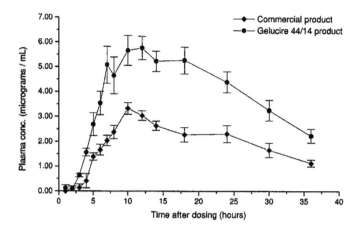

Figure 7   Comparison of mean plasma concentration versus time profiles of α-tocopherol after oral administration of a commercial product or in a formulation containing Gelucire 44/14 to six healthy male volunteers in the fasted state. Two capsules, each containing 300 IU of α-tocopherol, were given to each subject in a cross-over study design. *Source*: From Ref. 33.

He et al. (35) used Gelucire 44/14 in combination with *N,N*-dimethyl acetamide (DMA) to enhance solubility, stability, and bioavailability of a poorly water-soluble antiviral agent that was chemically unstable and poorly soluble in aqueous media. It was, however, soluble and stable in DMA and incorporating Gelucire 44/14 resulted in a stable, semi-solid formulation that could be easily filled into soft gelatin capsules. Solid dispersion formulations of flurbiprofen (36) and piroxicam (37) prepared in a mixture of Gelucire 44/14 and Labrasol (caprylocaproyl macrogolglycerides) demonstrated an improved dissolution rate in vitro and a corresponding higher bioavailability as compared to conventional formulations (38,39).

Polyethylene Glycol-Polysorbate 80 Mixtures

Among all the excipients available for use in solid dispersions, the polyethylene glycols with molecular weights ranging from 1000 to 8000 and which exist in a waxy, semi-solid state at ambient temperature, have probably been the most thoroughly studied. Serajuddin et al. (40) demonstrated that solid dispersion formulations prepared from mixtures of PEG and polysorbate 80 may perform similarly to Gelucire 44/14. Although polysorbate 80 is liquid at room temperature, it forms a semi-solid matrix when mixed with PEG in up to a 4:1 ratio of polysorbate 80 and PEG (Fig. 8). It was hypothesized that polysorbate 80 was incorporated within the amorphous region of the PEG solid structure, and that the crystalline structure of solid PEG was minimally affected by polysorbate 80, because the two excipients were poorly miscible with one another (41).

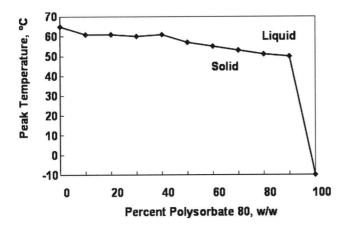

Figure 8 Phase behavior of PEG 8000 and polysorbate 80 mixtures. Mixtures of PEG 8000 containing up to 90% of polysorbate 80 remain in the solid state at room temperature. *Abbreviation*: PEG, polyethylene glycol. *Source*: From Ref. 41.

Joshi et al.(42) prepared solid dispersions of a poorly water-soluble and weakly basic drug (pK$_a$ ~ 5.5) in neat Gelucire 44/14 and in a 1:3-mixture of polysorbate 80 and PEG3350. The highest drug solubility (100 μg/mL) was observed at pH 1.5; the solubility dropped to <1 μg/mL between pH 3.5 and 5.5, and the drug was practically insoluble (<0.02 μg/mL) at pH > 5.5. The solid dispersion formulations were prepared by dissolving the drug in the molten excipients at 65°C, which was filled into size 0 hard gelatin capsules and allowed to congeal, with each capsule containing either 25 mg or 50 mg of the drug in a total fill weight of 600 mg. The dissolution profiles of the two formulations were similar and, based on dissolution rate and other formulation physicochemical considerations, such as the higher melting point of the PEG-polysorbate mixture compared to Gelucire 44/14, the solid dispersion containing the mixture of polysorbate 80 and PEG3350 was selected for in vivo evaluation. The absolute bioavailability of the drug in dogs from the PEG-polysorbate 80 solid dispersion was 21-fold higher than that of a capsule containing micronized bulk drug blended with lactose and microcrystalline cellulose. It was hypothesized that polysorbate 80 ensured complete release of drug from the solid dispersion in a finely divided metastable amorphous (oily) state, which led to an increase in the drug dissolution rate.

Using in silico modeling with GastroPlus software, Dannenfelser et al. (16) predicted that the bioavailability of a highly permeable, poorly water-soluble (aqueous solubility ~0.17 μg/mL at 25°C), neutral compound would be dependent on its apparent solubility in the GI fluids and on the drug particle size. Three different formulations of the drug were prepared: (*i*) a solution in a solvent-surfactant mixture, (*ii*) a solid dispersion in a 1:3-mixture of polysorbate 80 and PEG3350, and (*iii*) a dry blend of micronized drug with microcrystalline cellulose filled in hard gelatin capsules. The solid dispersion was prepared by dissolving the drug in the melted

PEG3350 at 65°C ± 5°C and filling (as the molten mixture) into hard gelatin capsules; the formulation congealed at room temperature, forming solid plugs in the capsules. The extents of absorption of the solid dispersion and the micronized drug, relative to the solution formulation, were 99% and 10%, respectively; absolute bioavailability could not be determined since a parenteral reference formulation was not available. Once again, this study demonstrated the utility of surfactant-containing solid dispersion formulation for enhancing the bioavailability of a poorly soluble drug and, in this instance, the solid dispersion formulation was selected for testing in Phase I clinical studies.

Other investigators have also reported enhanced dissolution (43) and bioavailability (44) of drugs from PEG-polysorbate mixtures. PEG solid dispersions containing varying amounts of the ionic and nonionic surfactants, sodium dodecyl sulfate (SDS), and polysorbate 80, respectively, were described by Sjökvist et al. (45). In this instance, instead of directly filling the molten formulations into hard gelatin capsules, the congealed formulation was first pulverized and then filled into capsules as the waxy, solid material. In another study, Owuso-Ababio et al. (46) prepared solid dispersions of mefenamic acid in neat PEG3350 or in a mixture of PEG3350 and polysorbate 20. Relative to the neat PEG solid dispersion, an increase in the dissolution rate of mefenamic acid was seen, when polysorbate 20 was incorporated.

Lipid-Polysorbate Mixtures

Polysorbates have proven useful in preparing solid dispersion formulations of poorly water-soluble drugs in combination with excipients other than PEGs. One interesting formulation approach was reported by Attama et al. (47), who described the preparation of homogeneous dispersions of up to 30% w/w of diclofenac in molten mixtures of polysorbate 65 and goat fat (melting point 51°C). Molded tablets were prepared by allowing the molten formulation to congeal at ambient room temperature. The in vitro dissolution rate of the drug from this formulation was proportional to the surfactant concentration.

Tocopheryl Polyethylene Glycol 1000 Succinate (TPGS)

Another lipid-based excipient useful for preparing solid dispersion formulations is d-α-tocopheryl polyethylene glycol 1000 succinate (TPGS; Vitamin E TPGS, Eastman Chemical, Tennessee, U.S.A.). This excipient, which is listed in the United States Pharmacopoeia, is a water-soluble, surface-active, and self-emulsifying derivative of vitamin E that is capable of solubilizing many poorly water-soluble drugs. Because of its relatively low melting point (~40°C), molten TPGS formulations are suitable for filling into both soft and hard gelatin capsules; however, hard gelatin capsules require band-sealing in order to prevent leakage of the contents. Koo et al. (48) compared the bioavailability of solid dispersions of the antimalarial drug, halofantrine, formulated in PEG600, TPGS, Gelucire 44/14, or a 1:1 mixture of TPGS and Gelucire 44/14. The drug was dissolved in a molten excipient at 70°C to 80°C, and the solution was either poured into precooled suppository molds or filled directly into hard gelatin capsules and allowed to solidify. Each dosage unit contained 100 mg of halofantrine and 600 mg of an excipient. When administered to fasted beagle dogs, the solid dispersion formulations produced a uniform, five- to seven-fold improvement in halofantrine bioavailability relative to the commercial tablet formulation. In vitro dissolution studies in aqueous media revealed that both TPGS and Gelucire 44/14 formulations dispersed the drug in the solubilized state, whereas the PEG600 formulation dispersed the drug in the solid state. However, in this instance, no significant difference in oral bioavailability was observed among these three formulations, leading the investigators to conclude that optimal halofantrine bioavailability could be achieved either by full solubilization in the formulation or by particle size reduction.

In another study conducted in rats, the bioavailability of paclitaxel was improved four- to six-fold by coadministration with TPGS due to its effect on the solubility and permeability of the drug (49). Other investigators have studied the role of TPGS in enhancing the absorption of drugs, which are both poorly soluble and poorly permeable (50,51). Sokol et al. (52) reported enhanced absorption of cyclosporine from vitamin E TPGS formulations administered to pediatric patients, as compared to formulations without vitamin E TPGS. Formulations including TPGS allowed a 40% to 72% reduction in the cyclosporine dosage required to maintain therapeutic plasma drug concentrations. Similarly, Chang et al. (53) reported a significant increase in cyclosporine bioavailabilty in healthy volunteers when administered with TPGS. In both of these instances, the authors suggested not only drug solubilization, but also inhibition of the intestinal P-glycoprotein transporter as a contributing factor to the enhanced cyclosporine bioavailability.

TPGS is the primary excipient used in the soft gelatin capsule formulation of aprenavir (Agenerase®, GSK, North Carolina, U.S.A.), which was also shown to improve the drug bioavailability through a combination of increased solubility and permeability enhancement due to excipient-mediated P-glycoprotein efflux inhibition (54).

Block Copolymers

Another surface active lipid excipient class that has shown significant promise for application in solid dispersion formulations is the block copolymer (55–59), various grades of which are commercially available as poloxamers (Pluronics®). Ho et al. (56) reported that the dissolution rate of nifedipine from a solid dispersion in Pluronic F-68 was positively correlated with the Pluronic F-68:nifedipine concentration ratio. In another study, the in vitro dissolution rate in pH 6.8 buffer and the bioavailability in dogs of a poorly water-soluble drug, ABT-963, were increased relative to a conventional capsule formulation containing drug-excipient granules by a solid dispersion formulation Pluronic-F68 prepared by solvent evaporation or filled into capsules in the molten state (58). At a concentration of approximately 7.5% w/w, the drug formed a eutectic mixture with Pluronic F-68, which thermal analysis, powder X-ray diffraction (XRD), scanning electron microscopy (SEM), and elemental mapping demonstrated to be comprised of crystalline ABT-963 and Pluronic F-68. More recently, Yin et al. (59) prepared a spray-dried formulation of the water-insoluble drug, BMS-347070, which resulted in rapid drug absorption and bioavailability in dogs comparable to that of a solution formulation. The drug was dissolved in acetone or methylene chloride along with Pluronic F-127 and spray-dried to form a dispersion of nanosized crystalline drug material within a crystalline, water-soluble matrix. The authors hypothesized that the polyethylene oxide segments of Pluronic F-127 crystallized, while the polypropylene oxide segments of the excipient remained amorphous, creating a size-restricted domain in which the drug substance formed physically stable nanocrystals.

Gels

Fluid-filled hard gelatin capsules can be prepared from thixotropic gel formulations, the viscosity of which is lowered by adding suitable excipients or through the application of pressure during the filling process. While this technique has proven useful in certain instances, it has found only limited application due to the difficulty of identifying appropriate excipients from which these formulations can be prepared.

A thixotropic, lipid-based formulation of the poorly water-soluble drug, propantheline bromide, which was suitable for hard gelatin encapsulation at room temperature was prepared by first dissolving the drug in Miglyol 829. Subsequent incorporation of colloidal silicon dioxide increased the viscosity of the fill material in proportion to the amount added, while simultaneously increasing the in vitro dissolution rate of the drug (60). In another study, colloidal silicon dioxide was used as a gelling agent to formulate a SEDDS from a mixture of an oil (diesters of caprylic/capric acids; Captex 200), a surfactant (polysorbate 80) and a cosurfactant (C8/C10 mono-/diglycerides; Capmul MCM) (61).

Jirby et al. (62) described the preparation of semi-solid "amphiphilogel" formulations of poorly water-soluble drugs from combinations of solid and liquid surfactants or amphiphiles. The semi-solid surfactants, Span 40 (sorbitan monopalmitate) or Span 60 (sorbitan monostearate), were used as solid gelators and combined with the liquid surfactants, Span 20 (sorbitan monolaurate) or a Tween (polysorbate 20 or polysorbate 80). The solid and liquid components were heated together to 60°C to enable homogeneous mixing and gels were formed when mixtures were cooled to room temperature. The authors reported that bioavailability of poorly water-soluble drugs could be enhanced by incorporating them in such gels.

Pellets

Lipid and surfactant excipients have been used to prepare self-emulsifying pellets that are suitable for direct filling into hard gelatin capsules or for preparing tablets by direct compression. Franceschinis et al. (63) produced self-emulsifying pellets with improved drug dissolution and enhanced permeability of the model drug, nimesulide, by wet granulation with microcrystalline cellulose, lactose, mono-, and diglycerides and polysorbate 80. In another study, a self-emulsifying pellet formulation of progesterone was prepared by extrusion and spheronization (64). A 50:50 mixture of oil (mono- and diglycerides) and polysorbate 80 was prepared by melting the glycerides at 50°C, adding the surfactant, and cooling the mixture to room temperature, yielding a liquid in which the progesterone was dissolved. The solution was combined with microcrystalline cellulose and small amounts of water and ethanol, resulting in solidified mass that was extruded, spheronized and filled into hard gelatin capsules. A three-way randomized crossover study was conducted in beagle dogs comparing progesterone bioavailability from hard gelatin capsules containing the extruded pellets, the liquid formulation (pre-extrusion), and an aqueous suspension. At a constant dose of 16 mg, the area under the curve (AUC) and maximum plasma concentration (C_{max}) of the extruded pellets and the liquid formulations were both found to be seven- to nine-fold higher than those of the aqueous suspension, clearly demonstrating that the bioavailability-enhancing properties of the liquid formulation were not lost following conversion to an extruded semi-solid formulation capable of being dry-filled into capsules or compressed into tablets.

Phospholipids

Phosphatidylcholine (PC) and its derivatives, dipalmitoylphosphatidylcholine (DPPC) or dimyristoylphosphatidylcholine (DMPC), have also been used to enhance the dissolution rate and bioavailability of poorly water-soluble drugs. Law et al. (65) demonstrated that the in vitro dissolution and in vivo absorption of nifedipine was enhanced 2.6-fold and 3.4-fold, respectively, when 5% PC was incorporated into nifedipine-PEG solid dispersions. The increase in bioavailability was hypothesized to have resulted from the formation of phospholipid vesicles, which entrapped a fraction of the nifedipine dose during dissolution in aqueous media and prevented precipitation of the drug. To test the assumption, one part of the turbid dissolution medium containing the dissolved nifedipine-PEG-PC solid dispersion in water was filtered through a 1.2 μm membrane filter and centrifuged. The supernatant was analyzed under a microscope to confirm absence of drug particles or lipid vesicles. Likewise, an aliquot of the turbid dissolution medium was filtered though a 1.2 μm membrane filter and was analyzed without centrifugation for absence of drug particles. Passing the media through the filter did not disrupt the lipid vesicles. Nifedipine concentrations were determined in both the turbid medium and the clear supernatant (Fig. 9).

As seen in Figure 9, the nifedipine concentration in the supernatant was significantly less than that in the uncentrifuged dissolution medium, indicating that the presence of lipidic vesicles might have contributed to higher entrapment of nifedipine. The formulations were administered orally to rats and the plasma concentrations of nifedipine were significantly higher from solid dispersions containing PC (Fig. 10).

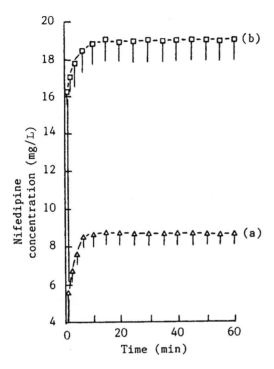

Figure 9 Dissolution profiles of a nifedipine/phosphatidylcholine (PC)/polyethylene glycol (5:5:90) solid dispersion in water. Nifedipine concentrations were determined after (a) centrifuging and analyzing the clear supernatant, and (b) analyzing the turbid layer containing lipid vesicles of PC. Nifedipine appeared to be entrapped in lipid vesicles during dissolution, based on microscopic and chromatographic analysis. *Abbreviation*: PC, phosphatidylcholine. *Source*: From Ref. 65.

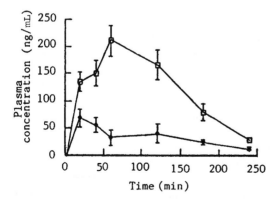

Figure 10 Comparison of mean plasma concentration versus time profiles of nifedipine in rats after oral administration of solid dispersion formulations consisting of nifedipine-PEG (5:95) (♦) or nifedipine-PC-PEG (5:5:90) (□). *Abbreviations*: PC-PEG, phosphatidylcholine-polyethylene glycol; PEG, polyethylene glycol. *Source*: From Ref. 65.

The derivatives of PC, DPPC, and DMPC have also been shown to enhance the dissolution rate of nifedipine. Yamamura et al. (66) demonstrated that comilled mixtures of nifedipine with either DPPC or DMPC had higher dissolution rates when compared with their corresponding solid dispersions or simple physical mixtures. Solid dispersions, in turn, had higher dissolution rates than the physical mixtures. A possible explanation for the superior nifedipine dissolution rate produced by cogrinding could be the result of distortion in the crystal lattice of the phospholipid excipient resulting in the generation of an amorphous form of the excipient that was not observed in solid dispersions or the comilled physical mixtures.

Incorporation of 5% to 20% w/w of various phospholipids has also been reported to enhance the dissolution rates and enhance the absorption of poorly water-soluble drugs such as griseofulvin, fludrocortisone, and carbamezapine (67–69), while ~5% w/w cholesterol has been shown to reduce the age-related changes in the dissolution rates of solid dispersions of poorly water-soluble drugs, though the mechanism is not fully understood (70,71).

CHALLENGES IN DEVELOPMENT OF LIPID-BASED SOLID DISPERSIONS

One of the major hurdles in developing a lipid-based solid dispersion formulation involves the selection of a suitable excipient. An ideal excipient should

- be safe, inert, and available at a purity level suitable for human use,
- not degrade during manufacturing or storage,
- be capable of solubilizing the drug dose in a volume not exceeding that of an oral capsule,
- (preferably) possess surface active properties to enable self-emulsification or complete dissolution of the drug dose,
- reliably and reproducibly enhance the oral bioavailability of the drug relative to a conventional formulation,
- be physically and chemically stable, and compatible with a wide range of drugs and other excipients,
- be nonhygroscopic and inert to the capsule shell or other packaging components,
- allow simple and efficient dosage form manufacture and permit ready scale-up from bench top to production-sized batches.

Some important aspects and challenges that need to be addressed during selection of a suitable excipient will now be discussed in greater detail.

Drug Solubility in Carrier

The amount of a drug released from a lipid-based solid dispersion formulation is often determined by the solubility of the drug in the excipient matrix, which should be sufficient to allow complete solubilization of the drug dose in the volume of a single oral capsule. In instances where the drug cannot be fully solubilized in the formulation, a properly chosen surfactant can improve the dissolution rate of a poorly soluble drug. In one instance, the authors showed that the dissolution rate of a poorly soluble compound, SB-210661, was higher in the presence of 0.5% polysorbate 40, as compared to 0.5% SDS, despite the fact that contact angle measurements indicated better wettability with SDS. The superior dissolution rate from the polysorbate 40-containing formulation was attributed to its 100-fold lower critical micelle concentration, which may have solubilized a higher fraction of the dispersed drug during dissolution (72).

Compared to a fully-solubilized solid dispersion formulation of a drug, a suspension formulation requires more stringent manufacturing controls on parameters, such as concentration and particle size of the dispersed phase and formulation viscosity. Rowley et al. (73) studied the rheology and capsule filling properties of molten PEG6000, 8000, 10000, and 20000 dispersions of lactose monohydrate, which was selected as a model drug compound due to its low solubility in PEG. Hard gelatin capsules were filled with the molten formulations at 70°C using a semi-automatic filling machine. Satisfactory capsule filling was achievable, but was constrained by the apparent viscosity of the formulation, which was dependent upon the concentration and particle size of the dispersed phase (lactose) and the molecular weight of the PEG continuous phase.

Thus, preliminary solubility screening studies should seek to identify those excipients that are not only physically and chemically compatible with one another, but also those which can provide the maximum solubilizing power for the drug as well. The solubility of a drug in surfactant or polymer excipients, which are semi-solid at ambient room temperature, can be estimated by extrapolation from solubilized concentrations obtained from temperatures at which the excipients are molten. However, it is necessary to confirm preliminary solubility estimates with multiple analytical techniques and construction of phase diagrams for assessing phase miscibility (74–76). Microscopic detection of crystalline drug material in the excipient matrix is useful for detecting concentrations $\geq 2\%$ crystalline drug in the polymer matrix, but may not be reliable when the excipient matrix itself is crystalline in nature (77). DSC and XRD have also been used to detect the existence of crystalline drug in the excipient matrix (25,26,78). However, when using DSC to study a semi-solid drug dispersion, a control consisting of a simple physical admixture of drug and excipient at identical composition should be run before drawing phase miscibility diagrams, since the drug could dissolve in the excipient during heating, leading to erroneous conclusions (79). Confocal Raman spectroscopy has also been used to assess the physical state and distribution of drugs in solid dispersions. Using this technique, Breitenbach et al. (80) determined that the physical state of ibuprofen, dispersed in a solid matrix of polyvinylpyrrolidone, was equivalent to that of a solution of the drug in dimeric vinylpyrrolidone.

Drug Stability in Carrier

The physicochemical stability of a drug in a lipid-based formulation is dependent on drug loading and solubility in the excipient matrix, specific mechanism(s) of drug degradation, and formulation hygroscopicity. In some cases, solubilization of the drug in the lipid matrix can be maintained; in others, however, precipitation could occur during storage due to moisture sorption or enhanced molecular mobility. Serajuddin et al. (81) studied the crystallization of REV5901 due to water migration into the excipient matrix from the capsule shell. The drug was dissolved in either PEG400 or in a 6:1 mixture of Gelucire 44/14: PEG400, and 700 mg of formulation, containing 125 mg of the drug, was encapsulated in soft gelatin capsules. Following storage of the capsules under ambient conditions, the equilibrium water content of the PEG400 solution had increased to 6.3%, which reduced the initial solubility of the drug in the vehicle by 45%, leading to crystallization. On the other hand, the equilibrium water content in the Gelucire 44/14:PEG400 mixture after exposure to similar storage conditions was only 1.1%, with full solubility of the drug in the formulation being maintained.

Land et al. (82) investigated the impact of hydration levels of long- and medium-chain triglyceride oils on the solubility of the model hydrophobic compounds, progesterone, estradiol, and testosterone. While the solubility of progesterone was unaffected by the hydration level of the triglyceride, the solubilities of estradiol and testosterone were decreased by 30% to 40% in the presence of moisture. Such a decrease in solubility was attributed to conversion of estradiol and testosterone to their less soluble hydrate form in the presence of trace amount of water dissolved in the oil.

The impact of moisture on the molecular mobility and physical transformation of a drug from a metastable state to its stable form has been documented in the literature (83,84). In order to better understand the characteristics of lipids that could alter the physical stability of drugs in solid dispersions, changes in the properties of neat lipids subsequent to moisture uptake have been studied. In one such study (85), the impact of hydration on physical properties of Gelucire 44/14 was investigated. Because of its natural and semi-synthetic origin, Gelucire 44/14 consists of several chemical components; it was observed that moisture uptake initially resulted in partial deliquescence of glycerol, the most hydrophilic component, followed by PEG and its esters and lastly, the glycerides. It was suggested that the hydrophilic fraction of the excipient be controlled so as to minimize formulation deliquescence during storage and consequently minimize drug crystallization.

In another study, Gelucire 50/13 sustained release solid dispersion formulations containing 10% w/w of either caffeine or paracetamol were stored at 20°C and 37°C, and the drug release in distilled water was monitored periodically over 180 days using the United States Pharmacopea (USP) rotating basket method (86). While the release profiles for caffeine from the solid dispersion showed only a slight increase over time regardless of the storage temperature, a significant increase in the release of paracetamol was observed for samples stored at both 20°C and 37°C, although the increase was more significant at the higher temperature. The observed change in dissolution rate was associated with "blooming," or the formation of scales on the surface of the formulation matrix, which is indicative of a loss of physical integrity.

Damian et al. (87) studied the effect of temperature and aging on the release of the poorly soluble antiviral agent, UC-781, from solid dispersion formulations prepared from PEG6000, Gelucire 44/14, or PVP K30. The formulations that contained between 5% and 80% w/w of UC-781, were stored for up to 12 months at either 4°C to 8°C or 25°C under 25% RH. The dissolution rate of UC-781 from all of the formulations decreased as a function of storage time when tested with the USP paddle method at 50 rpm using purified water media containing 0.2% w/v polysorbate 80. When stored at 25°C, the drop in dissolution was the least from PVP solid dispersions, where the percent drug dissolved at 60 minutes decreased from 90% for freshly prepared samples to 80% following storage for 12 months. For the PEG6000 solid dispersion formulation, the percent of drug dissolved at 60 minutes dropped from 75% for freshly prepared samples to 23% for samples stored for 12 months. Under similar conditions, the dissolution rate of the Gelucire 44/14-based formulation decreased from 85% to 40%. The decrease in the drug dissolution rate upon storage was attributed to a change in the physical state of the excipient matrix, possibly reorganization of the polymer crystalline domain, as evidenced by a higher observed enthalpy of fusion.

Weuts et al. (88) monitored the dissolution behavior of loperamide from PEG solid dispersions stored under various stressed conditions (i.e., 40°C/0% RH, 25°C/52% RH, and 4°C/0% RH). The rate of loperamide dissolution in pH 4.5 aqueous buffer medium declined upon storage and, in this instance, was associated with increased crystallinity of the dispersed drug occurring during storage under conditions of elevated temperature and humidity.

Formation of reactive intermediates (e.g., peroxides) secondary to excipient degradation can result in chemical instability of the formulated drug. Lipid excipients containing unsaturated fatty acids and polyglycolzyed glycderides, which oxidize with aging, can be particularly problematic for drugs sensitive to oxidative degradation (89). For instance, oxidation of PEG400 over time was believed to generate formaldehyde, which led to degradation of a guanine derivative compound (90). In another study, the degradation of fenprostalene in a PEG400 solution was attributed to a reaction between the drug and peroxide intermediates formed from PEG400 in the presence of atmospheric oxygen (91). Oxidation of polyoxyethylene surfactants under stressed conditions has also led to the formation of peroxides as well as formaldehyde (92–94), both of which are capable of leading to gelatin cross-linking in capsule shells resulting in a slower dissolution rate (89). A decrease in the in vitro drug dissolution rate was observed over time for a capsule formulation of gemfibrozil (95) and was associated with the formation of a tough, water-insoluble film on the inner surface of the capsule shell, which prevented release of the formulation. The observed film was attributed to denaturation of the inner capsule surface by formaldehyde that was formed subsequent to auto-oxidation of polysorbate 80 present in the formulation. Although the concentration of formaldehyde formed was less than 0.08%, it had a significant impact on the release rate of the drug substance in vitro but did not effect drug bioavailability relative to control capsules in which gelatin cross-linking was not present.

In summary, certain types of lipid and surfactant excipients can have deleterious effects on both drug stability and release rate due to formation of reactive degradants or changes in the physical state of the excipient upon aging. Therefore, careful monitoring of not only the drug, but also the excipient, is needed during stressed stability studies to ensure adequate drug stability and reproducible formulation performance during the shelf life of the product.

DRUG RELEASE

Drug release from a solid dispersion formulation may be broadly described by the following sequence:

- dissolution of water-soluble excipient components,
- exposure of lipid and/or drug to aqueous media,
- lipid micellization or emulsification,
- equilibrium partitioning of drug from the oily phase to the aqueous phase, and
- in some cases, digestion of lipid.

The released drug is absorbed either from the aqueous phase or, possibly to a lesser extent, directly from the finely dispersed, intact or digested oil droplets. The percent drug release and absorption from capsules containing lipid-based solid dispersions is therefore largely dependent upon factors including emulsification rate, particle size, and polarity of the resulting oily droplets, and the partitioning of drug from the oily phase or micelles into the aqueous media (96). Establishing a bio-relevant in vitro dissolution testing method that can be indicative of such a complex drug release process from lipid-based solid dispersion is therefore challenging.

In this section, some advances in the evaluation of drug release from lipid-based solid dispersions are discussed.

Modified Two-Step Partitioning Process

Fassihi et al. (97) described a modified two-phase dissolution method to monitor the release of nifedipine from capsules containing solid dispersion formulation of drug in a mixture of Gelucire 44/14 and Labrasol. Formulation was prepared by dissolving nifedipine in a molten mixture of Gelucire 44/14 and Labrasol, which was then filled into size 00 hard gelatin capsules and allowed to solidify. Each capsule contained 30 mg of nifedipine dissolved in the formulation. Drug release was determined using either USP I (basket) or modified USP II (paddle) methods. In the modified paddle method, a size 16 screen (opening of 1.2 mm) was inserted horizontally in the dissolution vessel, to prevent the capsule or nondisintegrated lipid excipient matrix from floating on the dissolution medium. A layer of octanol was spread on the surface of aqueous dissolution medium (simulated gastric fluid containing enzymes), and samples were withdrawn from the octanol layer during testing. Fresh octanol was added to replace the amount removed during sampling. The octanol/water partition coefficient of nifedipine is 1000:1, which minimizes the lag time for partitioning of released drug into the octanol layer. The authors studied the effects of various dissolution apparatus designs to select the optimum hydrodynamic conditions for ensuring complete release of nifedipine from the formulation. While this particular dissolution methodology helps to prevent issues typically encountered during dissolution testing of lipid dosage forms (e.g., floating of capsules and lipid fractions, drug loss during sampling and analysis of turbid emulsions, and lack of sink conditions), it could potentially overestimate drug release due to the high solvent capacity of the octanol layer, which would readily solubilize any recrystallized or undissolved drug that was released into the aqueous phase of the dissolution medium.

Measuring Particle Size of Undissolved Drug

In vitro formulation performance can be assessed not only by evaluating the drug dissolution rate, but also by determining the particle size of the released, but undissolved, drug in the dissolution medium. For instance, drug particle sizes in the sub-micron range increase the chances of complete dissolution of the dose in vivo during GI transit because of the relatively high drug particle surface area. In one study (98), solutions of REV5901 were prepared in PEG400, polysorbate 80, or peanut oil. The relative bioavailabilities of these three formulations were evaluated in rats in comparison to a 10% w/v aqueous suspension of the micronized drug (5–10 μm) in 0.5% HPMC. During in vitro dissolution testing of the peanut oil dispersion, it was observed that the neat drug precipitated and settled at the bottom of the dissolution vessel, whereas the drug released from PEG 400 and polysorbate 80 solutions separated as metastable oily globules with a mean droplet sizes of approximately 1.64 micron and 0.66 micron, respectively. The bioavailabilities from these two latter formulations were approximately 30% to 40% greater than that seen with the aqueous suspension formulation. The improved REV5901 bioavailability from the polysorbate 80 formulation, relative to the aqueous suspension formulation, was attributed to the ability of the surfactant to promote the formation of a finely divided, more rapidly dissolving form of the drug substance.

In another study (42), two solid dispersion formulations of a weakly basic, poorly water-soluble drug were prepared in either Gelucire 44/14 or in a mixture of PEG3350 and polysorbate 80. Based on preliminary in vitro evaluation, the solid dispersion in the PEG-polysorbate mixture was selected for further testing in dogs in comparison to a capsule formulation of micronized drug (5–10 μm) and an oral solution in a mixture of PEG400, polysorbate 80, and water. The relative bioavailability of the solution, the solid dispersion, and the powder-filled capsule were 60:36:1.7, thus demonstrating a 21-fold improvement in bioavailability by solid dispersion as compared to micronized drug. During in vitro dissolution testing of the solid dispersions, it was observed that part of the drug dissolved rapidly and the remaining, undissolved drug was dispersed as sub-micron particles. The presence of surfactant in the solid dispersion formulations may have prevented coalescence of the undissolved drug particles, thereby favoring rapid dissolution through maintenance of a high particle surface area. On the other hand, capsules containing micronized drug did not show complete in vitro release. Differences in the effective particle sizes of micronized drug and drug dispersed as sub-micron particles from solid dispersions could possibly explain the differences in the observed bioavailabilities. Particle size measurement of unfiltered sample aliquots of the dissolution media obtained during testing could therefore help in assessing relative in vivo absorption potential.

Soliman et al. (99) used particle size and turbidity measurements to optimize solid dispersion formulations of flurbiprofen prepared in a mixture of Gelucire 44/14 and Labrasol. A relationship between the mean diameter of the dispersed drug particles and the rate and cumulative percent of drug release during dissolution testing was observed.

Serajuddin et al. (16,42) believe that measuring the dissolved drug concentration as well as the drug particle size in unfiltered dissolution media as a function of time could be useful tools for evaluating the performance of lipid-based solid dispersion formulations. Either simulated gastric or simulated intestinal fluid (whichever has the lower solubilization capacity for the drug) should be chosen for testing the particle size of released drug, with purified water serving as a third, suitable alternative.

MANUFACTURING TECHNIQUES

In this section, an overview of various techniques suitable for large scale manufacturing of lipid-based solid dispersions will be presented.

Direct Capsule-Filling Technique

Solid dispersion formulations have traditionally been prepared by fusion method, wherein the drug substance is added to the molten excipient, the mixture is cooled and solidified, pulverized into fine powder and either filled into capsules or compressed as tablets (100). For lipid-based solid dispersions, the above steps could pose several manufacturing limitations, due to waxy nature of the material. Such challenges can be addressed by directly filling hard gelatin capsules with the molten formulation and allowing the molten mass to solidify.

Although the filling of molten formulations into hard gelatin capsules dates back to 1978 (101), the application of this technique for filling PEG-based solid dispersions into hard gelatin capsules was not described until 1987 (102). Since melting an excipient can alter its crystallinity by converting to metastable crystalline or amorphous states, Hawley et al. (103) evaluated the effects of melting and subsequent congealing on the rheology and crystalline structure of various poloxamers, polyethelene glycols, myristic acid, triglycerides, and selected block copolymers of polyethylene oxide/polypropylene oxide. It was observed that these manufacturing unit operations did not substantially change the crystalline structure of the studied excipients.

For a successful scale-up, excipients selected for direct filling operations and the drugs dissolved in the molten formulation should remain physically and chemically stable for the duration of the capsule filling operation. In addition, the viscosity of the molten fill can not change and must be within a range that allows accurate filling by the liquid handling apparatus. In one study, Robinson (104) successfully scaled-up a capsule filling process using either a Qualifill semi-automated or H&H capsule filler. Glyceride bases, such as Gelucire 50/12 or Precirol, a wax comprised of mono-, di-, and triglycerides of palmitostearic acid, were filled into size two capsules at a fill weight of 269 mg and at a filling temperature between 50°C and 52°C. Qualifill capsule filler was used to yield capsules with highly uniform fill weights (less than 1% RSD).

Some basic requirements for capsule liquid-filling machines include:

- provisions for thermal control of the bulk fill reservoir, for maintaining the product in the molten state prior to dosing,
- provisions for agitation of the bulk fill reservoir to prevent phase separation or settling of dispersed drug material prior to dosing,
- accurate dosing of liquid volumes ranging from 0.1 to 1.0 mL,
- ability to eject a filled capsule body, in the absence of cap, without spilling the molten or semi-solid contents, and
- surveillance systems to halt dosing when the absence of a capsule body is detected.

The filling of liquids and semi-solids into hard gelatin capsules and recent developments in this technique has been reviewed by Rowley (105).

Hot Melt Extrusion

While hot melt extrusion has been used as a continuous manufacturing process in the chemical and food industry for over a century (106,107), its commercial application in the pharmaceutical industry has been very limited. During hot melt extrusion, a mixture of drug substance and one or more excipients is continuously fed into a heated extruder barrel containing rotating horizontal screw(s). The elevated temperature and high shear mixing in the barrel typically results in softening of one or more of the formulation components and creates a fine dispersion of the drug substance in the excipient(s), which is continuously extruded through an orifice at the opposite end of the barrel (108,109). The extrudate is cooled, pulverized, and compressed into tablets or filled into hard gelatin capsules. Alternatively, the hot extrudate can be molded into tablets using calendering or injection molding techniques (110). Being a continuous manufacturing process, this technology offers minimal or no scale-up risks and provides flexibility in altering product quality by regulating process parameters such as the processing temperature, screw speed, and the material feed rate.

When manufacturing lipid-based solid dispersions using hot melt extrusion, excipients such as polyethylene glycols, fatty acids, polyglycolyzed glycerides, and low melting surfactants have commonly been used. In one study (111), melt extrusion was used to prepare solid dispersions of 17β-estradiol hemihydrate (17β-E2) with excipients such as PEG 6000, PVP (Kollidon 30), a vinylpyrrolidone-vinylacetate-copolymer (Kollidon VA 64), Sucroester WE15 and Gelucire 44/14. Melt extrusion was performed with an 18-mm single screw extruder equipped with three heating zones (Allrounder 100U, Arburg, Loβburg, Germany). Drug and excipient mixed in a mortar and pestle were introduced into the extruder barrel, which was maintained at 60°C, a temperature well below the melting point of the drug. Cooled extrudates were pulverized and mixed with microcrystalline cellulose, corn starch and magnesium stearate before compressing into tablets. The in vitro dissolution rate of 17β-E2 from the solid dispersion tablets in 0.1M HCl was enhanced 30-fold, as compared to simple physical admixtures of the neat drug and corresponding excipients. X-ray diffraction studies confirmed that the drug remained in the crystalline state in both solid dispersion and physical admixtures formulations, which led the investigators to conclude that the enhanced drug dissolution rate seen with solid dispersion could be the result of superior wetting of finely dispersed drug particles in solid dispersion by the surfactant during dissolution.

Melt Pelletization

Melt pelletization is a process in which a meltable binder is mixed with drug substance and excipients under high shear in a granulating bowl to produce pellets or granules of desired particle size. The binder is added either in its molten state or as a solid, which is subsequently softened or liquefied during processing. Examples of meltable binders include polyethylene glycols, lipid fatty acids, fatty alcohols, and polyglycolized glycerides.

A high shear jacketed granulator is typically used for melt pelletization processing to create the high shear force necessary to produce granules of uniform size distribution (112–114). During processing, temperatures inside the granulator are maintained above the melting point of the binder allowing the binder to melt and induce pellet formation. At the end of the process, dry agglomerates are obtained by cooling the product to ambient temperature.

Using melt pelletization, solid dispersions of diazepam were prepared with PEG3000 and Gelucire 50/13 as the thermo-softening binders (115). Binders were added by two different methods: "pump-on" and "melt-in." When the pump-on procedure was applied, diazepam was dissolved in the molten binder and then added to lactose in the jacketed mixing bowl. With the melt-in method, solid binder was added to preheated diazepam and lactose mixture, and the processing temperature was increased to at least 5°C above the melting temperature of the binder. The in vitro dissolution rate in pH 6.8 phosphate buffer was determined as a function of the drug concentration in solid dispersion, the binder type, processing temperature and cooling rate. It was found that the dissolution rate of diazepam from pellets containing either binder was significantly greater than that of neat diazepam. Also, Gelucire 50/13 provided a higher dissolution rate than PEG3000, possibly due to the surfactant properties of the former (116,117). The release rate was higher from solid dispersions containing lower drug levels, where the drug was believed to exist as a molecular dispersion in the polymer. Neither the processing temperature, nor the cooling rate, affected the in vitro dissolution rate.

Melt pelletization has been used not only to enhance, but also to retard the release rate of drug candidates. In a study conducted by Robinson (104), Gelucire 50/13 and Precirol were used to formulate sustained release dosage forms of a water soluble drug. High-shear mixing in a Becomix RW 15 mixer was used to manufacture batches ranging from 5 to 8 kg in size at a processing temperature of 80°C for 30 minutes. Excellent batch content uniformity (<1% RSD) and comparable dissolution profiles were observed for seven batches of product prepared using this technique. Dissolution testing was conducted using 900 mL of hydrochloric acid (pH 1.5) containing sodium chloride, which was adjusted to pH 7.4 after two hours by addition of aqueous sodium dodecyl sulfate (SDS) and a solution of sodium acetate and tris(hydroxymethyl)methylamine.

Although melt-pelletization technique is well suited for process scale-up, it is critical to define the process variables for successful and reproducible product manufacturing. Parameters such as impeller speed, mixing time during granulation, processing temperature, binder type, and nature (i.e., molten vs. solid binder), and cooling rate have been shown to influence the physicochemical properties, drug release profiles and potentially, the in vivo performance of the formulation, and must be addressed on a case-by-case basis (118–120).

CONCLUSIONS

In recent years, significant advances have been made in the area of oral drug delivery with regard to bioavailability enhancement and subsequently, the therapeutic efficacy of poorly soluble drugs. These advances have been made possible through a greater understanding of the interaction of the dosage form with the GI environment and through the application of physicochemical principles to dosage form development. While dietary oils, fats and other lipids have been considered to be suitable vehicles for the formulation of such drugs, a review published in 2004 showed that there are only four significant products on the market for which lipids are used as carriers and two of these products are for the same active pharmaceutical ingredient (12). Obviously, many challenges to the widespread application of lipid-based formulations still remain. This chapter has discussed recent advances, as well as challenges and opportunities, in the development of lipid-based solid dispersion systems and has provided several examples from the literature. It is hoped that lipid-based solid dispersions will provide new opportunities as they yield convenient solid dosage forms, which are capable of maintaining formulated drugs in the molecularly dispersed or amorphous state and subsequently release drugs as either solutions or finely divided and rapidly dissolving particles, thus leading to improved bioavailability.

REFERENCES

1. Pudipeddi M, Serajuddin ATM, Mufson D. Integrated drug product development—from lead candidate selection to life-cycle management. In: Smith CG, O'Donnell JT, eds. The Process of New Drug Discovery and Development. 2nd ed. New York: Informa Healthcare USA, Inc., 2006:15–51.
2. Horter D, Dressman JB. Influence of physicochemical properties on dissolution of drugs in the gastrointestnial tract. Adv Drug Delivery Rev 1997; 25:3–14.
3. Li S, He H, Parthiban LJ, Yin H, Serajuddin ATM. IV-IVC considerations in the development of immediate-release oral dosage form. J Pharm Sci 2005; 94:1396–1417.
4. Chiou WL, Riegelman S. Pharmaceutical application of solid dispersion systems. J Pharm Sci 1971; 60:1281–1302.
5. Ford JL. The current status of solid dispersions. Pharm Acta Helv 1986; 61:69–88.
6. Leuner C, Dressman J. Improving drug solubility for oral delivery using solid dispersions. Eur J Pharm Biopharm 2000; 50:47–60.
7. Serajuddin ATM. Solid dispersion of poorly water-soluble drugs: early promises, subsequent problems, and recent breakthroughs. J Pharm Sci 1999; 88:1058–1066.
8. Chokshi R, Zia H. Hot-melt extrusion technique: a review. Iranian J Pharm Res 2003; 3:3–16.
9. Hauss DJ, Fogal SE, Ficorilli JV, et al. Lipid-based delivery systems for improving the biovailability and lymphatic transport of a poorly water-soluble LTB4 inhibitor. J Pharm Sci 1998; 87:164–169.
10. Humberstone AJ, Charman WN. Lipid-based vehicles for the oral delivery of poorly water soluble drugs. Adv Drug Delivery Rev 1997; 25:103–128.
11. Pouton CW. Lipid formulations for oral administration of drugs: non-emulsifying, self-emulsifying and "self-microemulsifying" drug delivery systems. Eur J Pharm Sci 2000; 11(Suppl 2):S93–S98.
12. Gursoy RN, Benita S. Self-emulsifying drug delivery systems (SEDDS) for improved oral delivery of lipophilic drugs. Biomed Pharmacother 2004; 58:173–182.
13. Cole ET. Liquid-filled hard gelatin capsules. Pharm Technol 1989; September issue, 124–140.
14. Johnson KC, Swindell AC. Guidance in the setting of drug particle size specification to minimize variability in absorption. Pharm Res 1996; 13:1795–1798.
15. Chiou WL, Ma C, Chung SM, Wu TC, Jeong HY. Similarity in the linear and non-linear oral absorption of drugs between human and rat. Int J Clin Pharmacol Ther 2000; 38:532–539.
16. Dannenfelser RM, He H, Joshi Y, Bateman S, Serajuddin ATM. Development of clinical dosage forms for a poorly water soluble drug I: application of polyethylene glycol-polysorbate 80 solid dispersion carrier system. J Pharm Sci 2004; 93:1165–1175.

17. Savchenko PS. The nature of eutectics. Russian J Inorg Chem 1959; 4:186–189.
18. Rastogi RP, Bassi PS. Mechanism of eutectic crystallization. J Phys Chem 1964; 68:2398–2406.
19. Rai US, Mandal KD. Some physicochemical studies on organic eutectics and 1:2 addition compounds. Mol Cryst Liq Cryst 1990; 182B:387–404.
20. Hancock BC, Parks M. What is the true solubility advantage for amorphous pharmaceuticals? Pharm Res 2000; 17:397–404.
21. Chiou WL. Pharmaceutical applications of solid dispersion systems: X-ray diffraction and aqueous solubility studies on griseofulvin-poly(ethylene glycol) 6000 systems. J Pharm Sci 1977; 66:989–991.
22. Ford JL, Rubinstein MH. Ageing of indomethacin-polyethylene glycol 6000 solid dispersion. Pharm Acta Helv 1979; 54:353–358.
23. Matsumoto T, Zografi G. Physical properties of solid molecular dispersions of indomethacin with poly(vinylpyrrolidone) and poly(vinylpyrolidone-co-vinylacetate) in relation to indomethacin crystallization. Pharm Res 1999; 16:1722–1728.
24. Coleman M, Graf J, Painter P. The thermodynamics of mixing. In: Coleman M, Graf J, Painter P, eds. Specific interactions and the miscibility of polymer blends. Lancaster: Technomic Publication, 1991:1–47.
25. Vasanthavada M, Tong WQ, Joshi Y, Kislalioglu MS. Phase behavior of amorphous molecular dispersions I: determination of the degree and mechanism of solid solubility. Pharm Res 2004; 9:1598–1606.
26. Vasanthavada M, Tong WQ, Joshi Y, Kislalioglu MS. Phase behavior of amorphous molecular dispersions II: role of hydrogen bonding in solid solubility and phase separation kinetics. Pharm Res 2005; 22:440–448.
27. Vippagunta SR, Maul KA, Tallavajhala S, Grant DJW. Solid-state characterization of nifedipine solid dispersions. Int J Pharm 2002; 236:111–123.
28. Serajuddin ATM, Shen PC, Mufson D. Bernstein DF, Augustine MA. Effect of vehicle amphiphilicity on the dissolution and bioavailability of a poorly water-soluble drus from solid dispersions. J Pharm Sci 1988; 77:414–417.
29. Serajuddin ATM, Sheen PC, Mufson D, Bernstein D, Augustine MA. Preformulation study of a poorly water-soluble drug, α-pentyl-3-(2-quinolinylmethoxy)benzenemethanol: selection of the base for dosage form development. J Pharm Sci 1986; 75:492–496.
30. Sheen PC, Kim SI, Petillo JJ, Serajuddin ATM. Bioavailability of a poorly water-soluble drug from tablet and solid dispersion in man. J Pharm Sci 1991; 80:712–714.
31. Aungst BJ, Nguyen NH, Roger NJ, et al. Amphiphilic vehicles improve the oral bioavailability of a poorly soluble HIV protease inhibitor at high doses. Int J Pharm 1997; 156:79–88.
32. Al-Razzak LA, Dias L, Kaul D, Ghosh S. Lipid based systems for oral delivery: physiological mechanistic and product development perspectives. Symposia abstracts and biographies, AAPS Annual Meeting, Boston, MA, November 6, 1997; Alexandria, VA: AAPS, 1997:18.
33. Barker SA, Yap SP, Yuen KH, McCoy CP, Murphy JR, Craig DQM. An investigation into the structure and bioavailability of α-tocopherol dispersions in Gelucire 44/14. J Controlled Release 2003; 91:477–488.
34. Vippagunta SR, Maul KA, Tallavajhala S, Grant DJW. Solid-state characterization of nifedipine solid dispersions. Int J Pharm 2002; 236:111–123.

35. He Y, Johnson JLH, Yalkowsky SH. Oral formulation of a novel antiviral agent, PG301029, in a mixture of Gelucire 44/14 and DMA (2:1, wt/wt). AAPS Pharm Sci Tech 2005; 6:E1–E5.

36. Soliman MS, Khan MA. Preparation and in vitro characterization of a semi solid dispersion of flurbiprofen with Gelucire 44/14 and Labrasol. Pharmazie 2005; 60:288–293.

37. Nilufer Y, Aysegul K, Yalcin O, Ayhan S, Sibel AO, Tamer B. Enhanced bioavailability of piroxicam using Gelucire 44/14 and Labrasol: in vitro and in vivo evaluation. Eur J Pharm Biopharm 2003; 235:247–265.

38. Hu Z, Prasad YV, Tawa R, et al. Diethylether fraction of Labrasol having a stronger absorption enhancing effect on gentamicin than Labrasol itself. Int J Pharm 2002; 234:223–235.

39. Chang RK, Shojaei AH. Effect of a lipoid excipient on the absorption profile of compound UK 81252 in dogs after oral administration. J Pharm Pharm Sci 2004; 7:8–12.

40. Serajuddin ATM, Sheen PC, AugustineMA. Improved dissolution of a poorly water-soluble drug from solid dispersions in poly(ethylene glycol):polysorbate 80 mixtures. J Pharm Sci 1990; 79:463–464.

41. Morris KR, Knipp GT, Serajuddin ATM. Structural properties of poly(ethylene glycol)-polysorbate 80 mixture, a solid dispersion vehicle. J Pharm Sci 1992; 81:1185–1188.

42. Joshi HN, Tejwani RW, Davidovich M, et al. Bioavailability enhancement of a poorly water-soluble drug by solid dispersion in polyethylene glycol-polysorbate 80 mixture. Int J Pharm 2004; 269:251–258.

43. Veiga MD, Escobar C, Bernard MJ. Dissolution behavior of drugs from binary and ternary systems. Int J Pharm 1993; 93:215–220.

44. Sheen PC, Khetarpal VK, Cariola CM, Rowlings CE. Formulation studies of a poorly water-soluble drug in solid dispersions to improve bioavailability. Int J Pharm 1995; 18:221–227.

45. Sjökvist E, Nyström C, Alden M, Caram-Lelham N. Physico-chemical aspects of drug release. XIV. The effects of some ionic and non-ionic surfactants on properties of a sparingly soluble drug in solid dispersions. Int J Pharm 1992; 79:23–33.

46. Owusu-Ababio G, Ebube NK, Reams R, Habib M. Comparative dissolution studies for mefenamic acid-polyethylene glycol solid dispersion systems and tablets. Pharm Dev Technol 1998; 3:405–412.

47. Attama AA, Nzekwe IT, Nnamani PO, Adikwu MU, Onugu CO. The use of solid self-emulsifying systems in the delivery of diclofenac. Int J Pharm 2003; 262:23–28.

48. Khoo SM, Porter CJH, Charman WN. The formulation of halofantrine as either non-solubilising PEG6000 or solubilising lipid based solid dispersion: physical stability and absolute bioavailability assessment. Int J Pharm 2000; 205:65–78.

49. Varma MV, Panchagnula R. Enhanced oral paclitaxel absorption with vitamin E-TPGS: effect on solubility and permeability in vitro, in situ and in vivo. Eur J Pharm Sci 2005; 25:445–453.

50. Wu SH. Vitamin E TPGS as a vehicle for drug delivery system. Paper presented at AAPS short course "Formulation with Lipids," Parsippany, NJ, June 3, 1998. Alexandria, VA: AAPS, 1998.

51. Boudreaux JP, Hayes DH, Mizrahi S, Maggiore P, Blazek J, Dick D. Use of water-soluble liquid vitamin E to enhance cyclosporine absorption in children after liver transplant. Transplant Proc 1993; 25:1875.

52. Sokol RJ, Butler-Simon N, Connor C, et al. Multicenter trial of d-α-tocopheryl polyethylene glycol 1000 succinate for treatment of vitamin E deficiency in children with chronic choleostasis, Gastroenterology 1993; 104:1727–1735.

53. Chang T, Benet LZ, Hebert MF. The effect of water-soluble vitamin E on cyclosporine pharmacokinetics in healthy volunteers. Clin Pharmacol Ther 1996; 59:297–303.

54. Yu L, Bridgers A, Polli J, et al. Vitamin-E TPGS increases absorption flux of an HIV protease inhibitor by enhancing its solubility and permeability. Pharm Res 1999; 16:1812–1817.

55. Shin SC, Cho CW. Physicochemical characterization of piroxicam-poloxamer solid dispersion. Pharm Dev Technol 1997; 2:403–407.

56. Ho HO, Chen CN, Sheu, MT. Influence of pluronic F-68 on dissolution and biavailability characteristics of multiple-layer pellets of nifedipine for controlled release delivery. J Controlled Release 2000; 68:433–440.

57. Passerini N, Albertini B, Gonzalez-Rodriguez ML. Preparation and characterization of ibuprofen-poloxamer 188 granules obtained by melt granulation. Eur J Pharm Sci 2002; 15:71–78.

58. Chen Y, Zhang GGZ, Neilly J, Marsh K, Mawhinney D, Sanzgiri, YD. Enhancing the bioavailability of ABT-963 using solid dispersion containing pluronic F-68. Int J Pharm 2004; 286:69–80.

59. Yin SX, Franchini M, Chen JL, et al. Bioavailability enhancement of a COX-2 inhibitor, BMS-347070, from nanocrystalline dispersion prepared by spray-drying. J Pharm Sci 2005; 94:1598–1707.

60. Walters PA, Rowley G, Pearson JT, Taylor CJ. Formulation and physical properties of thixotropic gels for hard gelating capsules. Drug Dev Ind Pharm 1992; 18:1613–1631.

61. Patil P, Joshi J, Paradkar P. Effect of formulation variables on preparation and evaluation of gelled self-emulsifying drug delivery systems (SEDDS) of ketoprofen. AAPS PharmSciTech 2004; 5:1–8.

62. Jibry N, Heenan RK, Murdan S. Amphiphilogels for drug delivery: formulation and characterization. Pharm Res 2004; 21:1852–1861.

63. Franceschinis E, Voinovich D, Grassi M, et al. Self-emulsifying pellets prepared by wet granulation in high-shear mixer: influence of formulation variables and preliminary study on the in vitro absorption. Int J Pharm 2005; 291:87–97.

64. Tuleu C, Newton M, Rose J, et al. Comparative bioavailability study in dogs of a self-emulsifying formulation of progesterone presented in a pellet and liquid form compared with an aqueous suspension of progesterone. J Pharm Sci 2004; 93:1495–1502.

65. Law SL, Lo WY, Lin FM, Chiang CH. Dissolution and absorption of nifedipine in polyethyleneglycol solid dispersion containing phosphatidylcholine. Int J Pharm 1992; 84:161–166.

66. Yamamura S, Rogers JA. Characterization and dissolution behavior of nifedipine and phosphatidylcholine binary systems. Int J Pharm 1996; 130:65–73.

67. Venkatram S, Rogers JA. Characteristics of drug:phospholipids coprecipitates I: physical properties and dissolution behavior of griseofulvin-dimyristoylphosphatidycholine systems. J Pharm Sci 1984; 73:757–761.

68. Vudathala GK, Rogers JA. Dissolution of fludrocortisone from phospholipids coprecipitates. J Pharm Sci 1992; 81:282–286.

69. Biswas M, Akogyeram CO, Scott KR, Potti GK, Gallelli JF, Habib MJ. Development of carbamazepine: phospholipids solid dispersion formulations. J Controlled Release 1993; 23:239–245.
70. Vudathala GK, Rogers JA. Effect of cholesterol on the aging of griseofulvin-phospholipid coprecipitates. Int J Pharm 1991; 69:13–91.
71. Vudathala G, Roger J. Oral bioavailability of griseofulvin from aged griseofulvin: lipid coprecipitates: in vivo studies in rats. J Pharm Sci 1992; 81:1166–1169.
72. Perng CY, Kearney AS, Patel K, Palepu NR, Zuber G. Investigation of formulation approaches to improve the dissolution of SB-210661, a pooly water soluble 5-lipoxygenase inhibitor. Int J Pharm 1998; 176:31–38.
73. Rowley G, Hawley AR, Dobson CL, Chatham S. Rheology and filling characteristics of particulate dispersions polymer melt formulations for liquid fill hard gelatin capsules. Drug Dev Ind Pharm 1998; 24:605–611.
74. Ford JL, Rubinstein MH. Phase equilibria and dissolution rates of indomethacin-polyethylene glycol 6000 solid dispersions. Pharm Acta Helv 1978; 53:327–332.
75. Suzuki H, Sunada H. Comparison of nicotinamide, ethylurea and polyethylene glycol as carriers for nifedipine solid dispersion systems. Chem Pharm Bull 1997; 45:1688–1693.
76. Fernandez M, Rodriguez IC, Margarit MV, Cerezo A. Characterization of solid dispersions of piroxicam/polyethylene glycol 4000. Int J Pharm 1992; 84:197–202.
77. Shi HG, Farber L, Michaels JN, et al. Characterization of crystalline drug nanoparticles using atomic force microscopy and complementary techniques. Pharm Res 2003; 20:479–484.
78. Vippagunta SR, Maul KA, Tallavajhala S, Grant DJW. Solid-state characterization of nifedipine solid dispersions. Int J Pharm 2002; 236:111–123.
79. Mura P, Faucci MT, Manderioli A, Furlanetto S, Pinzauti S. Thermal analysis as a screening technique in preformulation studies of picotamide solid dosage forms. Drug Dev Ind Pharm 1998; 24:747–756.
80. Breitenbach J, Schrof W, Neumann J. Confocal Raman-spectroscopy: analytical approach to solid dispersions and mapping of drugs. Pharm Res 1999; 16:1109–1113.
81. Serajuddin ATM, Sheen PC, Augustine MA. Water migration from soft gelatin capsule shell to fill material and its effect on drug solubility. J Pharm Sci 1986; 75:62–64.
82. Land LM, Li P, Bummer PM. The influence of water content of triglyceride oils on the solubility of steroids. Pharm Res 2005; 22:784–788.
83. Andronis V, Zografi G. The molecular mobility of supercooled amorphous indomethacin as a function of temperature and relative humidity. Pharm Res 1998; 15:835–842.
84. Shamblin SL, Zografi G. The effects of absorbed water on the properties of amorphous mixtures containing sucrose. Pharm Res 1999; 16:1119–1124.
85. Svensson A, Nevec C, Cabane B. Hydration of an amphiphilic excipient, Gelucire® 44/14. Int J Pharm 2004; 281:107–118.
86. Khan N, Craig DQM. Role of blooming in determining the storage stability of lipid-based dosage forms. J Pharm Sci 2004; 93:2962–2971.
87. Damian F, Blaton N, Kinget R, Mooter GV. Physical stability of solid dispersions of the antiviral agent UC-781 with PEG 6000, Gelucire 44/14 and PVP K30. Int J Pharm 2002; 244:87–98.

88. Weuts I, Kempen D, Verreck G, et al. Study of the physicochemical properties and stability of solid dispersions of loperamide and PEG6000 prepared by spray drying. Eur J Pharm Biopharm 2005; 59:119–126.

89. Chen GL, Hao WH. Factors affecting zero-order release kinetics of porous gelatin capsules. Drug Dev Ind Pharm 1998; 24:557–562.

90. Bindra DS, Williams TD, Stella VJ. Degradation of O-6-benzylguanine in aqueous polyethylene glycol 400 (PEG 400) solutions: concerns with formaldehyde in PEG 400. Pharm Res 1994; 11:1060–1064.

91. Johnson DM, Taylor WF. Degradation of feprostalene in polyethylene glycol 400 solution. J Pharm Sci 1984; 73:1414–1417.

92. Bergh M, Magnusson K, Lars J, Nilson G, Karlberg AT. Formation of formaldehyde and peroxides by air oxidation of high purity polyoxyethylene surfactants. Contact Dermatitis 1998; 39:14–20.

93. Frontini R, Mielck JB. Formation of formaldehyde in polyethyleneglycol and in poloxamer under stress conditions. Int J Pharm 1995; 114:121–123.

94. Bergh M, Shao LP, Hagelthorn G, Gafvert E, Nilsson JLG, Karlberg AT. Contact allergens from surfactants. Atmospheric oxidation of polyoxyethylene alcohols, formation of ethoxylated aldehydes, and their allergenic activity. J Pharm Sci 1998; 87:276–282.

95. Chafetz L, Hong WH, Tsilifonis DC, Taylor AK, Philip J. Decrease in the rate of capsule dissolution due to formaldehyde from polysorbate 80 autoxidation. J Pharm Sci 1984; 73:1186–1187.

96. Shah NH, Carvajal MT, Patel CI, Infeld MH, Malick AW. Self-emulsifying drug delivery systems (SEDDS) with polyglycolyzed glycerides for improving in vitro dissolution and oral absorption of lipophilic drugs. Int J Pharm 1994; 106:15–23.

97. Pillay V, Fassihi R. A new method for dissolution studies of lipid-filled capsules employing nifedipine as a model drug. Pharm Res 1999; 16:333–337.

98. Serajuddin ATM, Sheen PC, Mufson D, Bernstein DF, Augustine MA. Physicochemical basis of increased bioavailability of a poorly water soluble drug following oral administration as organic solutions. J Pharm Sci 1988; 77:325–329.

99. Soliman MS, Khan MA. Preparation and in vitro characterization of a semi solid dispersion of flurbiprofen with Gelucire 44/14 and Labrasol. Pharmazie 2005; 60:288–293.

100. Sekguchi K, Obi N. Studies on absorption of eutectic mixture. I. A comparison of the behavior of eutectic mixture of sulfathiazole and that of ordinary sulfathiazole in man. Chem Pharm Bull 1961; 9:866–872.

101. Cuine A, Mathis C, Stamm A, Francois D. Mis en gelules de solutions visqueuses de principes actifs. I. Etudes preliminarie—excipients. Labo-Pharma Probl Tech 1978 ; 274:222–227.

102. Chatham SM. The use of bases in SSM formulations. STP Pharma 1987; 3:575–582.

103. Hawley AR, Rowley G, Lough WJ, Chatham S. Physical and chemical characterization of thermosoftened bases for molten filled hard gelatin capsule formulations. Drug Dev Ind Pharm 1992; 18:1719–1793.

104. Robinson LF. Physical characterization and scale-up manufacture of Gelucire 50/13 based capsule formulations. Bulletin Technique Gattefosse 2004; 97:97–111.

105. Rowley G. Filling of liquids and semi-solids into hard two-piece capsules. In: Podczeck F, Jones BE, eds. Pharmaceutical Capsules. 2nd ed. Bath: The Batch Press, 2004:169–194.

106. Bruin S, Van Zuilichem DJ, Stolp W. A review of fundamental and engineering aspects of extrusion of biopolymers in a single-screw extruder. J Food Process Eng 1978; 2:1–37.
107. Rossen JL, Miller RC. Food extrusion. Food Technol 1973; 45–63.
108. Breitenbach J. Melt extrusion from process to drug delivery technology. Review article. Eur J Pharm Biopharm 2002; 54:107–117.
109. Dreiblatt A. Process design. In: Ghebre-Sellassie I, Martin C, eds. Pharmaceutical Extrusion Technology. New York: Taylor & Francis, 2003:153–169.
110. Cuff G, Raof F. A preliminary evaluation of injection molding as a technology to produce tablets. Pharm Technol 1998; 22:96–106.
111. Hulsmann S, Backensfeld T, Keitel S, Bodmeier R. Melt extrusion—an alternative method for enhancing the dissolution rate of 17β-estradiol hemihydrate. Eur J Pharm Biopharm 2000; 49:237–242.
112. Schaeffer T. Pelletisation with meltable binders. In Sustained release formulations with lipid based excipient. Bulletin Technique Gattefosse 2004; 97:113–124.
113. Voinovich D, Moneghini M, Perissutti B, Franceschinis E. Melt pelletization in high shear mixer using a hydrophobic melt binder: influence of some apparatus and process variables. Eur J Pharm BioPharm 2001; 52:305–313.
114. Schaefer T, Taagegaard B, Thomsen LJ, Kristensen HG. Melt pelletization in a high shear mixer. IV. Effects of process variables in a laboratory scale mixer. Eur J Pharm Sci 1993; 1(3):125–131.
115. Seo A, Holm P, Kristensen HG, Schaefer T. The preparation of agglomerates containing solid dispersions of diazepam by melt agglomeration in a high shear mixer. Int J Pharm 2003; 259:161–171.
116. Dordunoo SK, Ford JL, Rubinstein. Preformulation studies on solid dispersions containing triamterene or temazepam in polyethylene glycols or Gelucire 44/14 for liquid filling of hard gelatin capsules. Drug Dev Ind Pharm 1991; 17:1685–1713.
117. Damian F, Balton N, Naesens L, Kinget R, Augustijns P, Van den Mooter G. Physicochemical characterization of solid dispersions of the antiviral agent UC-781 with polyethylene glycol 6000 and Gelucire 44/14. Eur J Pharm Sci 2003; 10:311–322.
118. Thies R, Kleinebudde P. Melt pelletisation of a hygroscopic drug in a high shear mixer. Part 1. Influence of process variables. Int J Pharm 1999; 188:131–143.
119. Voinovich D, Moneghini M, Perissutti B, Filipovic-Grcic J, Grabnar I. Preparation in high-shear mixer of sustained-release pellets by melt pelletisation. Int J Pharm 2000; 203:235–244.
120. Schaefer T, Mathiesen C. Melt pelletization in a high shear mixer. VIII. Effects of binder viscosity. Int J Pharm 1996; 139:125–138.

8

Oral Lipid-Based Formulations: Using Preclinical Data to Dictate Formulation Strategies for Poorly Water-Soluble Drugs

Christopher J. H. Porter and William N. Charman

Department of Pharmaceutics, Victorian College of Pharmacy, Monash University, Parkville, Victoria, Australia

INTRODUCTION: LIPID-BASED FORMULATIONS AND ORAL DRUG DELIVERY

The use of formulations containing natural and/or synthetic lipids as a potential strategy for improving the oral bioavailability of poorly water-soluble, highly lipophilic drug candidates has received increasing interest in recent years. For poorly water-soluble compounds, lipids are believed to assist absorption by reducing the inherent limitations of slow and incomplete dissolution and by facilitating the formation of colloidal species within the intestine that are capable of maintaining otherwise poorly water-soluble drugs in solution. Importantly, the formation of these solubilizing species does not necessarily arise directly from the administered lipid, but more frequently results from the intraluminal processing of these lipids (via digestion and dispersion) prior to absorption (1–3).

The coadministration of drugs with lipids can also influence the drug absorption pathway. Whilst most orally administered drugs gain access to the systemic circulation via the portal blood, some highly lipophilic drugs are transported to the systemic circulation via the intestinal lymphatics, thereby avoiding hepatic first-pass metabolism) (1,4–6). In addition, lipids can delay gastric transit and enhance passive intestinal permeability (7–10). More recently, certain lipids and lipidic excipients have been suggested to improve drug absorption through mitigation of presystemic drug metabolism associated with gut membrane-bound cytochrome P-450 enzymes or via inhibition of the P-glycoprotein efflux transporter (11–18).

Lipid-based formulations have been successfully and commercially applied to the formulation of cyclosporine, saquinavir, ritonavir, dutasteride, and amprenavir. The more widespread application of lipid-based formulations has, however, been hampered by the incorrect perception that these types of products are difficult and time-consuming to develop. This chapter briefly outlines some of the issues involved with in vitro assessment of lipid-based formulations, but will concentrate primarily on those issues pertaining to the use of in vivo preclinical data to

- identify the potential utility of lipid-based formulations,
- assess the relative importance of lymphatic transport in drug absorption, and
- screen for and develop effective lipid-based formulation strategies.

Since the performance of lipid-based formulations is often influenced by gastrointestinal lipid digestion and dispersion, these processes will be briefly described in the next section.

DIGESTION AND ABSORPTION OF LIPIDS

The digestion and absorption of lipids has been extensively reviewed in the literature and is also covered elsewhere in this volume (19–22). Briefly, lipid digestion involves three main sequential steps: (*i*) dispersion of fat globules into a coarse emulsion, (*ii*) enzymatic hydrolysis of triglyceride (TG) at the oil/water interface, and (*iii*) dispersion of the digestion products into a fine emulsion of high surface area from which absorption can readily occur (23). Digestion of dietary lipids that are predominantly in the form of poorly water-soluble, neutral TG, begins in the stomach where lingual and gastric lipases secreted by the salivary gland and gastric mucosa, respectively, initiate the hydrolysis of TG to its component diglyceride (DG) and free fatty acid (FA) components. Liberation of these more water soluble lipid digestion products, in combination with the shear force encountered during antral contraction and gastric emptying, facilitates the formation of a coarse emulsion, which upon entry into the duodenum, stimulates the secretion of bile salts and biliary lipids from the gall bladder and the release of lipase enzymes from the pancreas (24–26). Biliary-derived phospholipid and cholesterol adsorb to the surface of the oil droplets comprising the crude emulsion, resulting in improved colloidal stability and a reduction in the oil droplet size with an attendant increase in surface area. These changes facilitate lipid hydrolysis, which occurs at the oil/water interface through the combined actions of colipase and pancreatic lipase enzymes, and results in the production of one molecule of 2-monoglyceride (MG) and two molecules of FA for each TG molecule hydrolyzed. As lipolysis proceeds, these digestion products collect at the surface of the lipid droplets, typically forming liquid crystalline structures, which slough off from the droplet surface and, in conjunction with bile salts and phospholipids, form multilamellar and unilamellar vesicles and ultimately, bile salt-lipid mixed micelles (24,27). While the specific mechanisms controlling the gastrointestinal absorption of lipids have not been fully elucidated, it is known that bile salt mixed micelles are not absorbed intact but must dissociate and release the emulsified lipid digestion products prior to absorption into the enterocyte (28,29). Dissociation of mixed micelles may be triggered by a microclimate of lower pH associated with the intestinal brush border membrane (30,31).

In addition to passive diffusion, there is now evidence to suggest that specific membrane bound carrier proteins may facilitate the transport of lipid digestion products across the apical membrane of the enterocyte (32–34). Once within the enterocyte, the cytosolic FA binding proteins L-FABP and I-FABP bind to FA and facilitate FA solubilization and distribution to the cell nucleus and endoplasmic reticulum (35–38).

POSTABSORPTIVE PROCESSING OF LIPID DIGESTION PRODUCTS: LYMPH VS. PORTAL BLOOD

After absorption into the enterocyte, the lipid FA chain length dictates the specific transport pathway to the systemic circulation. Typically, short- and medium-chain lipids (carbon chain length <12), which account for approximately 10% of dietary lipid (but are common formulation components), are transported primarily by the portal blood (39). In contrast, long-chain lipids (>12 carbons) migrate to the endoplasmic reticulum where re-esterification to TG and subsequent incorporation into chylomicrons occurs prior to secretion into mesenteric lymph. However, the relationship of the lipid transport pathway to the FA chain length is not absolute. For example, up to 30% to 40% of the absorbed amount of long chain FA may pass directly into the portal blood and some lymphatic transport of medium-chain FA is also possible (40–42).

Lymphatic vessels from both the small and large intestine originate as a plexus of lymphatic capillaries in the mucosa and submucosa underlying the absorptive cells and these capillaries join to form larger mesenteric lymph collecting vessels. Mesenteric lymph subsequently drains into the cisterna chyli, where it mixes with hepatic and lumbar lymph prior to entry into the thoracic duct, which drains directly into the systemic circulation at the junction of the left subclavian and internal jugular veins, bypassing the liver and avoiding any potential drug loss through hepatic first-pass metabolism (1,5,6,43–45). The direct drainage of lymph from the gastrointestinal tract into the systemic circulation therefore dictates that drugs absorbed via the intestinal lymphatics will avoid hepatic first-pass metabolism (1,5,6,45).

LIPOPHILIC DRUG DISPOSITION DURING DIGESTION AND ABSORPTION OF LIPID-BASED FORMULATIONS

The complexities associated with obtaining intestinal fluid samples have often limited the study of the interaction of a drug in a lipid-based formulation with the gastrointestinal milieu to in vitro models. To this end several studies from our laboratories (46–51) and others (52–54) have utilized in vitro lipid digestion methodologies to examine the relative proclivity of drugs of varying physicochemical characteristics to

- remain associated with the undigested lipid phase of a formulation,
- partition into the colloidal species formed on interaction of the lipid formulation or its digestion products with biliary derived lipids, and
- precipitate during intestinal processing of the lipid formulation.

While a detailed discussion of these possibilities is beyond the scope of this chapter, it is clear that avoidance of precipitation in vivo and transfer of the drug into the dispersed colloidal species from which absorption is assumed to occur is paramount to optimal absorption. Depending on the physicochemical characteristics of the particular drug and the excipients contained in the formulation, drug precipitation may occur upon initial dispersion of the dosage form in the stomach. This is particularly apparent for formulations containing large quantities of water soluble surfactants, cosurfactants, and cosolvents. These formulations, classified as "Type III" by Pouton, (55,56), are those in which dispersion of the water soluble excipients may reduce the overall solubilizing capacity of the formulation. In contrast, those formulations containing a larger proportion of poorly water-soluble components, such as low hydrophilic–lipophilic balance (HLB) surfactants and lipids (Type I and Type II formulations) are less likely to be affected by dispersion in the gut contents. The performance of this latter group of formulations, however, is more susceptible to influence by lipid digestion. In this regard, recent studies from our laboratories have highlighted the possibility of drug precipitation following digestion of formulations comprised primarily of medium chain lipids. Since the digestion products of these lipids are considerably more water soluble than those comprised of long chain lipids, digestion may substantially reduce the solubilizing capacity of formulations incorporating medium chain lipid excipients (49,50).

After absorption, the majority of lipophilic drugs diffuse through the enterocyte and gain access to the systemic circulation by way of the portal blood. However, a number of highly lipophilic drugs, including cyclosporine (57), probucol (58), mepitiostane (59), naftifine (60), penclomedine (61), halofantrine (62,63), ontazolast (64), CI-976 (65), MK-386 (66), lipophilic vitamins, and vitamin derivatives (1), xenobiotics including dichloro-diphenyl-trichloroethane (DDT) and associated analogs (67,68), benzo(a)pyrene (69) and numerous lipophilic prodrugs (70) have been shown to be transported primarily by the intestinal lymphatics.

Although the precise mechanism(s) by which lipophilic drugs gain access to the intestinal lymph is not fully understood, the majority of lymphatically transported lipophilic compounds are solubilized within the TG core of chylomicrons. Small quantities of transported drug may also be associated with the very low density lipoprotein (VLDL) fraction of lymph. Promotion of lymphatic drug transport therefore requires an appropriate lipid source to stimulate lipoprotein synthesis by the enterocyte. Whilst dietary intake often provides the necessary lipid source required to support chylomicron formation, lipid-based formulations may also promote intestinal lymphatic drug transport by stimulating the turnover of lipoproteins through the enterocyte (71).

Charman and Stella have previously established an apparent relationship between the physicochemical properties of an administered drug and the extent of intestinal lymphatic drug transport (72). They suggested that candidate drug molecules should have a log octanol/water partition coefficient (log P) of at least 5 and significant TG solubility (>50 mg/mL) before intestinal lymphatic transport is likely to become a significant contributor to oral bioavailability. As a caveat, these criteria were based on the assumption that the drug is well absorbed and metabolically stable in the intestinal lumen and within the enterocyte, a situation, which is often not the case for highly lipophilic drug candidates.

The requirement for a high log P value takes into consideration the differences in the flow rate between portal blood and intestinal lymph (approximately 500-fold in the rat) and the maximum lipid content of lymph (1–2%). Since the transport of lipophilic drugs in intestinal lymph is associated with the chylomicron lipid fraction, simple mass terms dictate that for a drug to be equally transported by the portal blood and the intestinal lymph, a partition coefficient of at least 50,000:1 in favor of chylomicron lipid is required, which translates to a log P of 4.7.

Appreciable solubility of a drug in a lipid such as a long chain triglyceride (LCT) is an important corequisite for lymphatic drug transport as this reflects the solubility of the drug in the lipid core of the chylomicron. By way of example, the cumulative lymphatic transport of two high log P compounds, with varying lipid solubilities, hexachlorobenzene (HCB, log P 6.53) and DDT (log P 6.19) has previously been studied in an anesthetized rat model. In this case after intraduodenal administration, the lymphatic transport of DDT (the solubility of which in peanut oil is 13-fold higher than HCB) was substantially greater (33.5% dose) than the corresponding lymphatic transport of HCB (2.3% dose) (72). A recent study assessing the potential for bile salt micelle-mediated conversion of the hydrochloride salt of halofantrine to the corresponding lipophilic free base, as a prelude to lymphatic absorption, also highlights the need to consider the potential for lymphatic transport of lipophilic (and lipid soluble) free acids or free bases after administration as the corresponding salt (73).

It is therefore clear that lipid based formulations can influence a drug's biopharmaceutical profile via a number of different mechanisms, including changes in gastric transit time, solubility in the intestinal lumen, intestinal membrane permeability, and lymphatic transport. In vitro models have been developed to evaluate the potential capacity of lipids and lipidic excipients to enhance drug absorption and bioavailability via changes to both drug solubility and permeability. These aspects are well addressed elsewhere in this volume, and a considerable number of recent publications have explored the utility of both dispersion and simulated digestion testing (46,47,49–53) and the impact of lipids and lipidic excipients on permeability using a range of in vitro permeability models (8,9,74–76). However, neither of these assessments is capable of fully representing the overall range of potential effects that lipids can have on the biopharmaceutical profile of a coadministered drug. Therefore, at some stage during preclinical development of a lipid-based formulation, in vivo evaluation in an appropriate animal species is required.

IN VIVO EVALUATION OF LIPID-BASED FORMULATIONS

Several factors need to be taken into account when selecting the appropriate study design for assessing the in vivo performance of a lipid-based drug formulation. These include animal species, use of anesthesia, route of dosing (oral vs. intraduodenal), dosing volumes (absolute volume and volume per kg of body weight), ability to administer a human-size clinical dosage unit, the type and number of samples required (e.g., lymph, blood, bile, urine, multiple vs. single samples), study cost and relative simplicity. The importance of each of these factors is likely to vary depending on the stage of development and whether the purpose of the study is to simply demonstrate initial proof of concept or rather to provide a more structured evaluation of potential clinical formulations. When deciding on the particular animal model or study design, a clear understanding of the questions that need to be answered is paramount. A discussion of the specific advantages and disadvantages of different animal models is given below and is structured in the form of questions that those models might be used to answer.

Will Lipid-Based Formulations Enhance the Delivery of This Drug Candidate?

When initially confronted with a poorly water-soluble compound for which conventional formulation approaches aimed at improving absorption (e.g., salt or crystal form selection, particle size reduction, solid dispersions, or the addition of surfactants) has failed, the first question typically raised is, "what type of formulation strategy is going to allow further development of this drug?" For compounds in which the primary limitation to absorption is poor aqueous solubility and slow dissolution rate, and where intestinal permeability is not a limiting factor, (e.g., BCS II drugs) (77), a lipid-based formulation should be considered.

An indication of the potential utility of a lipid-based formulation can be gained from knowledge of the drug physicochemical properties (e.g., water solubility, log P, and solubility in lipids) and pharmacological properties (e.g., target and anticipated dose) coupled with a reasonable understanding of the barriers to drug absorption. However, before embarking on a series of studies to evaluate specific lipid-based formulations, an initial proof-of-concept study is warranted. Since the primary mechanism by which lipid-based formulations enhance drug absorption stems from the solubilization of the drug, either directly or following interaction of the lipid excipients and their digestion products with endogenous lipids and surfactants (e.g., phospholipids and bile salts), proof of concept can often be demonstrated from a simple fed-fasted relative bioavailability (food effect) study. In such a study, dietary lipid is often sufficient to produce solubilizing conditions within the gastrointestinal tract (GIT) and, in the majority of cases, will be sufficient for assessing the maximum potential of a lipid-based formulation to improve drug absorption.

There are, however, a limited number of situations where lipidic formulations may provide advantage over and above that indicated by a food effect study. These include instances where specific components of a lipidic formulation, most commonly surfactants (which will not be present in a typical meal), may interfere with intestinal efflux or metabolism processes thereby improving oral bioavailability (11–18). It is also possible that the beneficial utility of food (or a lipidic formulation) in terms of stimulation of drug solubilization, may be masked by an opposing reduction of bioavailability resulting from a "negative" food–drug interaction, such as drug complexation with a food component. Conversely, for drugs subject to extensive hepatic first-pass metabolism, food may increase oral bioavailability via increased hepatic blood flow, a mechanism unlikely to be replicated by the use of a lipid-based formulation. Food has also been shown to alter the clearance and volume of distribution of highly lipophilic drugs, although the changes are typically not very large (78,79). Finally, a key consideration when assessing the utility of a lipid-based formulation is that of maximum drug-loading capacity. An indication of drug solubility in the lipids and surfactants being considered in the prototype formulation(s) is therefore an important early indicator of the feasibility of a lipid-based formulation approach.

Notwithstanding the aforementioned considerations, food effect data gives a quick and relatively facile first look at the potential utility of a lipid-based formulation, prior to expending resources on formulation development studies. In some instances, clinical data may be available (e.g., where the decision to explore alternative formulation approaches has arisen as a result of bioavailability problems encountered, or confirmed during the early phases of a clinical program). However, this will not often be the case, and an initial estimation of the likely impact of food (and potential utility of lipid-based formulations) should occur during preclinical development.

The most useful preclinical food effect data is likely to be obtained in non-rodent species since most small rodent species used in laboratory investigations will not typically eat on command, and generally consume a relatively low fat diet. Hence, food effect data is most readily generated in beagle dogs. There is a relatively small historical data base of food effect data in dogs, but in many cases the available data well reflects food effect data in humans. In some instances, however, food effects in dogs may be more pronounced that in humans due to the higher luminal bile salt concentrations in dogs (80), resulting in greater increases in postprandial solubilization and absorption. In our laboratory, the oral bioavailability of danazol, a poorly water-soluble steroid derivative, was increased approximately 7.5-fold in fed beagle dogs (50), whereas previous human data (81) demonstrated a more modest (three-fold) difference between pre- and postprandial administration (Fig. 1A). Similarly, the oral bioavailability of halofantrine, a lipophilic antimalarial, was increased 10-fold in fed beagle dogs (82) and only three-fold after postprandial administration to healthy human volunteers (Fig. 1C) (83). In the case of celecoxib, a poorly water-soluble nonsteroidal

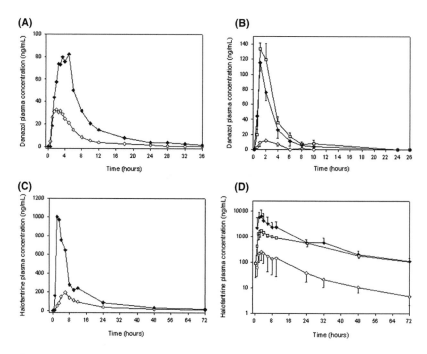

Figure 1 Examples of the ability of food effect studies in both humans and dogs to indicate the potential utility of lipid-based formulations. (**A**) Mean (n = 12) plasma profiles for danazol after oral administration of a commercial 100 mg danazol capsule to healthy volunteers after eight hours fasting (◇) or postprandially (◆). *Source*: From Ref. 81. (**B**) Plasma profiles (mean ± SE, n = 4) for danazol after oral administration of 15 mg of danazol as a powder-in-capsule formulation to beagle dogs after an overnight fast (◇) or postprandially (◆), or after administration of 15 mg of danazol in a self-microemulsifying formulation containing soybean oil, Maisine® 35-1 and Cremophor® EL (□). *Source*: From Ref. 50. (**C**) Mean (n = 6) plasma profiles for halofantrine (Hf) after oral administration of 250 mg Hf HCl as a simple tablet formulation to healthy volunteers after an overnight fast (◇) and postprandially (◆). *Source*: From Ref. 83. (**D**) Plasma profiles (mean ± SE, n = 4) for Hf after oral administration of 250 mg of Hf HCl as a simple tablet formulation to beagle dogs after an overnight fast (◇) or postprandially (◆) (*Source*: From Ref. 82) or after administration of 233 mg of Hf base (molar equivalent to 250 mg Hf HCl) in a self-emulsifying formulation containing peanut oil and Tagat® TO (surfactant) (□). *Source*: From Ref. 105.

anti-inflammatory, a similar trend was also reported where feeding increased oral bioavailability three-fold in the dog, but only marginally in humans (84). In this instance, however, these differences were ascribed to the lower drug dose administered to human subjects and also to the fact that intestinal transit times in humans are approximately twice as long as those in dog, thereby resulting in improved drug dissolution in the fasted state and a correspondingly lower impact of food on absorption.

Examples from the literature where positive food effect data has been indicative of the potential utility of lipid-based formulations include cyclosporine (79,85), saquinavir (86,87), and vitamin E (88–90), although in each case the relative impact of formulation components on solubility, permeability, and lymphatic transport are unclear. In our hands, the positive food effect data described above led to evaluation of the utility of lipid-based formulations for danazol and halofantrine (Fig. 1). In the case of danazol, the positive food effect was reflected in enhanced oral bioavailability after oral administration to dogs of a lipid-based microemulsion preconcentrate (50). However, the low solubility of danazol in the tested formulation precluded the development of a practical clinical formulation (Fig. 1B). Interestingly, the lipid formulation employed appeared capable of matching the bioavailability-enhancing effect of food, suggesting achievement of maximal bioavailability.

In the case of halofantrine, lipid-based formulations have been shown to enhance oral bioavailability (Fig. 1D) (91–93), and in general, lipid-based formulations incorporating excipients comprised of long chain FA substituents appear to be more effective than those comprised of short or medium chain FA. These effects appear to reflect advantages of long chain FA on both drug solubilization and lymphatic transport (49,93,94), but with either excipient class, enhanced bioavailability is predicted by the large positive food effect seen both clinically and preclinically.

Is Intestinal Lymphatic Transport a Factor in the Biopharmaceutical Profile of This Drug Candidate?

Although intestinal lymphatic transport may not contribute significantly to the overall transport of drug from the intestine to the systemic circulation for many currently marketed oral drug products, there are a number of highly lipophilic molecules, and an increasing number of newly discovered, candidate drug compounds for which lymphatic transport does play a significant role in drug transport following oral administration. From a drug development perspective, early information as to the possible role of lymphatic transport and its formulation dependence is important for several reasons. Firstly, drug transported lymphatically avoids hepatic first-pass metabolism and may lead to significant improvements in oral bioavailability for high hepatic extraction ratio drugs. A good example of this is the use of the highly lipophilic undecanoate ester of testosterone to promote intestinal lymphatic transport and improve delivery of testosterone to the systemic circulation. In this example, while the proportion of the testosterone undecanoate dose delivered systemically via the intestinal lymph is low (2–3%), recent studies from our group, in collaboration with colleagues at NV Organon, have shown that this accounts for greater than 80% of the systemically available testosterone (95). Thus, lymphatic transport of even a relatively modest proportion of the drug dose may be clinically relevant when hepatic first pass metabolism is significant (95). Secondly, if the proposed site of drug action is in the lymph (e.g., immunodulatory or antineoplastic agents), enhanced delivery to the lymphatics and exposure of the lymphatic capillaries to relatively high drug concentrations may be therapeutically advantageous. Finally, data from our laboratories and those of others have suggested that the clearance of drugs delivered to the systemic circulation associated with lymph chylomicrons may be different from that of the same drug absorbed via the portal blood (65,93). This has significant implications for the design and conduct of preclinical safety studies, particularly if the formulation used results in a different proportion of the absorbed drug dose being delivered lymphatically as compared to the clinical formulation. This may be especially pertinent for the highly lipophilic, poorly water-soluble compounds that are likely candidates for significant lymphatic transport, as these are often dissolved or suspended in lipids to achieve maximal exposures, and to facilitate identification of target organ toxicities and assignment of safety margins.

It should be clear that an early indication of whether lymphatic transport is likely to play a significant role in drug uptake is important. Recently, a number of animal models for estimating intestinal lymphatic drug transport [based on the original surgical preparation described in (99)] have been described and reviewed (93,96–98), and the majority of studies have been conducted either in rats or dogs. Drugs or drug candidates that are transported to the systemic circulation via the intestinal lymphatics are highly lipophilic, and possess very low aqueous solubilities. In order to assess the relative propensity for lymphatic transport, therefore, conditions and models should be sought, which first maximize drug absorption into the enterocyte and subsequently, enhance the fraction of the total amount absorbed that is transported into the intestinal lymph. Since postprandial administration often enhances absorption of lipophilic drugs and also provides a ready supply of lipids to drive chylomicron formation and intestinal lymphatic drug transport, coadministration with food may, in many cases, represent a simple means for overcoming luminal solubility and dissolution limitations to drug absorption. As described above, useful postprandial drug absorption data is most readily gathered in larger, nonrodent animal species and as such, our preference is to use a dog model to provide initial proof of concept data for intestinal lymphatic transport. The triple cannulated dog model has been described in detail in the literature (94,96) and has recently been applied to examine the lymphatic transport of halofantrine (71,94) (Fig. 2A), testosterone undecanoate (95), and several experimental drug candidates (100). Assuming that the quantity of dietary lipid is known, by monitoring TG levels in the lymph the efficiency of

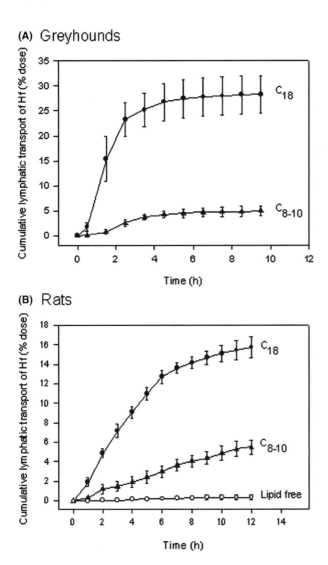

Figure 2 Lymphatic transport of halofantrine (Hf) after administration to greyhounds and rats in lipid-based formulations comprised of lipids with different fatty acid chain lengths. (**A**) Cumulative recovery (expressed as % Hf dose, mean ± SD, n = 3/4) of Hf in greyhound thoracic lymph after oral administration of 50 mg Hf in self-emulsifying formulations of Hf containing Cremophor® EL and either long chain lipids (●), or medium chain lipids (▲). *Source*: From Ref. 71. (**B**) Cumulative recovery (expressed as % Hf dose, mean ± SE, n = 4) of Hf in rat mesenteric lymph after oral administration of 2.5 mg Hf dissolved in long chain triglyceride lipid (●), medium chain triglyceride lipid (▲) or as a simple lipid-free aqueous suspension (□). *Source*: From Ref. 93.

lipid absorption and lymphatic transport can be readily monitored and used as a quality control indicator of the health and absorptive status of the test animal. This study design allows reasonably accurate assessment of the relative contribution of lymphatic transport to overall drug exposure, often with as little as two test animals. Practical considerations for this dog model, however, involve the relatively high study cost and procedural complexity, and the attendant ethical issues involved in conducting terminal studies in large animals. Consequently, screening studies examining the impact of various formulation approaches on the extent of lymphatic transport are most appropriately conducted in smaller species such as rats. However, data from these studies should be interpreted with care since methodologies employed for the study of lymphatic drug transport often differ between research groups, making cross-comparison of results difficult. The most common differences include the sites of lymph fistulation and exteriorization of the cannula (101), the extent of hydration and fasting/fed state of the animal subsequent to fistulation (102), whether the experiment is performed in conscious or anesthetized animals (62,63), and the site of drug/lipid administration (62). For example, we have previously examined the impact of anesthesia, degree of formulation dispersion and administration route on the lymphatic transport of halofantrine in rats (62,63). In anesthetized animals, where the drug was administered by intraduodenal infusion, a clear relationship was seen between formulation performance in vivo and the extent of lipid dispersion. Thus, the lymphatic transport of halofantrine increased from as low as 3.9% of the administered dose after administration of a simple lipid solution, to 11.8% after administration of an emulsion formulation, and finally to 17.7% after administration of a highly-dispersed, micellar formulation (63). In all cases, the type (2:1 molar mixture of oleic acid:glyceryl monooleate) and volume of lipid administered (50 µl) was identical. In contrast, when the same formulations were administered orally to conscious animals the dependence of absorption on lipid dispersion was not observed and the extent of lymphatic transport of halofantrine was similar for both the lipid and micellar solutions (19.1% and 20.0% respectively) (62). These data suggest that the reduction in intestinal processing inherent in anesthetized animals, coupled with intraduodenal administration of the formulation, allowed the degree of lipid dispersion to dictate the relative extent of drug absorption. Conversely, following oral administration to conscious animals, improved gastrointestinal processing of the lipid solution formulation most likely led to efficient in vivo lipid dispersion via bile salt/phospholipid mixed micelles, thereby lessening the influence of initial formulation dispersion on drug absorption.

Figure 2B illustrates how data generated in conscious rats can be used to screen for formulation-related changes in lymphatic transport, and that the rank order data are comparable to that obtained in dogs (Fig. 2A). In this example, the lymphatic transport of halofantrine after oral administration of a simple lipid-solution formulation to conscious rats was increased after administration as a medium chain lipid solution, when compared to a lipid-free suspension formulation (93). Considerably more lymphatic transport was seen, however, after administration of halofantrine formulated in a long chain (C_{18}) lipid solution vehicle. These data presumably reflect the resynthesis of long chain FA to TG within the enterocyte and subsequent transfer into chylomicrons, thereby providing a "lipid sink" into which the drug may partition. In contrast, medium chain lipids typically diffuse through the enterocyte and are absorbed into the portal blood, limiting the extent of lymphatic transport. Except in the case of liquid dosage forms, a limitation to the use of rats for screening the performance of prospective formulations is the inability to administer clinical dosage forms due to the size of the individual capsule or tablet dosage units. However, the data in Figure 2 suggest that the relative patterns of lymphatic transport seen in conscious rats are reflective of results obtained in dogs following administration of a clinical dosage unit (in this case soft gelatin encapsulated, self-emulsifying liquid formulations based on medium and long chain lipids) (71).

Which Lipid Based Formulation Is the Most Useful for This Drug Candidate?

Once it has been established that a lipid-based formulation is of potential value and following evaluation of the contribution of lymphatic transport to overall drug exposure, the next phase of development is identification of a commercializable formulation. These activities represent the most complex and costly phase of formulation development and therefore, have stimulated considerable interest in identifying rapid and relatively inexpensive in vitro methodologies for guiding formulation development. Whilst ourselves and others have had some recent successes with in vitro dissolution and dispersion tests and models of lipid digestion (46,47,49–53) as methods for optimizing lipid-based formulations, the complex dynamics of the interaction of these formulations with the gastrointestinal milieu mandates in vivo evaluation for clearly establishing proof-of-concept.

The complexities and costs of lymphatic surgery are such that the majority of formulation development studies, where an indication of intestinal lymphatic transport is required, are typically conducted in rats prior to final confirmatory studies in dogs (although initial proof-of-concept studies in dogs may replace those conducted in rats). However, for drugs where lymphatic transport is unlikely to play a significant role in bioavailability, the in vivo studies to support formulation development may be conducted in either rats or dogs. In this case, studies in rats provide time and cost savings, but the same complexities as those described before with reference to lymphatic transport studies, such as the impact of anesthesia, and method of administration are equally important when addressing absorption into the blood. A further consideration in interpreting the data from rat studies is that rat bile flow is continuous and thought to be independent of food intake, whereas in the dog, the presence of food or lipid in the GIT is required to stimulate gall bladder contraction and bile release, and the cascade of events that eventually lead to the digestion and absorption of lipids. While the constant stream of bile in the fasted rat may be sufficient to process a small quantity of formulation lipid, a mass of lipid larger than that commonly used in oral formulations may be required to stimulate optimal bile production and the related digestive events in dogs. Therefore, results obtained in the fasted rat may not always be mirrored in higher species, suggesting the need for evaluation of the clinical prototype formulation in the dog. The capacity to dose prototype clinical formulations and to examine the utility of this relatively small quantity of formulated lipid (on a mg dose/kg body weight basis) is a significant advantage of the dog model over smaller animals such as the rat, where clinical formulations are too large to be administered and the quantities of lipid that can practically be dosed is still relatively large. Thus a 50 μl dose of formulation to a 300 g rat provides the equivalent load to administration of more than 10 mL of lipid to a human. Particularly when assessing lipidic formulations, this final point becomes extremely important. It is becoming increasingly clear that the principle design criteria for efficient lipid-based formulations involve maintenance of the drug in solution. That may be as a simple lipid solution or as a dispersion of any of a number of colloidal particles, such as emulsion droplets, vesicles, micelles, or microemulsions. By so doing, drug dissolution as a barrier to absorption is reduced, thereby maximizing bioavailability. Under these circumstances, the degree of dilution that the formulation undergoes in the GIT and the quantity of lipid administered on a mg/kg basis can have a significant impact on drug solubilization/precipitation patterns. For example, we have recently shown that in the presence of a combination of bile salt, phospholipids, and relatively high concentrations of lipid digestion products derived from medium chain TG, a vesicular phase is formed, which has a very high solubilizing capacity for lipophilic drugs, including halofantrine and danazol (46,103). In contrast, at lower lipid concentrations a phase change occurs resulting in the production of a micellar system with significantly reduced solubilizing capacity (49,104). The estimation of absorption using in vivo models, which accurately reflect the likely relative luminal concentrations of drug and formulation-derived lipid is therefore of particular significance for lipid-based formulations, and will most accurately reflect drug absorption in humans.

SUMMARY

In summary, while advances in the in vitro assessment of lipid formulations have been made, few of these approaches are, as of yet, robustly predictive of performance in vivo. As such, in vivo assessment of lipid formulations still remains the mainstay by which decisive data can be generated. Under these circumstances, the key to efficient development of a useful formulation is to minimize the number of relatively costly and time-consuming preclinical in vivo studies that need to be conducted, to simplify those studies wherever possible, and to maximize the quantity and quality of information flowing from each study. In this chapter, we have described one strategic and stepwise approach to the in vivo evaluation of lipidic formulations, starting with proof-of-concept studies in postprandial dogs that suggest both the potential downstream utility of lipidic formulations, and the potential role of intestinal lymphatic transport in the drug absorption/transport pathway. These proof-of-concept studies are followed by early formulation development work and identification of appropriate lipidic excipients in either rats or dogs (conducted in parallel with in vitro solubility, dispersion, digestion, and stability studies), and finally confirmation that full size clinical formulations perform as predicted by early preclinical screens—the latter studies typically conducted in beagle dogs.

Integration of this preclinical information with knowledge of the basic biopharmaceutical (permeability and metabolism) and physicochemical (aqueous and lipid solubility, pKa, log P, etc.) properties of the drug candidate allows a measured and justifiable approach to be taken in the identification of a prototype clinical lipid-based formulation.

REFERENCES

1. Charman WN. Lipid vehicle and formulation effects on intestinal lymphatic drug transport. In: Charman WN, Stella VJ, eds. Lymphatic Transport of Drugs. Boca Raton: CRC Press, 1992:113–179.
2. Humberstone AJ, Charman WN. Lipid based vehicles for the oral delivery of poorly water soluble drugs. Adv Drug Deliv Rev 1997; 25:103–128.
3. Porter CJ, Charman WN. Lipid-based formulations for oral administration: opportunities for bioavailability enhancement and lipoprotein targeting of lipophilic drugs. J Recept Signal Transduct Res 2001; 21:215–257.
4. Porter CJ, Edwards GA, Charman SA. Lymphatic transport of proteins after s.c. injection: implications of animal model selection. Adv Drug Deliv Rev 2001; 50:157–171.
5. Porter CJ, Charman WN. Intestinal lymphatic drug transport: an update. Adv Drug Deliv Rev 2001; 50:61–80.
6. O'Driscoll CM. Lipid-based formulations for intestinal lymphatic delivery. Eur J Pharm Sci 2002; 15:405–415.
7. Anderberg EK, Lindmark T, Artursson P. Sodium caprate elicits dilatations in human intestinal tight junctions and enhances drug absorption by the paracellular route. Pharm Res 1993; 10:857–864.
8. Lindmark T, Nikkila T, Artursson P. Mechanisms of absorption enhancement by medium chain fatty acids in intestinal epithelial Caco-2 cell monolayers. J Pharmacol Exp Ther 1995; 275:958–964.
9. Lindmark T, Schipper N, Lazorova L, de Boer AG, Artursson P. Absorption enhancement in intestinal epithelial Caco-2 monolayers by sodium caprate: assessment of molecular weight dependence and demonstration of transport routes. J Drug Target 1998; 5:215–223.
10. Hunt JN, Knox MT. A relation between the chain length of fatty acids and the slowing of gastric emptying. J Physiol (Lond) 1968; 194:327–336.
11. Cornaire G, Woodley J, Hermann P, Cloarec A, Arellano C, Houin G. Impact of excipients on the absorption of P-glycoprotein substrates in vitro and in vivo. Int J Pharm 2004; 278:119–131.

12. Cornaire G, Woodley JF, Saivin S, et al. Effect of polyoxyl 35 castor oil and Polysorbate 80 on the intestinal absorption of digoxin in vitro. Arzneimittelforschung 2000; 50:576–579.

13. Hugger ED, Novak BL, Burton PS, Audus KL, Borchardt RT. A comparison of commonly used polyethoxylated pharmaceutical excipients on their ability to inhibit P-glycoprotein activity in vitro. J Pharm Sci 2002; 91:1991–2002.

14. Nerurkar MM, Ho NF, Burton PS, Vidmar TJ, Borchardt RT. Mechanistic roles of neutral surfactants on concurrent polarized and passive membrane transport of a model peptide in Caco-2 cells. J Pharm Sci 1997; 86:813–821.

15. Nerurkar MM, Burton PS, Borchardt RT. The use of surfactants to enhance the permeability of peptides through Caco-2 cells by inhibition of an apically polarized efflux system. Pharm Res 1996; 13:528–534.

16. Shono Y, Nishihara H, Matsuda Y, et al. Modulation of intestinal P-glycoprotein function by cremophor EL and other surfactants by an in vitro diffusion chamber method using the isolated rat intestinal membranes. J Pharm Sci 2004; 93:877–885.

17. Wacher VJ, Wong S, Wong HT. Peppermint oil enhances cyclosporine oral bioavailability in rats: comparison with D-alpha-tocopheryl poly(ethylene glycol 1000) succinate (TPGS) and ketoconazole. J Pharm Sci 2002; 91:77–90.

18. Batrakova EV, Han HY, Alakhov V, Miller DW, Kabanov AV. Effects of pluronic block copolymers on drug absorption in Caco-2 cell monolayers. Pharm Res 1998; 15:850–855.

19. Phan CT, Tso P. Intestinal lipid absorption and transport. Front Biosci 2001; 6:D299–D319.

20. Nordskog BK, Phan CT, Nutting DF, Tso P. An examination of the factors affecting intestinal lymphatic transport of dietary lipids. Adv Drug Deliv Rev 2001; 50:21–44.

21. Ros E. Intestinal absorption of triglyceride and cholesterol. Dietary and pharmacological inhibition to reduce cardiovascular risk. Atherosclerosis 2000; 151:357–379.

22. Nutting DF, Kumar NS, St Hilaire RJ, Mansbach CM, II. Nutrient absorption. Curr Opin Clin Nutr Metab Care 1999; 2:413–419.

23. Carey MC, Small DM, Bliss CM. Lipid digestion and absorption. Annu Rev Physiol 1983; 45:651–677.

24. Hernell O, Staggers JE, Carey MC. Physical-chemical behaviour of dietary and biliary lipids during intestinal digestion and absorption. 2. Phase analysis and aggregation states of luminal lipids during duodenal fat digestion in healthy adult human beings. Biochemistry 1990; 29:2041–2056.

25. Ladas SD, Isaacs PE, Murphy GM, Sladen GE. Comparison of the effects of medium and long chain triglyceride containing liquid meals on gall bladder and small intestinal function in normal man. Gut 1984; 25:405–411.

26. Borgstrom B, Hildebrand H. Lipase and co-lipase activities of human small intestinal contents after a liquid test meal. Scand J Gastroenterol 1975; 10:585–591.

27. Staggers JE, Hernell O, Stafford R.J, Carey MC. Physical-chemical behaviour of dietary and biliary lipids during intestinal digestion and absorption. 1. Phase behaviour and aggregation states of model lipid systems patterned after aqueous duodenal contents of healthy adult human beings. Biochemistry 1990; 29:2028–2040.

28. Hoffman NE. The relationship between uptake in vitro of oleic acid and micellar solubilization. Biochim Biophys Acta 1970; 196:193–203.

29. Simmonds WJ. The role of micellar solubilization in lipid absorption. Aust J Exp Biol Med Sci 1972; 50:403–421.
30. Shiau YF. Mechanism of intestinal fatty acid uptake in the rat: the role of an acidic microclimate. J Physiol 1990; 421:463–474.
31. Thomson AB, Schoeller C, Keelan M, Smith L, Clandinin MT. Lipid absorption: passing through the unstirred layers, brush-border membrane, and beyond. Can J Physiol Pharmacol 1993; 71:531–555.
32. Stremmel W. Uptake of fatty acids by jejunal mucosal cells is mediated by a fatty acid binding membrane protein. J Clin Invest 1988; 82:2001–2010.
33. Stremmel W, Lotz G, Strohmeyer G, Berk PD. Identification isolation and partial characterization of a fatty acid binding protein from rat jejunal microvillus membranes. J Clin Invest 1985; 75:1068–1076.
34. Poirier H, Degrace P, Niot I, Bernard A, Besnard P. Localization and regulation of the putative membrane fatty-acid transporter (FAT) in the small intestine. Comparison with fatty acid-binding proteins (FABP). Eur J Biochem 1996; 238:368–373.
35. Ockner RK, Manning JA. Fatty acid-binding protein in small intestine. Identification, isolation, and evidence for its role in cellular fatty acid transport. J Clin Invest 1974; 54:326–338.
36. Besnard P, Niot I, Poirier H, Clement L, Bernard A. New insights into the fatty acid-binding protein (FABP) family in the small intestine. Mol Cell Biochem 2002; 239:139–147.
37. Huang H, Starodub O, McIntosh A, Kier AB, Schroeder F. Liver fatty acid-binding protein targets fatty acids to the nucleus. Real time confocal and multiphoton fluorescence imaging in living cells. J Biol Chem 2002; 277:29139–29151.
38. McArthur MJ, Atshaves BP, Frolov A, Foxworth WD, Kier AB, Schroeder F. Cellular uptake and intracellular trafficking of long chain fatty acids. J Lipid Res 1999; 40:1371–1383.
39. Kiyasu JY, Bloom B, Chaikoff IL. The portal transport of absorbed fatty acids. J Biol Chem 1952; 199:415–419.
40. McDonald GB, Saunders DR, Weidman M, Fisher L. Portal venous transport of long-chain fatty acids absorbed from rat intestine. Am J Physiol 1980; 239:G141–G150.
41. McDonald GB, Weidman M. Partitioning of polar fatty acids into lymph and portal vein after intestinal absorption in the rat. Quart J Exp Physiol 1987; 72:153–159.
42. Mansbach CM, II, Dowell RF, Pritchett D. Portal transport of absorbed lipids in rats. Am J Physiol 1991; 261:G530–G538.
43. Swartz MA. The physiology of the lymphatic system. Adv Drug Deliv Rev 2001; 50:3–20.
44. O'Driscoll CM. Anatomy and Physiology of the lymphatics. In: Charman WN, Stella VJ, eds. Lymphatic Transport of Drugs. Boca Raton: CRC Press, 1992.
45. Porter CJH. Drug delivery to the lymphatic system. Criti Rev Ther Drug Carrier Syst 1997; 14:333–393.
46. Kaukonen AM, Boyd BJ, Porter CJ, Charman WN. Drug solubilization behavior during in vitro digestion of simple triglyceride lipid solution formulations. Pharm Res 2004; 21:245–253.

47. Kaukonen AM, Boyd BJ, Charman WN, Porter CJ. Drug solubilization behavior during in vitro digestion of suspension formulations of poorly water-soluble drugs in triglyceride lipids. Pharm Res 2004; 21:254–260.

48. Sek L, Porter CJ, Kaukonen AM, Charman WN. Evaluation of the in-vitro digestion profiles of long and medium chain glycerides and the phase behaviour of their lipolytic products. J Pharm Pharmacol 2002; 54:29–41.

49. Porter CJ, Kaukonen AM, Taillardat-Bertschinger A, et al. Use of in vitro lipid digestion data to explain the in vivo performance of triglyceride-based oral lipid formulations of poorly water-soluble drugs: studies with halofantrine. J Pharm Sci 2004; 93:1110–1121.

50. Porter CJH, Kaukonen AM, Boyd BJ, Edwards GA, Charman WN. Susceptibility to lipase-mediated digestion reduces the oral bioavailability of danazol after oral administration as a medium-chain lipid based microemulsion formulation. Pharm Res 2004; 21:1405–1412.

51. Porter CJ, Charman WN. In vitro assessment of oral lipid based formulations. Adv Drug Deliv Rev 2001; 50(suppl 1):S127–S147.

52. Zangenberg NH, Mullertz A, Kristensen HG, Hovgaard L. A dynamic in vitro lipolysis model. I. Controlling the rate of lipolysis by continuous addition of calcium. Eur J Pharm Sci 2001; 14:115–122.

53. Zangenberg NH, Mullertz A, Kristensen HG, Hovgaard L. A dynamic in vitro lipolysis model. II: Evaluation of the model. Eur J Pharm Sci 2001; 14:237–244.

54. Reymond JP, Sucker H. In vitro model for ciclosporin intestinal absorption in lipid vehicles. Pharm Res 1988; 5:673–676.

55. Pouton CW. Key issues when formulating hydrophobic drugs with lipids. Bulletin Technique Gattefosse 1999; 92:41–49.

56. Pouton CW. Lipid formulations for oral administration of drugs: non-emulsifying, self emulsifying and "self microemulsifying" drug delivery systems. Eur J Pharm Sci 2000; 11(suppl 2):S93–S98.

57. Ueda CT, Lemaire M, Gsell G, Nussbaumer K. Intestinal lymphatic absorption of cyclosporin A following oral administration in an olive oil solution in rats. Biopharm Drug Dispos 1983; 4:113–124.

58. Palin KJ, Wilson CJ. The effect of different oils on the absorption of probucol in the rat. J Pharm Pharmacol 1984; 36:641–643.

59. Ichihashi T, Kinoshita H, Yamada H. Absorption and disposition of epithiosteroids in rats (2): avoidance of first-pass metabolism of mepitiostane by lymphatic absorption. Xenobiotica 1991; 21:873–880.

60. Grimus RC, Schuster I. The role of the lymphatic transport in the enteral absorption of naftifine by the rat. Xenobiotica 1984; 14:287.

61. Myers RA, Stella VJ. Factors affecting the lymphatic transport of penclomedine (NSC-338720), a lipophilic cytotoxic drug: comparison to DDT and hexachlorobenzene. Int J Pharmaceut 1992; 80:51–62.

62. Porter CJH, Charman SA, Humberstone AJ, Charman WN. Lymphatic transport of halofantrine in the conscious rat when administered as either the free base or the hydrochloride salt: effect of lipid class and lipid vehicle dispersion. J Pharm Sci 1996; 85:357–361.

63. Porter CJH, Charman SA, Charman WN. Lymphatic transport of halofantrine in the triple-cannulated anesthetized rat model: effect of lipid vehicle dispersion. J Pharm Sci 1996; 85:351–356.

64. Hauss DJ, Fogal SE, Ficorilli JV, et al. Lipid-based delivery systems for improving the bioavailability and lymphatic transport of a poorly water-soluble LTB4 inhibitor. J Pharm Sci 1998; 87:164–169.
65. Hauss DJ, Mehta S, Radebaugh GW. Targeted lymphatic transport and modified systemic distribution of CI-976, a lipophilic lipid-regulator drug, via a formulation approach. Int J Pharmaceut 1994; 108:85–93.
66. Kwei GY, Novak LB, Hettrick LH, et al. Lymphatic uptake of MK-386, a sterol 5-alpha reductase inhibitor, from aqueous and lipid formulations. Int J Pharmaceut 1998; 164:37–44.
67. Sieber SM. The lymphocytic absorption of p,p'-DDT and some structurally-related compounds in the rat. Pharmacology 1976; 14:443–454.
68. Sieber SM, Cohn VH, Wynn WT. The entry of foreign compounds into the thoracic duct lymph of the rat. Xenobiotica 1974; 4:265–284.
69. Laher JM, Rigler MW, Vetter RD, Barrowman JA, Patton JS. Similar bioavailability and lymphatic transport of benzo(a)pyrene when administered to rats in different amounts of dietary fat. J Lipid Res 1984; 25:1337–1342.
70. Charman WN, Porter CJH. Lipophilic prodrugs designed for intestinal lymphatic transport. Adv Drug Deliv Rev 1996; 19:149–169.
71. Khoo SM, Shackleford DM, Porter CJ, Edwards GA, Charman WN. Intestinal lymphatic transport of halofantrine occurs after oral administration of a unit-dose lipid-based formulation to fasted dogs. Pharm Res 2003; 20:1460–1465.
72. Charman WN, Stella VJ. Estimating the maximal potential for intestinal lymphatic transport of lipophilic drug molecules. Int J Pharmaceut 1986; 34:175–178.
73. Khoo SM, Prankerd RJ, Edwards GA, Porter CJ, Charman WN. A physicochemical basis for the extensive intestinal lymphatic transport of a poorly lipid soluble antimalarial, halofantrine hydrochloride, after postprandial administration to dogs. J Pharm Sci 2002; 91:647–659.
74. Udata C, Patel J, Pal D, Hejchman E, Cushman M, Mitra AK. Enhanced transport of a novel anti-HIV agent cosalane and its congeners across human intestinal epithelial (Caco-2) cell monolayers. Int J Pharm 2003; 250:157–168.
75. Brown JR, Collett JH, Attwood D, Ley RW, Sims EE. Influence of monocaprin on the permeability of a diacidic drug BTA-243 across Caco-2 cell monolayers and everted gut sacs. Int J Pharm 2002; 245:133–142.
76. Meaney CM, O'Driscoll CM. A comparison of the permeation enhancement potential of simple bile salt and mixed bile salt:fatty acid micellar systems using the CaCo-2 cell culture model. Int J Pharm 2000; 207:21–30.
77. Amidon GL, Lennernas H, Shah VP, Crison JR. A theoretical basis for a biopharmaceutic drug classification: the correlation of in vitro drug product dissolution and in vivo bioavailability. Pharm Res 1995; 12:413–420.
78. Humberstone AJ, Porter CJ, Edwards GA, Charman WN. Association of halofantrine with postprandially derived plasma lipoproteins decreases its clearance relative to administration in the fasted state. J Pharm Sci 1998; 87:936–942.
79. Gupta SK, Manfro RC, Tomlanovich SJ, Gambertoglio JG, Garovoy MR, Benet LZ. Effect of food on the pharmacokinetics of cyclosporine in healthy subjects following oral and intravenous administration. J Clin Pharmacol 1990; 30:643–653.
80. Kostewicz ES, Carlsson AS, Hanish G, et al. Comparison of dog and human intestinal fluid and its impact on solubility estimations. Eur J Pharm Sci 2002; 17:S111.

81. Charman WN, Rogge MC, Boddy AW, Berger BM. Effect of food and a monoglyceride emulsion formulation on danazol bioavailability. J Clin Pharmacol 1993; 33:381–386.

82. Humberstone AJ, Porter CJ, Charman WN. A physicochemical basis for the effect of food on the absolute oral bioavailability of halofantrine. J Pharm Sci 1996; 85:525–529.

83. Milton KA, Edwards G, Ward SA, Orme ML, Breckenridge AM. Pharmacokinetics of halofantrine in man: effects of food and dose size. Br J Clin Pharmacol 1989; 28:71–77.

84. Paulson SK, Vaughn MB, Jessen SM, Lawal Y, Gresk CJ, Yan B, Maziasz TJ, Cook CS, Karim A. Pharmacokinetics of celecoxib after oral administration in dogs and humans: effect of food and site of absorption. J Pharmacol Exp Ther 2001; 297:638–645.

85. Vonderscher J, Meinzer A. Rationale for the development of Sandimmune Neoral Transplant Proc 1994; 26:2925–2927.

86. Perry CM, Noble S. Saquinavir soft-gel capsule formulation. A review of its use in patients with HIV infection. Drugs 1998; 55:461–486.

87. Hoffmann-La-Roche F. Fortovase (saquinavir) Soft Gelatin Capsules. Product Information. 2003.

88. Iuliano L, Micheletta F, Maranghi M, Frati G, Diczfalusy U, Violi F. Bioavailability of vitamin E as function of food intake in healthy subjects: effects on plasma peroxide-scavenging activity and cholesterol-oxidation products. Arterioscler Thromb Vasc Biol 2001; 21:E34–E37.

89. Julianto T, Yuen KH, Noor AM. Improved bioavailability of vitamin E with a self emulsifying formulation. Int J Pharm 2000; 200:53–57.

90. Barker SA, Yap SP, Yuen KH, McCoy CP, Murphy JR, Craig DQ. An investigation into the structure and bioavailability of alpha-tocopherol dispersions in Gelucire 44/14. J Control Release 2003; 91:477–488.

91. Khoo SM, Porter CJ, Charman WN. The formulation of Halofantrine as either non-solubilizing PEG6000 or solubilizing lipid based solid dispersions: physical stability and absolute bioavailability assessment. Int J Pharm 2000; 205:65–78.

92. Khoo SM, Humberstone AJ, Porter CJH, Edwards GA, Charman WN. Formulation design and bioavailability assessment of lipid-based self emulsifying formulations of halofantrine. Int J Pharm 1998; 167:155–164.

93. Caliph SM, Charman WN, Porter CJ. Effect of short-, medium-, and long-chain fatty acid-based vehicles on the absolute oral bioavailability and intestinal lymphatic transport of halofantrine and assessment of mass balance in lymph-cannulated and non-cannulated rats. J Pharm Sci 2000; 89:1073–1084.

94. Khoo SM, Edwards GA, Porter CJ, Charman WN. A conscious dog model for assessing the absorption, enterocyte-based metabolism, and intestinal lymphatic transport of halofantrine. J Pharm Sci 2001; 90:1599–1607.

95. Shackleford DM, Faassen WA, Houwing N, et al. Contribution of lymphatically transported testosterone undecanoate to the systemic exposure of testosterone after oral administration of two andriol formulations in conscious lymph duct-cannulated dogs. J Pharmacol Exp Ther 2003; 306:925–933.

96. Edwards GA, Porter CJ, Caliph SM, Khoo SM, Charman WN. Animal models for the study of intestinal lymphatic drug transport. Adv Drug Deliv Rev 2001; 50:45–60.

97. Hauss DJ, Fogal SE, Ficorilli JV. Chronic collection of mesenteric lymph from conscious, tethered rats. Contemp Topics Lab Animal Sci 1998; 37:56–58.

98. Boyd M, Risovic V, Jull P, Choo E, Wasan KM. A stepwise surgical procedure to investigate the lymphatic transport of lipid-based oral drug formulations: cannulation of the mesenteric and thoracic lymph ducts within the rat. J Pharmacol Toxicol Methods 2004; 49:115–120.

99. Bollman JL, Cava JC, Grindley JH. Techniques for the collection of lymph from the liver. small intestine and thoracic duct of the rat. J Lab Clin Med 1948; 33:1349.

100. Shackleford DM, Porter CJH, Charman WN. Lymphatic absorption of orally-administered prodrugs. In prodrugs: Challanges and rewards. Stella VJ, Borchardt RT, Hageman MJ, Oliyai R, Tilley JW, Magg H. eds. Washington DC: AAPS Press, 2007:653–682.

101. Noguchi T, Charman WNA, Stella VJ. Lymphatic appearance of DDT in thoracic or mesenteric lymph duct cannulated rats. Int J Pharmaceut 1985; 24:185–192.

102. Charman WN, Noguchi T, Stella VJ. An experimental system designed to study the in situ intestinal lymphatic transport of drugs in anaesthetized rats. Int J Pharmaceut 1986; 33:155.

103. Kossena GA, Boyd BJ, Porter CJ, Charman WN. Separation and characterization of the colloidal phases produced on digestion of common formulation lipids and assessment of their impact on the apparent solubility of selected poorly water-soluble drugs. J Pharm Sci 2003; 92:634–648.

104. Kossena GA, Charman WN, Boyd BJ, Dunstan DE, Porter CJ. Probing drug solubilization patterns in the gastrointestinal tract after administration of lipid-based delivery systems: a phase diagram approach. J Pharm Sci 2004; 93:332–348.

105. Humberstone AJ. Physicochemical and biological factors which impact on the bioavailability and pharmacokinetics of halofantrine. PhD Thesis, Monash University, Australia, 1996.

9

Physiological Processes Governing the Gastrointestinal Absorption of Lipids and Lipophilic Xenobiotics

Rachna Gajjar, Chun-Min Lo, and Patrick Tso

Department of Pathology, University of Cincinnati Medical Center, Cincinnati, Ohio, U.S.A.

INTRODUCTION

The transport of orally-administered lipophilic drugs and xenobiotics into the systemic circulation relies, at least partially, on association with intestinal chylomicrons (CM) followed by lymphatic transport to the venous blood supply. This review discusses the digestion, uptake, and transport of dietary lipids by both passive and active processes, the role of bile salts in the solubilization of lipid digestion products and the impact these processes have on the absorption of lipophilic drugs and xenobiotics by the gastrointestinal tract. Finally, the intracellular trafficking and the resynthesis of complex lipids from lipid digestion products are explored, and the formation and secretion of CM are described. This chapter is intended to complement the discussion appearing elsewhere in this book describing the use of preclinical data to guide formulation development strategies for poorly water-soluble drugs.

TYPES OF DIETARY LIPIDS

In order to understand how fat absorption may affect the coincident absorption of drugs and xenobiotics by the gastrointestinal tract, we must first have a thorough understanding of the processes involved in the digestion, uptake, intracellular metabolism, and packaging of dietary lipids into CM which are the major lipoprotein particles carrying lipophilic compounds to the systemic circulation. As will become evident, the processes involved are complex and physiologically regulated. This review will include a thorough discussion on the possible role of intestinal brush border membrane lipid transporters in the uptake of lipids by the enterocytes, the physiological processes governing the formation and secretion of CMs into the lymphatic system and how these processes can be manipulated to control lymphatc drug uptake. We will also discuss the exciting findings by two independent research groups on the ABCG5 and ABCG8 (1,2) which are involved in the rare human genetic disorder of sitosterolemia and how they may play a role in the absorption of cholesterol and other lipophilic compounds. Readers interested in learning more about cholesterol absorption are referred to the excellent reviews by Dawson and Rudel (1) and the more recent review by Lammert and Wang (3).

Dietary fat can be defined as the part of the diet that can be extracted by organic solvents (2). Consequently, dietary fat is comprised of a wide array of compounds ranging from the nonpolar hydrocarbons to the relatively polar phospholipids (PL) and glycolipids. The classification of these various lipids and their behavior in an aqueous system have been clearly reviewed by Carey and Small (4). A lipid is classified as polar or nonpolar based on its interaction with water. Nonpolar lipids are insoluble in the bulk water phase and therefore will not interact with water (Fig. 1). Examples of nonpolar lipids include triglyceride, cholesteryl esters (CE), hydrocarbons, some xenobiotics, and carotene. The polar lipids can be classified into three categories: (I) insoluble nonswelling amphiphiles, (II) insoluble swelling amphiphiles, and (III) soluble amphiphiles. The class I insoluble nonswelling amphiphiles, which do not interact with water, include triacylglycerol (TG), diacylglycerol (DG), nonionized long-chain fatty acids (FA), cholesterol, and fat-soluble vitamins. When added to water, these water insoluble amphiphiles rise to the surface to form a lipid monolayer at the air-water interface. The class II lipids, or the insoluble swelling amphiphiles, include monoacylglycerols (MG), ionized FAs, and PLs. In addition to forming a monolayer on the surface of water, this group of lipids has the unique ability to interact with water to form a laminated, lipid–water structure known as a liquid crystal. In the liquid crystalline state, the polar and nonpolar portions of these amphiphilic molecules self-associate, thereby creating separate, ordered hydrophobic, and hydrophilic environments, the latter of which associate with water molecules from the bulk solution phase. This unique association of lipid and water is referred as "swelling," hence the classification of "swelling amphiphiles."

The class III lipid molecules, or the "soluble swelling amphiphiles," possess relatively strong polar groups that render these molecules soluble in water at low concentrations. The soluble swelling amphiphiles can be further sub-divided based on their propensity for lyotropic mesomorphism; when the aqueous

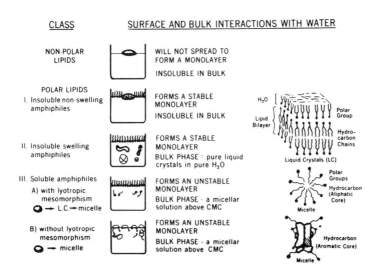

Figure 1 Classification of lipids based on their ability to interact with water. Nonpolar lipids: octadecane, carotene, squalene, cholesteryl oleate, cholesteryl linoleate, and paraffin oil. Polar lipids: (I) TGs, DGs, long-chain protonated fatty acids, and fat-soluble vitamins. (II) PLs, MGs, monoethers, and alpha-hydroxy fatty acids. (IIIA) Sodium salts of long-chain fatty acids, many anionic, cationic and nonionic detergents, and lysophosphatidylcholine. (IIIB) Bile salts, sulfated bile alcohols, and saponins. *Abbreviations*: DGs, diacylglycerols; MG, monoglycerols; PL, phospholipids; TG, triglycerols. *Source*: From Ref. 3.

concentration of these lipids approaches the critical micellar concentration, the monomers aggregate to form the liquid crystalline state prior to forming micelles. Sodium salts of long-chain FAs (e.g., sodium oleate) are examples of soluble swelling amphiphiles possessing lyotropic mesomorphism. Bile salts are examples of soluble swelling amphiphiles not possessing lyotropic mesomorphism; as such, they form micelles directly without passing through an intermediate, liquid crystalline state.

The recommended maximum daily amount of dietary fat consumption has been reduced over the years, and currently the USDA/HHS Dietary Guidelines recommend a diet that provides 30% or less of its total energy from fat and less than 10% of this energy from saturated FAs. The American Heart Association has also adopted this standard. These guidelines apply to individuals two years of age and older. Dietary fat constitutes a significant source of calories in the Western diet—as much as 30% of total caloric intake, or 90 to 100 g per day. Dietary intake of fat has received considerable attention in the last few decades since diets high in fat have been linked to high blood lipids, especially cholesterol and increased risk of coronary heart disease (5–7). It is generally accepted that diets rich in saturated FAs are more cholesterolemic (raising blood cholesterol) than diets rich in polyunsaturated

FAs (8). Trans-FAs, which have double bonds, behave more like saturated FAs and are considered to be just as atherogenic as saturated fat (9,10).

Over the past decade, there has been an increased effort to modify the FA profile of naturally occurring TGs in order to obtain a particular physical property or to influence a specific physiological function. This topic has been ably reviewed by Heird et al. (11), Bell et al. (12), and more recently by Chan et al. (13). These chemically modified TGs, also called structured triglycerides (STG), are produced by the selective esterification of both medium- and long-chain FAs on the TG glycerol backbone (14–19). From a drug delivery perspective, STGs that contain medium-chain FAs may facilitate rapid hydrolysis and absorption because of their smaller molecular size and greater water solubility as compared to long-chain TGs. Tso et al. (20) demonstrated that STGs promote greater lymphatic absorption of the vitamins A and E than a constituent physical mixture of similar FA composition. One interesting observation of this study was that the enhanced delivery of the vitamins A and E into lymph by STGs occurred in animals with normal gastrointestinal function as well as those in which gastrointestinal absorptive functions had been experimentally imparied by ischemia/reperfusion-induced injury. On this basis, Tso et al. (20) proposed that STGs can also be potentially used as a vehicle to enhance the lymphatic absorption of lipid soluble drugs. This possibility certainly warrants further investigation.

LUMINAL DIGESTION OF DIETARY LIPIDS

Gastric Lumen

Digestion of dietary lipids is initiated in the stomach by acid lipase, which is secreted by the gastric mucosa. The distribution of gastric lipase in different parts of the human stomach is shown in Figure 2 (21). The highest gastric lipase activity is detected in the fundus of the stomach, a finding that has been confirmed by an independent study conducted during the postmortem examination of two healthy human subjects (22). Human gastric lipase has a pH optimum

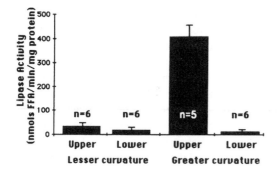

Figure 2 Localization of lipase in the human stomach—the level of lipolytic activity in the gastric mucosa of four sampling sites. *Source*: From Ref. 18.

ranging from 3.0 to 6.0 (21,23), and it exerts greater hydrolytic activity on medium-chain TGs as compared to long-chain TGs (24), yielding diglycerides and free FA as its primarly hydrolytic products (21,23,25); gastric lipase does not hydrolyze either PL or CE. Human gastric lipase has been cloned and found to contain 379 amino acid residues (26) and shows considerable sequence homology (78%) with rat lingual lipase (27) but minimal homology with pancreatic lipase from this species.

The digestion of TG by gastric lipase in the stomach plays an important role in lipid digestion, particularly in neonates, in whom the pancreatic lipase system is not fully functional (28). Milk fat, the primary source of nourishment for neonates, contains considerable medium-chain TG, and acid lipases work more efficiently with medium-chain TG than with long-chain TG.

Gastric lipases also play an important role in lipid digestion in adults. This is evident in patients with cystic fibrosis, who maintain their ability to absorb dietary lipid even though pancreatic lipase secretion is markedly or completely inhibited (29,30). Carriere et al. (31) demonstrated that although the gastric lipase activity observed is lower in vivo, it was sufficient to initiate the digestion of a significant portion of the ingested TG.

Preliminary emulsification of dietary fat in the stomach is an important prerequisite for the subsequent efficient hydrolysis by pancreatic lipase. The grinding action of the antrum, the retropulsion of antral contents back to the corpus and the controlled ejection of the antral contents into the duodenum provides most of the mechanical energy required for the initial emulsification of dietary TG. As shown in Figure 3, gastric chyme is propelled forward through the

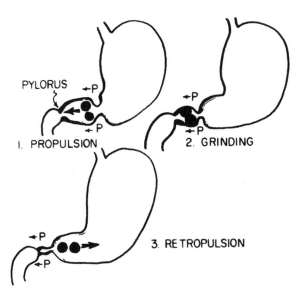

Figure 3 Diagrammatic representation of the consequences of antral peristalsis. *Source*: From Ref. 256.

antrum of the stomach, via the peristaltic waves of the corpus, to the pylorus, which controls the forceful ejection of liquid and small particles in the chyme into the duodenum. These contractions also cause repeated retropulsion of the unejected gastric contents from the the terminal antrum back into the corpus for further mixing and emulsification. The DG and FA that result from the action of acid lipases in the stomach and the PL that is normally present in the diet further aid in the subsequent, further emulsification of dietary fat.

Intestinal Lumen

The nascent, crude lipid emulsion formed in the stomach enters the small intestine as fine lipid droplets less than 0.5 mm in diameter (32,33). In the presence of bile, TG digestion occurs primarily through the action of pancreatic lipase, which acts at the interface between the oil and aqueous phases in the proximal portions of the small intestinal lumen (34–37).

Pancreatic lipase (EC 3.1.1.3) is abundantly present in pancreatic juice and its relatively high activity and concentration (approximately 2–3% of the total protein present in this secretion) ensures efficient digestion of dietary fat (49). Consequently, only very severe pancreatic deficiency results in fat malabsorption. The enzyme preferentially hydrolyzes the sn-1 and sn-3 positions of the TG molecule to yield 2-MG and FA (42,44–46). Although 2-MG can isomerize to form 1-MG in aqueous media, this process is slow relative to the rate of 2-MG absorption and thus, 2-MG is likely the predominant form in which MG is absorbed (47). Further hydrolysis of the 1- or 2-MG by pancreatic lipase results in the formation of glycerol and FA (48). Pancreatic lipase has been purified from a number of species, including humans (50–53). Porcine pancreatic lipase, which has been sequenced, is a glycoprotein of 449 amino acid residues (54) possessing a carbohydrate chain of approximately 2000 Daltons that is attached to an asparagine residue at position 166 of the protein (55,56). In order to manifest lipid hydrolytic activity, pancreatic lipase must first attach to the lipid droplet at the oil/water interface by a process which appears to be mediated by the serine residue at position 152 of the protein (57). Purification of pancreatic lipase from native pancreatic secretions dramatically reduces its lipolytic activity in bile salt–lipid mixtures. This interesting observation led to the discovery of colipase, which, Morgan et al. demonstrated in 1969 to be necessary for elicitation of the lipolytic activity of pancreatic lipase in the presence of bile salts (58). The surface of emulsified TG lipid droplets are highly enriched in bile salt molecules which sterically hinder the attachment of pancreatic lipase. However, the binding of colipase to the TG/aqueous interface provides a binding site allowing for the efficient secondary binding of pancreatic lipase in a 1:1 ratio with colipase, thereby allowing lipolysis to proceed (64). Most of our current understanding of the biochemistry of colipase and its interaction with pancreatic lipase comes from the laboratories of Professor Borgstrom in Lund, Belgium and Professor Desnuelle in Marseille, France. Colipase has been purified from a number of animal species

(59–62) and the mechanism by which pancreatic lipase hydrolyzes lipid is discussed in detail by Erlanson-Albertsson (63).

Monolayer technique, so elegantly championed by Verger (38), has greatly advanced our understanding of how the oil/water interface affects lipolysis. Using this technique, the lipid under study is spread as a monomolecular film at the air/water interface. This allows the investigtor to study the effects of the physico-chemical properties of the lipid-water interface, as well as the relative lipid surface area, on the rate of lipolysis. Only a small amount of lipid is required for study using the monolayer technique, an obvious advantage when studying rare synthetic lipids. A disadvantage of this technique, however, is that the lipolytic enzymes tend to denature at the lipid/water interface, thereby creating in vitro conditions that are not necessarily reflective of the actual conditions in the small intestine in vivo (39,40). Despite this potential limitation, the monolayer technique has greatly advanced our understanding of lipid digestion by pancreatic lipase (41–43).

Digestion of Phospholipids

The digestion of PL occurs primarily in the small intestine, as gastric lipase (secreted in the stomach) is incapable of digesting PL. Over 90% of the PL occuring in bile is phosphatidylcholine (PC) which distributes between bile-cholesterol mixed micelles and TG droplets, favoring the mixed-micellar phase over the TG oil phase (65). PC is then hydrolyzed by pancreatic phospholipase A_2 (PLA_2) (EC 3.1.1.4) at the sn-2 position, yielding one molecule each of a FA and lysophosphatidylcholine (LPC) (66,67). Some phospholipase A_1 (PLA_1) activity in pancreatic juice is probably due to pancreatic lipase (68). Pancreatic PLA_2 possesses a molecular weight of approximately 14 kDa and is secreted as an anionic zymogen which is activated by tryptic cleavage of an N-terminal heptapeptide (69,70,82) in the presence of calcium (71,72) and bile salts (73). It possesses multiple isoforms (74,75) and apparently requires a 2:1 bile salt to PC molar ratio for optimal activity (76). PLA_2 is heat stable and manifests maximum lipoloytic acitivity at pH 8 to 9 (73).

PLA_2 from porcine, canine, and human species has been sequenced (77–80). Richmond and Hui (81) described the genomic organization of the PLA_2 gene in the mouse and demonstrated high sequence homology for this enzyme in the mouse, rat, dog, and human. Although the bulk of intestinal PLA_2 activity is derived from pancreatic secretions, there is probably some contribution from the intestinal mucosa (83), where the enzyme is known to be concentrated in the brush border. Tojo et al. (84,85) reported the presence of another lipolytic enzyme, phospholipase B/lipase (PLB/LIP), in the jejunal brush border membrane. This interesting enzyme contains four tandem homologous domains and a carboxyl terminal membrane binding domain (86). The activity of the enzyme is located in domain 2 of the tandem repeats and contains PLA_2, lysophospholipase, and lipase activities. Although the biochemical characterization of this enzyme is quite complete, its physiological function is not clear.

Digestion of Cholesteryl Ester

The bulk of dietary cholesterol intake occurs as the absorbable, free sterol form, with only 10% to 15% occurring as CE, which must first be hydrolyzed to free cholesterol prior to absorption (87). Pancreatic cholesterol esterase (3.1.1.13), also known as carboxylic ester hydrolase or sterol ester hydrolase, has been purified from porcine (88,89), rat (90), and human pancreas (91,92) and rat, bovine, and human pancreatic cholesterol esterases have been cloned (93–95). Human and rat cholesterol esterases have molecular weights of about 100 kDa and 70 kDa, respectively, and share 78% structural homology (90,91). Using site-directed mutagenesis, DiPersio et al. (96) demonstrated that substitution of threonine or alanine for serine at position 194 in rat cholesterol esterase abolished enzymatic activity. Using a similar approach, DiPersio et al. (97) further demonstrated that, in addition to serine, histidine in position 435 and aspartic acid (98) at position 320 formed a triad of amino acids comprising the catalytic site of this enzyme.

Human cholesterol esterase can hydrolyze CEs as well and phosphoglycerides but has little activity against mono-, di-, or triglycerides (99). Its enzymatic activity is greatly enhanced in the presence of bile salts, particularly trihydroxy bile salts such as sodium cholate, which promote self-association of the enzyme into dimers and tetramers (90,92) thereby protecting it from proteolytic inactivation.

MICELLAR SOLUBILIZATION AND UPTAKE OF DIETARY LIPIDS BY ENTEROCYTES

Much of our current understanding of the role of micellar solubilization in the gastrointestinal absorption of dietary lipids and their digestion products comes from the work of Hofmann and Borgstrom (100,101). This concept was subsequently modified by Carey et al. (33), who discovered the coexistence of unilamellar liposomes, which also played a role in lipid absorption in the small intestine. The relative importance of these different vehicles in facilitating the uptake of lipids by the enterocytes will be discussed in the following section. While the uptake of lipid digestion products by enterocytes has been generally accepted to occur via a passive process, a number of different investigators have provided evidence that the absorption of cetrain lipids may occur via an energy-dependent, carrier-mediated process.

Importance of Micellar Solubilization

Understanding the role of micellar solubilization in the uptake of 2-MG and FA by enterocytes also requires an understanding of the intestinal unstirred water layer (UWL), a concept first introduced by Dietschy et al. (102–104). As illustrated in Figure 4, the UWL, which mixes poorly with the bulk fluid phase in the intestinal lumen, forms a hydrophilic barrier through which solutes must pass in order to gain access to the intestinal brush border membrane. Because the solubility of FA

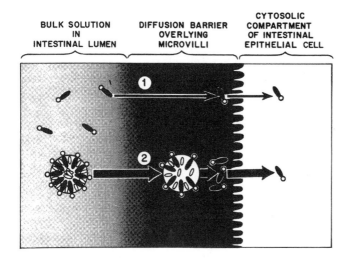

Figure 4 Diagrammatic representation of the effect of bile salt micelles (or vesicles) in overcoming the diffusion barrier resistance by the unstirred water layer. In the absence of bile acids, individual lipid molecules must diffuse across the barriers overlying the microvillus border of the intestinal epithelial cells (*arrow 1*). Hence, uptake of these molecules is largely diffusion limited. In the presence of bile acids (*arrow 2*), large amounts of these lipid molecules are delivered directly to the aqueous-membrane interface so that the rate of uptake is greatly enhanced. *Source*: From Ref. 97.

and MG in aqueous media is extremely low, very few of these molecules are able to penetrate the UWL unaided (Fig. 4, arrow 1). Micellar solubilization, by greatly increasing the aqueous solubility of FA and MG, promotes the diffusion of these substances across the UWL allowing contact with the brush border membrane and subsequent absorption by the enterocytes (Fig. 4, arrow 2).

Although bile salt mixed-micellar solubilization plays a central role in lipid absorption, the mechanism(s) by which bile salts facilitate the uptake of lipid soluble molecules and drugs by the small intestine may extend beyond their detergent properties. For instance, several investigators have reported that trihydroxy bile acids are more effective in promoting cholesterol absorption than dihydroxy bile acids; however, the degree of solubilization was not measured in these experiments (105–107). Watt and Simmonds (107) elegantly demonstrated the importance of micellar solubilization by bile salts in the uptake of cholesterol by the small intestine by showing that a linear relationship exists between the amount of absorbed cholesterol and the micellar cholesterol concentration. Their study demonstrated that cholesterol uptake by enterocytes is dependent on the specific planar structure of the bile acid by using Pluronic F-68, a nonionic surfactant with different molecular geometry that promotes the micellar solubilization of cholesterol (but not its uptake by enterocytes). A particularly important finding in this study was that the degree of nonspecific binding of cholesterol to silicone tubing was similar for micellar solutions of cholesterol, solubilized with either Pluronic F-68 or bile acids. This suggests that intestinal cholesterol absorption is an active process, possibly mediated by a transporter, and supports an earlier finding by Sylven (111), that both cholesterol and beta-sitosterol (plant sterol) are present in the human diet but that cholesterol, unlike beta-sitosterol, is well absorbed by the small intestine. Sylven found that the ability of the small intestine to discriminate between cholesterol and beta-sitosterol absorption is energy-dependent and compromised by deprivation of blood supply (111). The possibility that lipid transporters are present at the brush border membrane is further suggested in patients with beta-sitosterolemia, a condition where the intestine fails to discriminate between cholesterol and beta-sitosterol (112–114). This topic will be discussed in detail later in this chapter.

The dependence of cholesterol absorption on bile salt structure is further illustrated by the fact that chenodeoxycholyl taurine (CDC-tau), which is a better micellar solubilizer of cholesterol than cholyl taurine (C-tau), results in poorer cholesterol uptake than C-tau (108–110). Despite the knowledge gained from these studies and others, the manner in which bile salt structure affects its ability to promote the absorption of cholesterol and other lipid soluble drugs and xenobiotics is far from being clear.

Importance of Unilamellar Vesicles

When human jejunal contents obtained during digestion of a lipid meal were ultracentrifuged, three distinct layers were isolated and included a solid pellet at the bottom of the tube on which was layered an intermediate, micellar solution phase topped by an oily layer (101). The oily layer was found to consist primarily of TG, partial glycerides, and FAs; the intermediate micellar solution layer consisted of bile salts, FAs, and MGs; and the pellet was composed primarily of calcium salts of FAs (soaps). When Porter and Saunders (115) carefully compared the micellar solution phase obtained after ultracentrifugation of intestinal contents to that prepared by passing the unprocessed intestinal contents through a series of filters with progressively smaller pores (the smallest being 100 nm in diameter), mild turbidity was noted, regardless of the method of preparation; in addition, these investigators noted the existence of a lipid concentration gradient in these samples. The importance of these observations was not fully realized until subsequent studies of in vitro fat digestion, conducted under light microscopy by Patton and Carey (116), identified the existence of a "viscous isotropic phase" within the micellar solution phase, which consisted of a liquid crystalline mixture of MG and FA. Thus, in addition to disc-shaped, bile salt mixed micelles, the aqueous phase may contain liquid crystalline vesicles (121). However, Carey et al. (33) proposed that when lumenal bile salt concentrations exceed the critical micellar concentration, lipid digestion products are incorporated into lipid-saturated, disc-like mixed micelles with a hydrodynamic radius of approximately 200 Å in size. However, when the amount of lipid in the aqueous phase increases further, formation of liquid crystalline vesicles (liposomes) with a hydrodynamic radius of 400 to 600 Å occurs, a process which does not require bile (33,117). This finding may explain the reasonably good fat absorption seen in patients with low intraluminal bile salt concentration (118) or in patiens with bile fistulae (119). Thus, Carey et al. (33) proposed that the liquid crystalline vesicles play an important role in the uptake of FA and MG by enterocytes in these diseased states. Though it is generally assumed that absorption of highly lipophilic drug occurs solely through micellar solubilization, the possibility that liquid crystalline vesicles may also play a role in promoting the absorption of these drugs cannot be ruled out.

Because liquid crystalline vesicles and mixed micelles coexist in the small intestinal lumen and constantly exchange MG, FA, and bile salt molecules, their relative roles in the uptake of FA and MG was unresolved for quite some time. A recent investigation by Heubi et al. (120) using a combination of human and lymph fistula rat studies has clearly demonstrated that the absorption of FA can be mediated by bile salt–lipid vesicles but that the absorption of cholesterol is mediated solely by micelles.

Shoemaker and Nichols (122) observed that bile salts and lysophospholipids form submicellar aggregates. These submicellar aggregates coexist with artificial PL vesicles in an aqueous medium. Shortly thereafter, these investigators provided convincing evidence that these submicellar aggregates serve as an efficient shuttle mechanism for the transfer of lysophospholipids between membranes (123). The existence of these submicellar aggregates in the intestinal lumen and their role in delivering lysophospholipids as well as lipid soluble molecules and drugs to enterocytes for absorption remains to be explored.

Intestinal epithelial cells have an apical brush border membrane made up of many microvilli which impacts the uptake of lipid digestion products and lipophilic drugs. For example, the microvilli of the intestinal epithelial cells have a width of about 100 nm. The space between the microvilli is much smaller, ranging between 5 to 20 nm. Thus, to access the space between the microvilli, lipid carrying vehicles cannot be larger than the width of the gaps themselves. Consequently, the lipid vesicles and nanoparticles that are commonly used to transport drugs into the gastrointestinal tract are probably not able to enter the space between the microvilli. However, submicellar and micellar particles are able to penetrate the gap thereby facilitating the uptake and transfer of lipid soluble molecules from the vesicles to the membrane of the microvilli, implicating the inportant interaction that must occur between a lipid-based formulation the the endogenous lipid handling system in order for efficient drug absorption to occur.

MUCOSAL BRUSH BORDER MEMBRANE LIPID TRANSPORTERS

It has been generally accepted that FA and MG are absorbed by enterocytes via passive diffusion (124,125). This hypothesis was first challenged by Chow and

Hollander, who demonstrated that linoleate uptake by the small intestine is concentration-dependent, occuring via a carrier-mediated process at low concentration but predominantly by passive diffusion at high concentrations (127). Similar concentration-dependent absorption kinetics were found to apply to the intestinal absorption of the fat-soluble vitamin A, whereas the intestinal uptake of vitamins D and E and carotene occur by strictly passive processes (128).

Studies by Stremmel (126,129) suggested the existence of an intestinal brush border membrane FA-binding protein (FABP) that plays an apparent role in the uptake of FA by enterocytes. This FABP, which is predominantly localized in the apical and lateral areas of the villus membrane in the regions of the tight junction and crypt, is also capable of transporting cholesterol, but not CE, and it was shown that pretreatment of a jejunal loop with an anti-FABP antibody significantly reduced cholesterol uptake (129). Consequently, this FABP appears to be a plausible candidate as a transporter for not only cholesterol, but a whole array of lipophilic molecules, including drugs. This hypothesis have been challenged for two reasons: firstly, this transporter was subsequently demonstrated to be similar to mitochondrial glutamic oxaloacetic transaminase, which is not involved in lipid absorption (130); secondly, crypt cells, which are not involved in fat absorption, express this FABP.

More recent work has confirmed the presence of FA transporters in the intestinal brush border membrane, the expression of which appears to be the highest in the jejunum, followed by the duodenum and the ileum. Furthermore, a diet rich in long-chain, but not medium-chain, FAs results in increased transporter expression (144). Interested readers are referred to a review on this subject by Abumrad et al. (145).

Other lipid-binding proteins have been identified, including GP330 (also called megalin), CD36, SR-BI, caveolin, and more recently, the FATP4 (131). GP330 is a member of the low-density lipoprotein receptor gene family and is an endocytic receptor expressed in many absorptive epithelia, including the kidney proximal tubules, Type II pneumocytes, mammary epithelium, and thyroid follicular cells (132). It has been demonstrated that GP330 is involved in the renal uptake of polybasic drugs (132–134), vitamin B_{12} (134), cholesterol carrying lipoproteins (135), albumin (136), and proteases (133). Whether GP330 is expressed in the intestine is still uncertain (132).

Other potential FA transporters have been identified. Schaffer and Lodish (146) cloned a long-chain FA in adipocytes. Stahl et al. (131,147) identified the presence of FATP4, a member of the large family of FA transport proteins, in the small intestine. This finding was initially confirmed by Hermann et al. (148) who subsequently found that both FATP1 and FATP4 to be constituents of acyl-CoA synthetase, with substrate specificity for very long-chain FA (149). Caveolin, the first reported protein associated with caveolae, is another protein that binds cholesterol (150). Caveolae are nonclathrin-coated invaginations present on the surface of cells and are enriched with glycolipids (151), cholesterol (152), glycosyl-phosphatidylinositol-linked proteins (153), and other proteins involved in potocytosis (154). It is currently unknown if caveolin plays a role in the intestinal absorption of cholesterol, FAs, or lipid soluble drugs.

Several studies have reported that cholesterol absorption by the small intestine is regulated by the adenosine triphosphate (ATP)-binding casette-1 (ABC-1), a reverse cholesterol transporter (155). If, indeed, ABC transporters are reverse cholesterol transporters, are they as efficient in reversing intestinal cholesterol transport as plant sterols? Are ABC transporters involved in the reverse transport of other lipid soluble compounds such as lipid soluble drugs? Will the physiological and therapeutic manipulation of ABC transporters modify intestinal FA, cholesterol, sterol, and lipophilic drug absorption in animals and humans? These questions remain to be answered.

To date, the most convincing data supporting the existence of a transporter for cholesterol absorption is provided by studies of the hypocholesterolemic drug, ezetimibe (Zetia®, Schering-Plough) (158,159). After being metabolized in the liver, ezetimibe returns to the intestinal lumen to potently inhibit cholesterol absorption. Although the mechanism by which ezetimibe inhibits intestinal cholesterol absorption is far from clear, inhibition of Niemann-Pick C1-like protein (160), a lipid transporter which has been recently demonstrated to be a binding target for ezetimibe (161), has been suggested. Other possible mechanisms of action include disruption of sterol uptake by the brush border membrane (162) and inhibition of the endocytosis of cholesterol-rich microdomains secondary to binding of ezetimibe to the aminopeptidase, N(CD13) (163). A better understanding of how this drug inhibits cholesterol absorption could potentially provide new and useful information regarding the mechanism of absorption of lipophilic drugs and xenobiotics.

INTRACELLULAR TRAFFICKING OF TRIGLYCERIDE

While it is beyond the scope of this chapter to provide an in-depth account of intracellular lipid trafficking, a brief summary will be included as these processes may be involved in the intracellular trafficking of lipophilic drugs and xenobiotics and could play a role in their transport by CM.

It is not known how the various absorbed lipids migrate from the site of absorption in the intestine to the endoplasmic reticulum, where resynthesis of complex lipids and TG destined for CM takes place. In addition, chylomicron incorporation of lipophilic drugs absorbed by the enterocytes may involve some of these same pathways. A FABP present in the small intestine, first isolated and characterized by Ockner and Manning, has been suggested to play an important role in the intracellular transport of absorbed FA (164,165). We know there are at least two FABPs in enterocytes—the I-FABP (intestinal-FABP) and L-FABP (liver-FABP)—and that these FABPs differ in their binding specificity: I-FABP binds with high affinity to FA, whereas L-FABP binds to long-chain FAs, LPC, retinoids, bilirubin, carcinogens, and selenium (166–168). While the functioning of these FABP's has not yet been investigated in vivo, NMR binding studies conducted by Cistola et al. (169) suggested that I-FABP is involved in the intracellular transport of FA while L-FABP is involved in the intracellular transport of MG and LPC (169). A thorough review of this subject has been conducted by Storch and Thumser (170).

Investigating the functioning of FABPs and their role in intracellular lipid trafficking in living animals has proven extremely challenging for a number of reasons. Attempts at using "knock-out" animals, for which the gene encoding a specific FABP is absent, have failed to yield definitive results, since the absence of a specific FABP often results in the upregulation of other FABPs which are capable of compensating for functions of the absent FABP. For example, when Shaughnessy et al. (171) used the adipocyte FABP knockout mouse to study its function, the keratinocyte FABP functionally compensated for the absence of the adipocyte FABP. In other studies, investigators using I-FABP knock-out mice found that these animals have higher plasma TG and greater body weight than wild types (172), implying normal fat absorption in these genetically modified animals. Although the L-FABP knock-out animals have been generated, their ability to absorb lipid and lipid soluble drugs in the intestine has not been examined and certainly warrants further investigation (173).

Other intracellular lipid carrier proteins include the sterol carrier proteins, SCP-1 and SCP-2 (174,175). SCP-1 is involved in the intracellular transport of cholesterol from cytoplasmic lipid droplets to mitochondria and the translocation of cholesterol from the outer mitochondrial membrane to the inner mitochondrial membrane (178). It also appears to be involved in the intracellular trafficking of PC (179,180) and FAs (181). SCP-2, also known as the nonspecific lipid transfer protein, participates in the microsomal conversion of lanosterol to cholesterol (177) and has also been proposed to play a role in peroxisomal FA-CoA binding (182).

Monoglyceride and Fatty Acids

2-MG and FA are reconstituted in the enterocyte to form TG, the primary component of CM, via the MG pathway. As shown in Figure 5, 2-MG is reacylated into TG by the consecutive action of MG acyltransferase (MGAT) and DG acyltransferase (DGAT) (183,184). The enzymes involved in this MG pathway are present in a complex called "triglyceride synthetase" (183,185), which has been purified by Lehner and Kuksis (186). It is thought that the synthesis of TG from DG is catalyzed by the enzyme acyl CoA:DGAT. The gene for this enzyme has been isolated and a knockout mouse generated. Interestingly, this mouse can synthesize normal amounts of TG in the intestinal mucosa (187), thus raising the question as to whether another enzyme(s) is involved in the formation of TG from DG.

Wetterau and Zilversmit (195–197) demonstrated that a protein found in the liver, small intestine, and several other organs promotes the transfer of TG and cholesterol esterase between membranes. The small intestine and liver have the

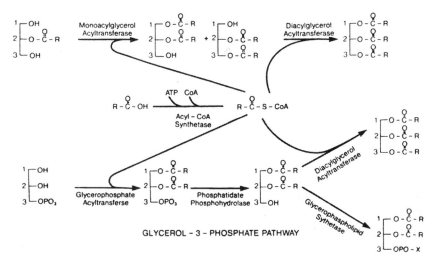

Figure 5   Pathways of triacylglycerol biosynthesis in the intestinal mucosa.

highest TG transfer activity, and both are active in packaging TG-rich lipoproteins. Therefore, Wetterau and Zilversmit proposed that this transfer activity plays a role in the intracellular packaging of lipoproteins, including CM, which are responsible for the transport of lipophilic drugs.

FORMATION OF INTESTINAL CM AND VLDLs

During fasting, very-low-density lipoproteins (VLDL) are the only lipoproteins produced by the enterocytes of the small intestine (239–241). Compared to CM, these lipoproteins are relatively small in size and contain proportionately lower amounts of TG. Hence, the ability of VLDL to carry lipid soluble drugs is limited in comparison to the substantially larger, TG-rich CM. In the fed state, however, the CM is the predominant lipoprotein species produced by the small intestine and it is this lipoprotein that is largely responsible for transporting the bulk of lipophilic drugs in the lymph (241–242). Currently, CM and VLDL are distinguished from one another based on the manner in which they separate following ultracentrifugation: lipoproteins that have a Svedberg flotation (S_f) rate exceeding 400 are classified as CMs whereas those with a S_f rate of 20 to 400 are defined as VLDLs (243).

Over the past decade, we have acquired a considerable amount of new information regarding the mechanism of the intracellular assembly, modification, and secretion of lipoproteins from the small intestinal epithelial cells. Using subcellular fractionation and pulse-chase techniques, Higgins et al. has provided new insight into the process by which CM are assembled within enterocytes. These researchers demonstrated that the first and rate-limiting step in the assembly of CM involves the formation of dense apo B48 PL-rich particles that accumulate within the lumen of the smooth endoplasmic reticulum. The second step, which occurs rapidly, results in the enrichment of the dense apo B48 PL-rich particles with TG and additional PLs (226,227). Mansbach et al. (228), using a cell-free system, has provided exciting new information showing that the transport of TGs and apo B48 from the endoplasmic reticulum to the Golgi apparatus is vectorial, temperature dependent (37°C) and requires ATP (a cytosolic protein) (228,229). Additionally, they have isolated 200 nm vesicles from the endoplasmic reticulum of enterocytes; presumably, these vesicles carry the TG-containing pre-CMs to the Golgi apparatus (229). In 2003, Siddiqi et al. demonstrated that the COPII proteins, Sar1, Sec23p, Sec24p, Sec13, and Sec31, are involved in the fusion of the endoplasmic reticulum vesicles with the Golgi apparatus (230,231). The importance of the COPII proteins in CM formation is further supported by the recent finding that patients with CM retention disorder involve mutation of the Sar1 GTPase of the COPII protein complex (232).

The differing FA composition of the TG contained in VLDL and CM has suggested that these lipoproteins are produced in the enterocytes by two distinct and separate pathways. Ockner et al. (239) demonstrated that intestinal VLDL secretion is markedly increased by intraduodenal infusion of palmitate; infusion of oleate and linoleate, however, had no effect on VLDL secretion but significantly increased CM secretion. Further evidence in support of separate biosynthetic pathways for VLDL and CM is provided by Vahouny et al. (245), who demonstrated in rats that puromycin had no significant effect on the incorporation of radiolabeled leucine into VLDL peptides but markedly inhibited the incorporation of the amino acid into CM peptides. In addition, an ultrastructural and biochemical study of enterocytes conducted by Mahley et al. (244) showed that CM and VLDL particles were contained in distinctly separate Golgi vesicles. Studies conducted by Tso et al. (246,247) have shown in rats that duodenal infusion of 0.5 mg/hr of the cationic surfactant, Pluronic L-81 (L-81), markedly impairs lymphatic transport of TG and cholesterol by inhibiting the formation of intestinal CMs; VLDL formation was not affected. Using this unique tool, Tso et al. (248) further showed that intraduodenal infusion of egg PC in rats resulted almost exclusively in the secretion of VLDL into intestinal lymph which was not affected by the administration of L-81. However, when triolein, which is a substrate for CM synthesis, was substituted for egg PC in the presence of L-81, the lymphatic transport of TG was inhibited (246,247). These results led Tso et al. (248) to propose separate pathways for the formation of CM and VLDL (Fig. 6). Moreover, Tso et al. (248) distinguished these biosynthetic pathways by demonstrating selective inhibition of the CM pathway by L-81 and the segregation of pre-VLDL and pre-CM particles into separate vesicles within the enterocytic Golgi apparatus, which supports the observations of Mahley et al. (244). Additional in vivo and in vitro studies have supported the existence of separate biosynthetic pathways for CM and VLDL. Nutting et al. (249) measured the time

EXIT

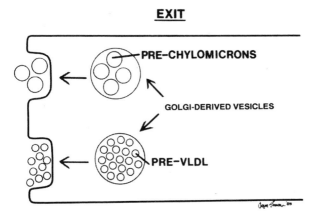

Figure 6 Packaging and secretion of intestinal CM and VLDL. The diagram depicts Golgi derived vesicles containing either pre-CM or pre-VLDL particles. Little mixing of pre-CM and pre-VLDL particles in these vesicles occurs. *Abbreviations*: CM, chylomicrons; VLDL, very low-density lipoproteins.

required for the appearance of radioactivity in the mesenteric lymph of rats following intestinal infusion of radiolabeled FA in control rats or those treated with L-81, which selectively inhibits CM secretion but does not affect VLDL secretion into the intestinal lymph. In the control rats, lymph radioactivity was detected 10.8 minutes following infusion of radiolabeled FA whereas radioactivity was not detected in the lymph of L-81 treated rats until 16.2 minutes after the FA infusion. Finally, using Caco-2 cells, Luchoomun and Hussain (250) demonstrated that L-81 inhibits CM but not VLDL formation in vitro.

From a drug delivery perspective, selective stimulation of VLDL or CM synthesis by coadministration of PC or TG, respectively, has implications for the amount of drug that could be transported by this route as well as for the distribution of the drug, which could potentially be influenced by the metabolic fate of the the lipoprotein with which it is associated.

In addition to their application as an in vitro model for assessing intestinal drug permeability, intestinal cell culture systems (e.g., Caco-2 cells) have been used extensively to study the formation and secretion of lipoproteins (233–237) and the genetic expression and post-translational modification of apolipoproteins (238). Using Caco-2 cells, a sequential assembly model for studying VLDL and CM formation was described by Hussain et al. (233) and provided information on the assembly of primordial lipoprotein particles, the synthesis of TG-rich lipid droplets, and the lipoprotein core expansion occuring following the fusion of primordial lipoproteins with nascent TG droplets (251).

Interpreting the results of studies employing Caco-2 cells, which are derived from a human colon carcinoma cell line, should be done cautiously as these cells differ from native small intestinal enterocytes in several important ways:

1. Caco-2 cells utilize the glycerol 3-phosphate pathway for the formation of TG from FAs and glycerol, which is of substantially lower capacity that the MG pathway used by native enterocytes for the formation of TG (252).
2. Enterocytes in the small intestine synthesize only apo B48, while Caco-2 cells synthesize apo B48 and apo B100.
3. Native enterocytes primarily secrete CM particles during active fat absorption, wheras Caco-2 cells secrete VLDL which, as described earlier, has significantly lower drug-carrying capacity as compared to CM.

PORTAL TRANSPORT OF FAS AND LIPOPHILIC COMPOUNDS

As described previously, the bulk of absorbed FA and an often significant fraction of lipophilic xenobiotics is transported by intestinal lymph in association with CM and VLDL. However, there is growing evidence for hepatic portal transport of these molecules in healthy individuals and in instances where the normal pathways for intestinal lipid absorption have been disrupted secondary to disease. Inhibition of CM synthesis, which is associated with abetalipoproteinemia in humans or can be induced experimentally in puromycin-treated rats (255,256) or following ischemia/reperfusion injury to the small intestine, has been shown to result in increased portal transport of FA secondary to compromised resynthesis of TG by the enterocytes. Similarly, increased portal transport of FA has been shown in bile fistula rats, again resulting from reduced TG by the enterocytes, which requires the presence of bile salts in the intestinal lumen (253,254). Reduction or elimination of intestinal bile and/or lipase would compromise the hydrolysis of TG to FA, thereby reducing the lumenal concentration of FA. Various studies have suggested an inverse relationship between the lumenal concentration of FA and the fraction of FA absorbed via the portal pathway. For example, McDonald et al. (259) demonstrated, in rats, that at low duodenal infusion (0.3 μmol/hr) of linoleic acid, a substantial amount of the absorbed FA (58%) was transported in the portal blood. Physiologically, it is unlikely to have such low FA concentration in the intestinal lumen. However, in humans with bile or lipase deficiency, this condition may prevail and the portal route may become important for intestinal FA transport by the intestinal mucosa. Using the rat as a model, Mansbach et al. reported that as much as 39% of the FA infused into the small intestinal lumen was absorbed via the portal circulation as TG (260).

      Likewise, while highly lipophilic drugs and xenobiotics exhibit significant transport in the intestinal lymph; these substances are often partially absorbed directly into the portal blood (261). In a recent paper, Cavret et al. (262) demonstrated that highly lipophilic, nonpolar compounds such as phenanthrene, benzo[*a*]pyrene, and tetrachlorodibenzo-*para*-dioxin are all absorbed by the small intestine and transported, in part, by the portal blood. Further studies are needed to determine the mechanisms governing the nonlymphatic transport of these highly lipophilic compounds as well as the specific carriers of these compounds in the blood.

CONCLUDING REMARKS

Many orally administered, lipophilic drugs are transported to the systemic circulation, at least in part, by the intestinal lymph in association with CMs and VLDL. Therefore, a thorough understanding of the processes by which the body assimilates hydrophobic molecules from the GIT, which includes the digestion, uptake, intracellular metabolism, and packaging of these substances into CMs, is critical to the design of effective oral delivery systems for hydrophobic, poorly water soluble drugs. It is hoped that this review will stimulate investigators working on theoretical and practical aspects of lipophilic drug delivery to further define the mechanisms that govern the gastrointestinal absorption and transport of these compounds. The next few years will be both exciting and challenging for investigators working in these areas as well as those involving the identification and characterization of the various transporters of lipid ligands and the transporters of the ABC family involved in the efflux of lipid ligands.

ACKNOWLEDGMENTS

This work was supported by the National Institutes of Health, grants DK-56910, DK-54504, and DK-56863.

REFERENCES

1. Dawson PA, Rudel LL. Intestinal cholesterol absorption. Curr Opin Lipidol 1999; 10:315–320.
2. Borgstrom B. Luminal digestion of fats. In: Go VL, ed., The Exocrine Pancreas. New York: Raven Press, 1986:361–373.
3. Lammert F, Wang DQ. New insights into the genetic regulation of intestinal cholesterol absorption. Gastroenterology 2005; 129:718–734.
4. Carey MC, Small DM. The characteristics of mixed micellar solution with particular reference to bile. Am J Med 1970; 49:590–608.
5. Kannel WB, Dawber TR, Friedman GD, Glennon WE, McNamara PM. Risk factors in coronary heart disease: an evaluation of several serum lipids as predictors of CHD. Ann Intern Med 1964; 49:888–899.
6. Levy D, Kannel WB. Cardiovascular risks: new insights from Framingham. Am Heart J 1988; 116:266–272.
7. Austin MA. Plasma triglyceride and coronary heart disease. Arterioscler Thromb Vasc Biol 1991; 11:2–14.
8. Beynen AC, Kritchevsky D. Dietary fat and serum cholesterol. In: Voorthuizen, ed., Nutritional Effects on Cholesterol Metabolism. Voorthuizen: Transmodial 1986:1–10.

9. Valenzuela A, Morgado N. Trans fatty acid isomers in human health and in the food industry. Biol Res 1999; 32:273–287.
10. Katan MB. Trans fatty acids and plasma lipoproteins. Nutr Rev 2000; 58:188–191.
11. Heird WC, Grundy SM, Hubbard VS. Structured lipids and their use in clinical nutrition. Am J Clin Nutr 1986; 43:320–324.
12. Bell SJ, Bradley D, Forse RA, Bistrian B. The new dietary fats in health and disease. J Am Diet Assoc 1997; 97:280–286.
13. Chan S, McCowen KC, Bistrian B. Medium-chain triglyceride and n-3 polyunsaturated fatty acid-containing emulsions in intravenous nutrition. Curr Opin Clin Nutr Metab Care 1998; 1:163–169.
14. McKenna MC, Hubbard VS, Bieri JG. Linoleic acid absorption from lipid supplements in patients with cystic fibrosis with pancreatic insufficiency and in control subjects. J Ped Gastroent Nutr 1985; 4:45–51.
15. Hubbard VS, McKenna MC. Absorption of safflower oil and structured lipid preparations in patients with cystic fibrosis. Lipids 1987; 22:424–428.
16. Mok KT, Maiz A, Yamazaki K, et al. Structured medium-chain and long-chain triglyceride emulsions are superior to physical mixtures in sparing body protein in the burned rat. Metabolism 1984; 33:910–915.
17. Swenson ES, Selleck KM, Babyan VK, Blackburn GL, Bistrian BR. Persistence of metabolic effects after long-term oral feeding of a structured triglyceride derived from medium-chain triglyceride and fish oil in burned and normal rats. Metabolism 1991; 40:484–490.
18. Babayan VK. Medium chain triacylglycerols and structured lipids. Lipids 1987; 22:417–420.
19. Mascioli EA, Babayan VK, Bistrian BR, Blackburn GL. Novel triacylglycerols for special medical purposes. J Par Ent Nutr 1988; 2:S127–S132.
20. Tso P, Lee T, DeMichele SJ. Randomized structure triglycerides increase lymphatic absorption of tocopherol and retinol compared with the equivalent physical mixture in a rat model of fat malabsorption. J Nutr 2001; 131:2157–2163.
21. Abrams CK, Hamosh M, Lee TC, et al. Gastric lipase: localization in the human stomach. Gastroenterology 1988; 95:1460–1464.
22. Moreau H, Laugier R, Gargouri Y, Ferrato F, Verger R. Human preduodenal lipase is entirely of gastric fundic origin. Gastroenterology 1988; 95:1221–1226.
23. Hamosh M, Scanlon JW, Ganot D, Likel M, Scanlon KB, Hamosh P. Fat digestion in the newborn: characterization of lipase in gastric aspirates of premature and term infants. J Clin Invest 1981; 67:838–846.
24. Liao TH, Hamosh P, Hamosh M. Fat digestion by lingual lipase: mechanism of lipolysis in the stomach and upper small intestine. Pediatr Res 1984; 18:402–409.
25. Cohen M, Morgan RGH, Hofmann AF. Lipolytic activity of human gastric and duodenal juice against medium- and long-chain triglycerides. Gastroenterology 1971; 60:1–15.
26. Bodmer MW, Angal S, Yarraton GT, et al. Molecular cloning of a human gastric lipase and expression of the enzyme in yeast. Biochim Biophys Acta 1987; 909:237–244.
27. Docherty AJP, Bodmer MW, Angal S, et al. Molecular cloning and nucleotide sequence of rat lingual lipase cDNA. Nucleic Acid Res 1985; 13:1891–1903.
28. Grand RJ, Watkins JB, Torti FM. Development of the human gastrointestinal tract: a review. Gastroenterology 1976; 70:790–810.

29. Ross CAC. Fat absorption studies in the diagnosis and treatment of pancreatic fibrosis. Arch Dis Child 1955; 30:316–321.

30. Armand M, Hamosh M, Philpott JR, et al. Gastric function in children with cystic fibrosis: effect of diet on gastric lipase levels and fat digestion. Pediatr Res 2004; 55:457–465.

31. Carriere F, Renou C, Lopez V, et al. The specific activities of human digestive lipases measured from the In vivo and In vitro lipolysis of test meals. Gastroenterology 2000; 229:949–960.

32. Senior JR. Intestinal absorption of fats. J Lipid Res 1964; 5:495–521.

33. Carey MC, Small DM, Bliss CM. Lipid digestion and absorption. Ann Rev Physiol 1983; 45:651–677.

34. Sarda L, Desnuelle P. Action de la lipase pancreatique sur les esters en emulsion. Biochim Biophys Acta 1958; 30:513–521.

35. Benzonana G, Desnuelle P. Etude cinetique de l'action de la lipase pancreatique sur des triglycerides en emulsion. Essai d'une enzymologie en milieu heterogene. Biochim Biophys Acta 1965; 105:121–136.

36. Desnuelle P. The lipase-colipase system. In: Rommel K, Goebell H, eds., Lipid Absorption: Biochemical and Clinical Aspects. Lancaster: MTP Press, 1976:23–37.

37. Schönheyder F, Volquartz K. Gastric lipase in man. Acta Physiol Scand 1946; 11:349–360.

38. Verger R. Enzyme kinetics of lipolysis. Methods Enzymol 1980; 64:340–392.

39. James LK, Augustein LG. Absorption of enzymes at interfaces: file formation and the effect on activity. Adv Enzymol 1966; 28:1–40.

40. McLaren AD, Packer L. Some aspects of enzyme reactions in heterogeneous systems. Adv Enzymol 1970; 33:245–308.

41. Brockerhoff H. Substrate specificity of pancreatic lipase. Biochim Biophys Acta 1968; 159:296–303.

42. Mattson FH, Beck LW. The specificity of pancreatic lipase on the primary hydroxyl groups of glycerides. J Biol Chem 1956; 219:735–740.

43. Simmonds WJ. Fat absorption and chylomicron formation. In: Nelson GJ, ed., Blood Lipids and Lipoproteins: Quantitation, Composition, and Metabolism. New York: Wiley (Interscience), 1972:705–743.

44. Borgstrom B. On the mechanism of the hydrolysis of glycerides by pancreatic lipase. Acta Chem Scand 1953; 7:557–560.

45. Mattson FH, Volpenhein RA. The digestion and absorption of triglycerides. J Biol Chem 1964; 239:2772–2777.

46. Mattson FH, Volpenhein RA. Hydrolysis of primary and secondary esters of glycerol by pancreatic juice. J Lipid Res 1968; 9:79–84.

47. Borgstrom B. Influence of bile salt, pH, and time on the action of pancreatic lipase; physiological implications. J Lipid Res 1964; 5:522–531.

48. Hofmann AF, Borgstrom B. Hydrolysis of long-chain monoglycerides in micellar solution by pancreatic lipase. Biochim Biophys Acta 1963; 70:317–331.

49. Patton JS. Gastrointestinal lipid digestion. In: Johnson LR, ed., Physiology of the Gastrointestinal Tract. New York: Raven Press, 1981:1123–1146.

50. Vandermeers A, Christophe J. Alpha-amylase et lipsae du pancreas de rat. Purification chromatographique, recherche du poids moleculaire et composition e acides amines. Biochim Biophys Acta 1968; 154:110–129.

51. Vandermeers A, Vandermeers-Piret MC, Rathe J, Christophe J. On human pancreatic triacylglycerol lipase: isolation and some properties. Biochim Biophys Acta 1974; 370:257–268.

52. Julien R, Canioni J, Rathelot J, Sarda L, Plummer TH Jr. Studies on bovine pancreatic lipase and colipase. Biochim Biophys Acta 1972; 280:215–224.

53. Rathelot J, Julien R, Bosc-Bierne P, Gargouri Y, Canioni P, Sarda L. Horse pancreatic lipase. Interaction with colipase from various species. Biochimie 1981; 63:227–234.

54. De Caro J, Boudouard M, Bonicel J, Guidoni A, Desnuelle P, Rovery M. Porcine pancreatic lipase. Completion of the primary structure. Biochim Biophys Acta 1981; 671:129–138.

55. Plummer TH, Sarda L. Isolation and characterization of the glycopeptides of porcine pancreatic lipases L_A and L_B. J Biol Chem 1973; 248:7865–7869.

56. Rathelot J, Canioni P, Bosc-Bierne I, et al. Limited trypsinolysis of porcine and equinine colipases. Biochim Biophys Acta 1981; 671:155–163.

57. Chapus C, Semeriva M. Mechanism of pancreatic lipase action. 1. Interfacial activation of pancreatic lipase. Biochemistry 1976; 15:4988–4991.

58. Morgan RGH, Barrowman J, Borgstrom B. The effect of sodium taurodeoxycholate and pH on the gel filtration behaviour of rat pancreatic protein and lipases. Biochim Biophys Acta 1969; 175:65–75.

59. Erlanson C, Borgstrom B. Purification and further characterization of colipase from porcine pancreas. Biochim Biophys Acta 1972; 271:400–412.

60. Sternby B, Borgstrom B. Purification and characterization of human pancreatic colipase. Biochim Biophys Acta 1979; 572:235–243.

61. Maylie MF, Charles M, Gache C, Desnuelle P. Isolation and partial identification of a pancreatic colipase. Biochim Biophys Acta 1971; 229:286–289.

62. Maylie MF, Charles M, Gache C, Desnuelle P. On porcine pancreatic colipase: large scale purification and some properties. Biochem Biophys Res Commun 1973; 52:291–297.

63. Erlanson-Albertsson C. Pancreatic colipase. Structural and physiological aspects. Biochim Biophys Acta 1992; 1125:1–7.

64. Patton JS, Albertsson PA, Erlanson C, Borgstrom B. Binding of porcine pancreatic lipase and colipase in the absence of substrate studies by two-phase partition and affinity chromatography. J Biol Chem 1978; 253:4195–4202.

65. Arnesjö B, Nilsson A, Barrowman J, Borgstrom B. Intestinal digestion and absorption of cholesterol and lecithin in the human. Scand J Gastroenterol 1969; 4:653–665.

66. Borgstrom B, Dahlqvist A, Lundh G, Sjövall J. Studies of intestinal digestion and absorption in the human. J Clin Invest 1957; 36:1521–1536.

67. Van den Bosch H, Postema NM, de Haas GH, Van Deenen LLM. On the positional specificity of phospholipase A from pancreas. Biochim Biophys Acta 1965; 98:657–659.

68. de Haas GH, Sarda L, Roger J. Positional specific hydrolysis of phospholipids by pancreatic lipase. Biochim Biophys Acta 1965; 106:638–640.

69. de Haas GH, Postema NM, Nieuwenhuizen W, Van Deenen LLM. Purification and properties of phospholipase A from porcine pancreas. Biochim Biophys Acta 1968; 159:103–117.

70. Arnesjö B, Barrowman J, Borgstrom B. The zymogen of phospholipase A_2 in rat pancreatic juice. Acta Chem Scand 1967; 21:2897–2900.

71. Verheij HM, Volwerk JJ, Jansen EH, et al. Methylation of histidine-48 in pancreatic phospholipase A2. Role of histidine and calcium ion in the catalytic mechanism. Biochemistry 1980; 19:743–750.

72. Fernandez MS, Mejia R, Zavala E. The interfacial calcium ion concentration as modulator of the latency phase in the hydrolysis of dimyristoylphosphatidylcholine liposomes by phospholipase A_2. Biochem Cell Biol 1991; 69:722–727.

73. Arnesjö B, Grubb A. The activation, purification, and properties of rat pancreatic juice phospholipase A_2. Acta Chem Scand 1971; 25:577–589.

74. Tsao FHC, Cohen H, Synder WR, Kezdy FJ, Law JH. Multiple forms of porcine pancreatic phospholipase A_2: isolation and specificity. J Supramol Structure 1973; 1:490–497.

75. Puijk WC, Verheij HM, Wietzes P, de Haas GH. The amino acid sequence of the phospholipase A_2 isoenzyme from porcine pancreas. Biochim Biophys Acta 1979; 580:411–415.

76. Nalbone G, Lairon D, Charbonnier-Augeire M, et al. Pancreatic phospholipase A2 hydrolysis of phosphatidylcholines in various physicochemical states. Biochim Biophys Acta 1980; 620:612–625.

77. de Haas GH, Slotboom AJ, Bonsen PPM, et al. Studies on phospholipase A and its zymogen from porcine pancreas. 1. The complete amino acid sequence. Biochim Biophys Acta 1970; 221:31–53.

78. Puijk WC, Verheij HM, de Haas GH. The primary structure of phospholipase A_2 from porcine pancreas. A reinvestigation. Biochim Biophys Acta 1977; 492:254–259.

79. O'Hara O, Tamaki M, Nakamura E, et al. Dog and rat pancreatic phospholipases A_2: complete amino acid sequences deduced from complementary DNAs. J Biochem 1986; 99:773–793.

80. Kerfelec B, LaForge KS, Vasiloudes P, Puigserver A, Scheele GA. Isolation and sequence of the canine pancreatic phospholipase A_2 gene. Eur J Biochem 1990; 190:299–304.

81. Richmond BL, Hui DY. Molecular structure and tissue-specific expression of the mouse pancreatic phospholipase A(2) gene. Gene 2000; 244:65–72.

82. Verheij HM, Slotboom AJ, de Haas GH. Structure and function of phospholipase A2. Rev Physiol Biochem Pharmacol 1981; 91:91–203.

83. Subbaiah PV, Ganguly J. Studies in the phospholipases of rat intestinal mucosa. Biochem J 1970; 118:233–239.

84. Tojo H, Ichida T, Okamoto M. Purification and characterization of a catalytic domain of rat intestinal phospholipase B/lipase associated with brush border membranes. J Biol Chem 1998; 273:2214–2221.

85. Tchoua U, Ito M, Okamoto M, Tojo H. Increased intestinal phospholipase A(2) activity catalyzed by phospholipase B/lipase in WBN/Kob rats with pancreatic insufficiency. Biochim Biophys Acta 2000; 1487:255–267.

86. Lu T, Ito M, Tchoua U, Takemori H, Okamoto M, Tojo H. Identification of essential residues for catalysis of rat intestinal phospholipase B/lipase. Biochemistry 2001; 40:7133–7139.

87. McIntyre N. Cholesterol absorption. In: Rommel K, Goebell H, Bohmer R, eds., Lipid Absorption: Biochemical and Clinical Aspects. London: MTP Press Ltd., 1976:73–84.

88. Albro PW, Thomas RO. Enzymatic hydrolysis of di-(2-ethylhexyl) phthalate by lipases. Biochim Biophys Acta 1973; 360:380–390.

89. Momsen WE, Brockman HL. Purification and characterization of cholesterol esterase from porcine pancreas. Biochim Biophys Acta 1977; 486:103–113.
90. Erlanson C. Purification, properties and substrate specificity of a carboxylesterase in pancreatic juice. Scand J Gastroenterology 1975; 10:401–408.
91. Lombardo D, Guy O, Figarella C. Purification and characterization of a carboxyl ester hydrolase from human pancreatic juice. Biochim Biophys Acta 1978; 527:142–149.
92. Meyer JG. Lipolytic enzymes of the human pancreas. II. Purification and properties of cholesterol ester hydrolase. Biochim Biophys Acta 1989; 1002:89–92.
93. Kyger EM, Wiegand RC, Lange LG. Cloning of the bovine pancreatic cholesterol esterase/lysophospholipase. Biochem Biophys Res Commun 1989; 164:1302–1309.
94. Kissel JA, Fontaine RN, Turck CW, Brockman HL, Hui DY. Molecular cloning and expression of cDNA for rat pancreatic cholesterol esterase. Biochim Biophys Acta 1989; 106:227–236.
95. Kumar BV, Aleman-Gomez JA, Colwell N, Lopez-Candales A. Structure of the human pancreatic cholesterol esterase gene. Biochemistry 1992; 31:6077–6081.
96. DiPersio LP, Fontaine RN, Hui DY. Identification of the active site serine in pancreatic cholesterol esterase by chemical modification and site-specific mutagenesis. J Biol Chem 1990; 265:16801–16806.
97. DiPersio LP, Fontaine RN, Hui DY. Site-specific mutagenesis of an essential histidine residue in pancreatic esterase. J Biol Chem 1991; 266:4033–4036.
98. DiPersio LP, Hui DY. Aspartic acid 320 is required for optimal activity of rat pancreatic cholesterol esterase. J Biol Chem 1993; 268:300–304.
99. Lombardo D, Fauvel J, Guy O. Studies on the substrate specificity of a carboxyl ester hydrolase from human pancreatic juice. I. Action on carboxyl esters, glycerides and phospholipids. Biochim Biophys Acta 1980; 611:136–146.
100. Hofmann AF, Borgstrom B. Physico-chemical state of lipids in intestinal content during their digestion and absorption. Fed Proc 1962; 21:43–50.
101. Hofmann AF, Borgstrom B. The intraluminal phase of fat digestion in man: The lipid content of the micellar and oil phases of intestinal content obtained during fat digestion and absorption. J Clin Invest 1964; 43:247–257.
102. Dietschy JM, Sallee VL, Wilson FA. Unstirred water layers and absorption across the intestinal mucosa. Gastroenterology 1971; 61:932–934.
103. Wilson FA, Sallee VL, Dietschy JM. Unstirred water layers in intestine: rate determinant of fatty acid from micellar solutions. Science 1971; 174:1031–1033.
104. Westergaard H, Dietschy JM. The mechanism whereby bile acid micelles increase the rate of fatty acid and cholesterol uptake into the intestinal mucosal cell. J Clin Invest 1976; 58:97–108.
105. Swell L, Flick DF, Field H Jr, Treadwell CR. Influence of dietary bile salts on blood cholesterol levels. Proc Soc Exp Biol Med 1953; 84:428–431.
106. Gallo-Torres HE, Miller ON, Hamilton JG. Further studies on the role of bile salts in cholesterol esterification and absorption from the gut. Arch Biochem Biophys 1971; 143:22–36.
107. Watt SM, Simmonds WJ. The specificity of bile salts in the intestinal absorption of micellar cholesterol in the rat. Clin Exp Pharmacol Physio 1976; 3:305–322.
108. Reynier MO, Montet JC, Gerolami A, et al. Comparative effects of cholic, chenodeoxycholic, and ursodeoxycholic acids on micellar solubilization and intestinal absorption of cholesterol. J Lipid Res 1981; 22:467–473.

109. Cohen RF, Raicht, Mosbach EH. Sterol metabolism studies in the rat. Effects of primary bile acids (sodium taurochenodeoxycholate and sodium taurocholate) on sterol metabolism. J Lipid Res 1977; 18:223–231.
110. Watt SM, Simmonds WJ. Effects of four taurine-conjugated bile acids on mucosal uptake and lymphatic absorption of cholesterol in the rat. J Lipid Res 1984; 25:448–455.
111. Sylven C. Influence of blood supply on lipid uptake from micellar solution by the rat small intestine. Biochim Biophys Acta 1970; 203:365–375.
112. Bhattacharyya AK, Connor WE. Beta-sitosterolemia and xanthomatosis. A newly described lipid storage disease in two sisters. J Clin Invest 1974; 53:1033–1043.
113. Shulman RS, Bhattacharyya AK, Connor WR, Fredrickson DS. Beta-sitosterolemia and xanthomatosis. N Engl J Med 1976; 294:482–483.
114. Salen G, Shefer S, Nguyen L, Ness GC, Tint GS, Batta AK. Sitosterolemia. Subcell Biochem 1997; 28:476.
115. Porter HP, Saunders DR. Isolation of the aqueous phase of human intestinal contents during the digestion of a fatty meal. Gastroenterology 1971; 60:997–1007.
116. Patton JS, Carey MC. Watching fat digestion. Science 1979; 204:145–148.
117. Stafford RJ, Carey MC. Physical-chemical nature of the aqueous lipids in intestinal content after a fatty meal: revision of the hofmann-borgstrom hypothesis. Clin Res 1981; 28:511 (Abstract).
118. Mansbach CM, Newton D, Stevens RD. Fat digestion in patients with bile acid malabsorption but minimal steatorrhea. Dig Dis Sci 1980; 25:353–362.
119. Porter HP, Saunders DR, Tytgat G, Brunster O, Rubin CE. Fat absorption in bile fistula man. A morphological and biochemical study. Gastroenterology 1971; 60:1008–1019.
120. Woollett LA, Buckley DD, Yao L, et al. Cholic acid supplementation enhances cholesterol absorption in humans. Gastroenterology 2004; 136:724–731.
121. Borgstrom B. The micellar hypothesis of fat absorption: must it be revisited? Scand J Gastroenterology 1985; 20:389–394.
122. Shoemaker DG, Nichols JW. Hydrophobic interaction of lysophospholipids and bile salts at submicellar concentrations. Biochemistry 1990; 29:5837–5842.
123. Shoemaker DG, Nichols JW. Interaction of lysophospholipid/taurodeoxycholate submicellar aggregates with phospholipid bilayers. Biochemistry 1992; 31:3414–3420.
124. Thomson ABR, Keelan M, Garg ML, Clandinin MT. Intestinal aspects of lipid absorption. Can J Physiol Pharmacol 1989; 67:179–191.
125. Strauss EW. Electron microscopic study of intestinal fat absorption in vitro from mixed micelles containing linolenic acid, monoolein, and bile salt. J Lipid Res 1966; 6:307–323.
126. Stremmel W. Uptake of fatty acids by jejunal mucosal cells is mediated by a fatty acid binding membrane protein. J Clin Invest 1988; 82:2001–2010.
127. Chow SL, Hollander D. A dual, concentration-dependent absorption mechanism of linoleic acid by rat jejunum in vitro. J Lipid Res 1979; 20:349–356.
128. Hollander D. Intestinal absorption of vitamins A, E, D, and K. J Lab Clin Med 1981; 97:449–462.
129. Stremmel W, Lotz G, Strohmeyer G, Berk PD. Identification, isolation, and partial characterization of a fatty acid binding protein from rat jejunal microvillous membranes. J Clin Invest 1985; 75:1068–1076.

130. Berk PD, Wada H, Horio Y, et al. Plasma membrane fatty acid-binding protein and mitochondrial glutamic-oxaloacetic transaminase of rat liver are related. Proc Natl Acad Sci USA 1990; 87:3484–3488.

131. Stahl A, Hirsch DJ, Gimeno RE, et al. Identification of the major intestinal fatty acid transport protein. Mol Cell 1999; 4:299–308.

132. Lundgren S, Carling T, Hjälm G, et al. Tissue distribution of human gp330/megalin, a putative Ca^{2+}-sensing protein. J Histochem Cytochem 1997; 45:383–392.

133. Farquhar MG. The unfolding story of megalin (gp330): now recognized as a drug receptor. J Clin Invest 1995; 96:1184.

134. Moestrup SK, Cui S, Vorum H, et al. Christensen, Evidence that epithelial glycoprotein 330/megalin mediates uptake of polybasic drugs. J Clin Invest 1995; 96:1404–1413.

135. Willnow TE, Goldstein JL, Orth K, Brown MS, Herz J. Low density lipoprotein receptor-related protein and gp330 bind similar ligands, including plasminogen activator-inhibitor complexes and lactoferrin, an inhibitor of chylomicron remnant clearance. J Biol Chem 1992; 267:26172–26180.

136. Cui S, Verroust PJ, Moestrup SK, Christensen EI. Megalin/gp330 mediates uptake of albumin in renal proximal tubule. Am J Physiol 1996; 271:F900–F907.

137. Hauser H, Dyer JH, Nandy A, et al. Identification of a receptor mediating absorption of dietary cholesterol in the intestine. Biochemistry 1998; 37:17843–17850.

138. Schulthess G, Compassi S, Werder M, Han CH, Phillips MC, Hauser H. Intestinal sterol absorption mediated by scavenger receptor is competitively inhibited by amphipathic peptides and proteins. Biochemistry 2000; 39:12623–12631.

139. Mardones P, Quinones V, Amigo L, et al. Hepatic cholesterol and bile acid metabolism and intestinal cholesterol absorption in scavenger receptor class B type I-deficient mice. J Lipid Res 2001; 42:170–180.

140. Harmon CM, Luce P, Beth AH, Abumrad NA. Labeling of adipocyte membranes by sulfo-N-succinimidyl derivatives of long-chain fatty acids: inhibition of fatty acid transport. J Membr Biol 1991; 121:261–268.

141. Abumrad NA, el-Maghrabi MR, Amri EZ, Lopez E, Grimaldi PA. Cloning of a rat adipocyte membrane protein implicated in binding or transport of long-chain fatty acids that is induced during preadipocyte differentiation. Homology with human CD36. J Biol Chem 1993; 268:17665–17668.

142. Van Nieuwenhoven FA, Verstijnen CPHJ, Abumrad NA, et al. Putative membrane fatty acid-translocase and cytoplasmic fatty acid-binding protein are co-expressed in rat heart and skeletal muscles. Biochem Biophys Res Commun 1995; 207:747–752.

143. Spitzberg VL, Matitashivili E, Gorewit RC. Association and coexpression of fatty-acid-binding protein and glycoprotein CD36 in bovine mammary gland. Eur J Biochem 1995; 230:872–878.

144. Poirier H, DeGrace P, Niot I, Bernard A, Besnard P. Localization and regulation of the putative membrane fatty-acid transporter (FAT) in the small intestine. Comparison with fatty acid-binding proteins (FABP). Eur J Biochem 1996; 238:368–373.

145. Abumrad NA, Sfeir Z, Connelly MA, Coburn C. Lipid transporters: membrane transport systems for cholesterol and fatty acids. Curr Opin Clin Nutr Metab Care 2000; 3:255–262.

146. Schaffer JE, Lodish HF. Expression cloning and characterization of a novel adipocyte long chain fatty acid transport protein. Cell 1994; 79:427–436.

147. Stahl A, Gimeno RE, Tartaglia LA, Lodish HF. Fatty acid transport proteins: a current view of a growing family. Trends Endocrinol Metab 2001; 12:331.

148. Hermann T, Buchkremer F, Gosch I, Hall AM, Bernlohr DA, Stremmel W. Characterization of the fatty acid transport protein 4 (FATP4) gene and functional assessment of FATP4 as very long chain acyl-CoA synthetase. Gastroenterology 2001; 120:A306.

149. Hermann T, Buchkremer F, Gosch I, et al. The fatty acid transport protein (FATP1) is a very long chain acyl-CoA synthetase. J Biol Chem 1999; 274:36300–36304.

150. Murata M, Peränen J, Schreiner R, Wieland F, Kurzchalia TV, Simons K. VIP21/caveolin is a cholesterol-binding protein. Proc Natl Acad Sci USA 1995; 92:10339–10343.

151. Parton RG. Ultrastructural localization of gangliosides; GM_1 is concentrated in caveolae. J Histochem Cytochem 1994; 42:155–166.

152. Rothberg KG, Ying Y-S, Kamen BA, Anderson RGW. Cholesterol controls the clustering of the glycophospholipid-anchored membrane receptor for 5-methyltetrahydrofolate. J Cell Biol 1990; 111:2931–2938.

153. Ying Y-S, Anderson RGW, Rothberg KG. Each caveola contains multiple glycosylphosphatidylinositol-anchored membrane proteins. Cold Spring Harb Symp Quant Biol 1992; 57:593–604.

154. Anderson RGW, Kamen BA, Rothberg KG, Lacey SW. Potocytosis: sequestration and transport of small molecules by caveolae. Science 1992; 255:410–411.

155. Repa JJ, Turley SD, Lobaccaro JMA, et al. Regulation of absorption and ABC-1 mediated efflux of cholesterol by RXR heterodimers. Science 2000; 289:1524–1529.

156. Berge KE, Tian H, Graf GA, et al. Accumulation of dietary cholesterol in sitosterolemia caused by mutations in adjacent ABC transporters. Science 2000; 290:1771–1775.

157. Lee MH, Lu K, Hazard S, et al. Identification of a gene ABCG5, important in the regulation of dietary cholesterol absorption. Nat Genet 2001; 27:79–83

158. van Heek M, Farley C, Compton DS, et al. Comparison of the activity and disposition of the novel cholesterol absorption inhibitor, SCH58235, and its glucuronide, SCH60663. Br J Pharacol 2000; 129:1748–1754.

159. van Heek M, Farley C, Compton DS, Hoos L, Davis HR. Ezetimibe selectivity inhibits intestinal cholesterol absorption in rodents in the presence and absence of exocrine pancreatic function. Br J Pharmacol 2001; 134:409–417.

160. Altmann SW, Davis HR Jr, Zhu LJ, et al. Niemann-Pick C1 Like 1 Protein is critical for intestinal cholesterol absorption. Science 2004; 303:1201–1204.

161. Garcia-Calvo M, Lisnock J, Bull HG, et al. The target of ezetimibe is Niemann-Pick C1-Like 1 (NPC1L!). Proc Natl Acad Sci U S A 2005; 102:8132–137.

162. Repa JJ, Dietschy JM, Turley SD. Inhibition of cholesterol absorption by SCH 58053 in the mouse is not mediated via changes in the expression on mRNA for ABCA1, ABCG5, or ABCG8 in the enterocyte. J Lipid Res 2002; 43:1864–1874.

163. Kramer W, Girbig F, Corsiero D, et al. Aminopeptidase N (CD13) is a molecular target of the cholesterol absorption inhibitor ezetimibe in the enterocyte brush border membrane. J Biol Chem 2005; 280:1306–1320.

164. Ockner RK, Manning JA. Fatty acid binding protein in small intestine. Identification, isolation and evidence for its role in cellular fatty acid transport. J Clin Invest 1974; 54:326–338.

165. Ockner RK, Manning JA, Poppenhausen RB, Ho WK. A binding protein for fatty acids in cytosol intestinal mucosa, liver, myocardium, and other tissues. Science 1972; 177:56–58.

166. Glatz JFC, Veerkamp JH. Intracellular fatty acid-binding proteins. Int J Biochem 1985; 17:13–22.

167. Bass MM. The cellular fatty acid-binding proteins: aspects of structure, regulation, and function. Int Rev Cytol 1988; 111:143–184.

168. Bansal MP, Cook RG, Danielson KG, Medina D. A 14-kilodalton selenium-binding protein in mouse liver is fatty acid-binding protein. J Biol Chem 1989; 264:13780–13784.

169 Cistola DP, Sacchettini JC, Banaszak LJ, Walsh MT, Gordon JI. Fatty acid interactions with rat intestinal and liver fatty acid-binding proteins expressed in Escherichia coli. A comparative 13C NMR study. J Biol Chem 1989; 264: 2700–2710.

170 Storch J, Thumser AE. The fatty acid transport function of fatty acid-binding proteins. Biochim Biophys Acta 2000; 1486:28–44.

171. Shaughnessy S, Smith ER, Kodukula S, Storch J, Fried SK. Adipocyte metabolism in adipocyte fatty acid binding protein knockout mice (aP2-/-) after short-term high-fat feeding: functional compensation by the keratinocyte fatty acid binding protein. Diabetes 2000; 49:904–911.

172. Vassileva G, Huwyler L, Poirier K, Agellon LB, Toth MJ. The intestinal fatty acid binding protein is not essential for dietary fat absorption in mice. FASEB J 2000; 14:2040–2046.

173. Newberry EP, Xie Y, Kennedy S, et al. Decreased hepatic triglyceride accumulation and altered fatty acid uptake in mice with deletion of the liver fatty acid-binding protein gene. J Biol Chem 2003; 278:51664–51672.

174. Nolan BJ, Arebalo RE, Hansburg E, Scallen TJ. Purification and properties of sterol carrier protein$_2$. J Biol Chem 1980; 255:4282–4289.

175. Scallen TJ, Seetharam B, Srikantaiah MV, Hansbury E, Lewis MK. Sterol carrier protein hypothesis: requirement for three substrate-specific soluble proteins in liver cholesterol biosynthesis. Life Sci 1975; 16:853–873.

176. Srikantaiah MV, Hansbury E, Loughram ED, Scallen TJ. Purification and proper-ties of sterol carrier protein 1. J Biol Chem 1976; 251:5496–5504.

177. Scallen TJ, Nolan BJ, Gavey KL, et al. Sterol carrier protein 2 and fatty acid-bind-ing protein. J Biol Chem 1985; 260:4733–4739.

178. Vahouny GV, Dennis P, Chanderbhan R, Fiskum RG, Nolan BJ, Scallen TJ. Sterol carrier protein 2 (SCP$_2$) mediated transfer of cholesterol to mitochondrial inner membranes. Biochem Biophys Res Commun 1984; 122:509–515.

179. Leonard AN, Cohen DE. Submicellar bile salts stimulate phosphatidylcholine transfer activity of sterol carrier protein 2. J Lipid Res 1998; 39:1981–1988.

180. Starodub O, Jolly CA, Atshaves BP, et al. Sterol carrier protein-2 localization in endoplasmic reticulum and role in phospholipid formation. Am J Physiol 2000; 279:C1259–C1269.

181. Murphy EJ. Sterol carrier protein-2 expression increases NBD-stearate uptake and cytoplasmic diffusion in L cells. Am J Physiol 1998; 275:G237–G243.

182. Wirtz KW, Wouters FS, Bastiaens PH, Wanders RJ, Seedorf U, Jovin TM. The non-specific lipid transfer protein (sterol carrier protein 2) acts as a peroxisomal fatty acid-CoA binding protein. Biochem Soc Trans 1998; 26:374–378.

183. Johnston JM. Triglyceride biosynthesis in the intestinal mucosa. In: Rommel K, Goebell H, Bohmer R, eds., Lipid Absorption: Biochemical and Clinical Aspects. Lancaster, UK: MTP Press, 1976:85–94.

184. Kuksis A, Manganaro F. Biochemical characterization and purification of intestinal acylglycerol acyltransferases. In: Kuksis A, ed., Fat Absorption. Boca Raton: CRC Press, 1986:233–259.

185. Rao GA, Johnston JM. Purification and properties of triglyceride synthetase from the intestinal mucosa. Biochim Biophys Acta 1966; 125:465–473.

186. Lehner R, Kuksis A. Triacylglycerol synthesis by purified triacylglycerol synthetase of rat intestinal mucosa. Role of acyl-CoA acyltransferase. J Biol Chem 1995; 270:13630–13636.

187. Smith SJ, Cases S, Jensen DR, et al. Obesity resistance and multiple mechanisms of triglyceride synthesis in mice lacking Dgat. Nat Genet 2000; 25:87–90.

188. Yen CE, Monetti M, Burry BJ, Farese RV Jr. The triacylglycerol synthesis enzyme DGAT1 also catalyzes the synthesis of diacylglycerols, waxes, and retinol esters. J Lipid Res 2005; 46:1502–1511.

189. Chen HC, Ladha Z, Farese RV Jr. Deficiency of acyl coenzyme A: diacylglycerol acyltransferase 1 increases leptin sensitivity in murine obesity models. Endocrinology 2002; 143:2893–2898.

190. Chen HC, Smith SJ, Laha Z, et al. Increased insulin and leptin sensitivity in mice lacking acyl CoA:diacylglycerol acyltransferase 1. J Clin Invest. 2002; 109:175–181.

191. Cases S, Zhou P, Shillingford JM, et al. Development of the mammary gland requires DGAT1 expression in stromal and epithelial tissues. Development 2004; 131:3047–3055.

192. Cao J, Burn P, Shi Y. Properties of the mouse intestinal Acyl-CoA: monoacylglycerol acyltransferase, MGAT2. J Biol Chem 2003; 278:25657–25663.

193. Cao J, Lockwood J, Burn P, Shi Y. Cloning and functional characterization of a mouse intestinal acyl-CoA: monoacylglycerol acyltransferase, MGAT2. J Biol Chem 2003; 278:13860–13866.

194. Cheng D, Nelson TC, Chen J, et al. Identification of acyl coenzyme A: monoacylglycerol acyltransferase 3, an intestinal specific enzyme implicated in dietary fat absorption. J Biol Chem 2003; 278:13611–13614.

195. Wetterau JR, Zilversmit DB. A triglyceride and cholesteryl ester transfer protein associated with liver microsomes. J Biol Chem 1984; 259:10863–10866.

196. Wetterau JR, Zilversmit DB. Purification and characterization triglyceride and cholesteryl ester transfer protein from bovine liver microsomes. Chem Phys Lipids 1985; 38:205–222.

197. Wetterau JR, Zilversmit DB. Localization of intracellular triacylglycerol and cholesteryl ester transfer activity in rat tissues. Biochim Biophys Acta 1986; 875:610–617.

198. Nilsson A. Intestinal absorption of lecithin and lysolecithin by lymph fistula rats. Biochim Biophys Acta 1968; 152:379–390.

199. Sato Y. The metabolic fate of lysolecithin administered into rat duodenal lumen. Tohuku J Exp Med 1970; 100:227–287.

200. Scow RO, Stein Y, Stein O. Incorporation of dietary lecithin and lysolecithin into lymph chylomicrons in the rat. J Biol Chem 1967; 242:4919–4924.

201. Subbaiah PV, Sastry PS, Ganguly J. Acylation of lysolecithin in the intestinal mucosa of rats. Biochem J 1970; 118:241–246.

202. Ottolenghi A. Estimation and subcellular distribution of lecithinase activity in rat intestinal mucosa. J Lipid Res 1964; 5:537.

203. Kim DL, Betzing H. Intestinal absorption of polyunsaturated phosphatidylcholine in the rat. Hoppe-Seylers Z Physiol Chem 1976; 357:1321–1331.

204. Erbland JF, Marinetti GV. The enzymatic acylation and hydrolysis of lysolecithin. Biochim Biophys Acta 1965; 106:128–138.

205. Thomson ABR, Dietschy JM. Intestinal lipid absorption: major extracellular and intracellular events. In: Johnson LR, ed., Physiology of the Gastrointestinal Tract. New York: Raven, 1981:1147–1220.

206. Bennett Clark S, Tercyak AM. Reduced cholesterol transmucosal transport in rats with inhibited mucosal acyl CoA: cholesterol acyltransferase and normal pancreatic function. J Lipid Res 1984; 25:148–159.

207. Gallo LL, Newbill T, Hyun J, Vahouny GV. Role of pancreatic cholesterol esterase in the uptake and esterification of cholesterol by isolated intestinal cells. Proc Soc Exp Biol Med 1977; 156:277–281.

208. Borja R, Vahouny GV, Treadwell CR. Role of bile and pancreatic juice in cholesterol absorption and esterification. Am J Physiol 1964; 206:223–228.

209. Norum KR, Helgerud P, Petersen LB, Groot PJE, Dejonge HR. Influence of diets on acyl-CoA: cholesterol acyltransferase in villous and crypt cells from rat small intestinal mucosa and in the liver. Biochim Biophys Acta 1983; 751:153–161.

210. Norum KR, Lilljeqvist AC, Drevon CA. Coenzyme-A-dependent esterification of cholesterol in intestinal mucosa from guinea-pig. Scand J Gastroenterol 1977; 12:281–288.

211. Field FJ, Cooper AD, Erickson SK. Regulation of rabbit intestinal acid acyl coenzyme A-cholesterol acyltransferase in vivo and in vitro. Gastroenterology 1982; 83:873–880.

212. Helgerud P, Saarem K, Norum KR. Acyl-CoA:cholesterol acyltransferase in human small intestine: its activity and some properties of the enzymic reaction. J Lipid Res 1981; 22:271–277.

213. Gallo LL, Chiang Y, Vahouny GV, Treadwell CR. Localization and origin of rat intestinal cholesterol esterase determined by immunocytochemistry. J Lipid Res 1980; 21:537–545.

214. Field FJ. Intestinal cholesterol esterase: intracellular enzyme or contamination of cytosol by pancreatic enzymes. J Lipid Res 1984; 25:389–399.

215. Helgerud P, Haugen R, Norum KR. The effect of feeding and fasting on the activity of acyl-CoA: cholesterol acyltransferase in rat small intestine. Eur J Clin Invest 1982; 12:493–500.

216. Watt SM, Simmonds WJ. The effect of pancreatic diversion on lymphatic absorption and esterification of cholesterol in the rat. J Lipid Res 1981; 22:157–165.

217. Fukushima H, Aono S, Nakamura Y, Endo M, Imai T. The effect of N-(alpha-methylbenzyl)linoleamide on cholesterol metabolism in rats. J Athero Res 1969; 10:403–414.

218. Harnett KM, Walsh CT, Zhang L. Effects of Bay o 2752, a hypocholesterolemic agent on intestinal taurocholate absorption and cholesterol esterification. J Pharmacol Exp Therap 1989; 251:502–509.

219. Tso P, Morshed KM, Nutting DF. Importance of acyl CoA-cholesterol acyltransferase (ACAT) in the esterification of cholesterol by enterocytes. FASEB J 1991; 5:A709.

220. Lee HT, Roark WH, Picard JA, et al. Inhibitors of acyl-CoA:cholesterol O-acyl-transferase (ACAT) as hypocholesterolemic agents: synthesis and structure-activity relationships of novel series of sulfonamides, acylphosphonamides and acylphosphoramidates. Bioorg Med Chem Lett 1998; 8:289–294.

221. Chang CC, Chen J, Thomas MA, et al. Regulation and immunolocalization of acyl-coenzyme A: cholesterol acyltransferase in mammalian cells as studied with specific antibodies. J Biol Chem 1995; 270:29532–29540.

222. Chang CC, Sakashita N, Ornvold K, et al. Immunological quantitation and localization of ACAT-1 and ACAT-2 in human liver and small intestine. J Biol Chem 2000; 275:28083–28092.

223 Miyazaki A, Sakashita N, Lee O, et al. Expression of ACAT-1 protein in human atherosclerotic lesions and cultured human monocyte-macrophages. Arterioscler Thromb Vas Biol 1998; 18:1568–1574.

224 Buhman KK, Accad M, Novak S, et al. Resistance to diet-induced hypercholesterolemia and gallstone formation in ACAT-2 deficient mice. Nat Med 2000; 6:1341–1347.

225. Rudel LL, Lee RG, Cockman TL. Acyl coenzyme A: cholesterol acyltransferase types 1 and 2: structure and function in atherosclerosis. Curr Opin Lipid 2001: 12:121–127.

226. Cartwright IJ, Plonne D, Higgins JA. Intracellular events in the assembly of chylomicrons in rabbit enterocytes. J Lipid Res 2000; 41:1728–1739.

227. Cartwright IJ, Higgins JA. Direct evidence for a two-step assembly of apoB48-containing lipoproteins in the lumen of the smooth endoplasmic reticulum of rabbit enterocytes. J Biol Chem 2001: 276:48048–48057.

228. Kumar NS, Mansbach CM. Determinants of triacylglycerol transport from the endoplasmic reticulum to the Golgi in intestine. Am J Physiol 1997: 273:G18–G30.

229. Kumar NS, Mansbach CM. Prechylomicron transport vesicle: isolation and partial characterization. Am J Physiol 1999; 276:G378–G386.

230. Siddiqi SA, Gorelick FS, Mahan JT, Mansbach CM. COPII proteins are required for Golgi fusion but not for endoplasmic reticulum budding of the prechylomicron transport vesicle. L Cell Sci 2002; 116:415–427.

231. Matsuoka K, Orci L, Amherdt M, et al. COPII-coated vesicle formation reconstituted with purified coat proteins and chemically defined liposomes. Cell 1998; 93:263–275.

232. Jones B, Jones EL, Bonney SA, et al. Mutations in a Sar1 GTPase of COPII vesicles are associated with lipid absorption disorders. Nat Genet 2003; 34:29–31.

233. Hussain MM. A proposed model for the assembly of chylomicrons. Atherosclerosis 2000; 148:1–15.

234. Murphy S, Albright E, Mathur SN, Field FJ. Effect of eicosapentaenoic acid on triacylglycerol transport in CaCo-2 cells. Biochim Biophys Acta 1990; 1045:147–155.

235. Kam NT, Albright E, Mathur SN, Field FJ. Inhibition of acylcoenzyme A:cholesterol acyltransferase activity in CaCo-2 cells results in intracellular triglyceride accumulation. J Lipid Res 1989; 30:371–377.

236. Kam NT, Albright E, Mathur SN, Field FJ. Effect of lovastatin on acyl-CoA: cholesterol acyltransferase (ACAT) activity and the basolateral-membrane secretion of newly synthesized lipids by CaCo-2 cells. Biochem J 1990; 272:427–433.

237. Traber MG, Kayden HJ, Rindler MJ. Polarized secretion of newly synthesized lipoproteins by the Caco-2 human intestinal cell line. J Lipid Res 1987; 28:1350–1363.

238. Murphy S, Albright E, Mathur SN, Davidson NO, Field FJ. Apolipoprotein B mRNA abundance is decreased by eicosapentaenoic acid in CaCo-2 cells. Effect on the synthesis and secretion of apolipoprotein B. Arterioscler Thromb 1992; 12:691–700.

239. Ockner RK, Hughes FB, Isselbacher KJ. Very low density lipoproteins in intestinal lymph: role in triglyceride and cholesterol transport during fat absorption. J Clin Invest 1969; 48:2367–2373.

240. Ockner RK, Manning JA. Fatty acid binding protein in small intestine. Identification, isolation and evidence for its role in cellular fatty acid transport. J Clin Invest 1974; 54:326–338.

241. Tso P, Drake DS, Black DD, Sabesin SM. Evidence for separate pathways of chylomicron and very low density lipoprotein assembly and transport by rat small intestine. Am J Physiol 1984; 247:G599–G610.

242. Zilversmit DB. The composition and structure of lymph chylomicrons in dog, rat, and man. J Clin Invest 1965; 44:1610–1622.

243. Lindgren FT, Jensen LC, Hatch FT. The isolation and quantitative analysis of serum lipoproteins. In: Nelson GJ, ed., Blood Lipids and Lipoproteins: Quantitation, Composition and Metabolism. New York: Wiley, 1972:181–274.

244. Mahley RW, Bennett BD, Morre DJ, Gray ME, Thistlethwaite W, LeQuire VS. Lipoproteins associated with golgi apparatus isolated from epithelial cells of rat small intestine. Lab Invest 1971; 25:435–444.

245. Vahouny GV, Blendermann EM, Gallo LL, Treadwell CR. Differential transport of cholesterol and oleic acid in lymph lipoproteins: sex differences in puromycin sensitivity. J Lipid Res 1981; 21:415–424.

246. Tso P, Balint JA, Bishop MB, Rodgers JB. Acute inhibition of intestinal lipid transport by Pluronic L-81 in the rat. Am J Physiol 1981; 241:G487–G497.

247. Tso P, Balint JA, Rodgers JB. Effect of hydrophobic surfactant (Pluronic L-81) on lymphatic lipid transport in the rat. Am J Physiol 1980; 239:G348–G353.

248. Tso P, Kendrick H, Balint JA, Simmonds WJ. Role of biliary phosphatidylcholine in the absorption and transport of dietary triolein in the rat. Gastroenterology 1981; 80:60–65.

249. Nutting D, Hall J, Barrowman JA, Tso P. Further studies on the mechanism of inhibition of intestinal chylomicron transport by Pluronic L-81. Biochim Biophys Acta 1989; 22:357–362.

250. Luchoomun J, Hussain MM. Assembly and secretion of chylomicrons by differentiated cells: Nascent triglycerides and preformed phospholipids are preferentially used for lipoprotein assembly. J Biol Chem 1999; 274:19565–19572.

251. Hussain MM, Kancha RK, Zhou Z, Luchoomun J, Zu H, Bakillah A. Chylomicron assembly and catabolism: role of apolipoproteins and receptors. Biochim Biophys Acta 1996; 1300:151–170.

252. Trotter PJ, Storch J. Fatty acid esterification during differentiation of the human intestinal cell line Caco-2. J Biol Chem 1993; 268:10017–10023.

253. Gallagher N, Webb J, Dawson AM. The absorption of ^{14}C oleic acid and ^{14}C triolein in bile fistula rats. Clin Sci 1965; 29:75–82.

254. Dawson AM. A review of fat transport. In: Burland WL, Samuel PD, eds., Transport Across the Intestine. London: Churchill Livingstone, 1965:210.

255. Sabesin SM, Isselbacher KJ. Protein synthesis inhibition: mechanism for production of impaired fat absorption. Science Washington DC 1965; 147:1149–1151.

256. Kayden HJ, Medick M. The absorption and metabolism of short and long chain fatty acids in puromycin-treated rats. Biochim Biophys Acta 1967; 176:37–43.

257. Ways PO, Paramentier CM, Kayden HD, Jones JW, Saunders DR, Rubin CE. Studies on the absorptive defect for triglyceride in abetalipoproteinemia. J Clin Invest 1967; 46:35–46.

258. Fujimoto K, Price VH, Granger DN, Specian R, Bergstedt S, Tso P. Effect of ischemia-reperfusion on lipid digestion and absorption in rat intestine. Am J Physiol 1991; 260:G595–G602.

259. McDonald GB, Saunders DR, Weidman M, Fisher L. Portal venous transport of long-chain fatty acids absorbed from rat intestine. Am J Physiol 1980; 239:G141–G150.

260. Mansbach CM II, Dowell RF, Pritchett D. Portal transport of absorbed lipids in rats. Am J Physiol 1991; 261:G530–G538.

261. Jandacek RJ, Tso P. Factors affecting the storage and excretion of toxic lipophilic xenobiotics. Lipids 2001; 36:1289–1305.

262. Cavret S, Laurent C, Feidt C, Laurent F, Rychen G. Intestinal absorption of 14C from 14C-phenanthrene, 14C-benzo[a]pyrene and 14C-tetrachlorodibenzo-para-dioxin: approaches with the Caco-2 cell line and with portal absorption measurements in growing pigs. Reprod Nutr Dev 2003; 43:145–154.

10

Characterizing Release from Lipid-Based Formulations

Jennifer Dressman, Karen Schamp, and Karen Beltz
Institute of Pharmaceutical Technology, Johann Wolfgang Goethe University, Frankfurt am Main, Germany

Jochem Alsenz
Preformulation F. Hofmann-LaRoche Grenzacherstrasse, Basel, Switzerland

RELEASE TESTING OF LIPID-BASED DOSAGE FORMS: WHAT DO WE HOPE TO ACHIEVE?

Characterizing the release of an active pharmaceutical ingredient (API) is usually performed for one or more of the following reasons:

- to compare formulation candidates during product development
- as a quality control procedure after manufacture
- to assure that quality is maintained throughout the product shelf-life
- to assure that quality is maintained from batch to batch
- to assure that quality is maintained after a change is made in the composition or manufacturing procedure
- to predict product performance in vivo.

According to the aims of the release test, the conditions may need to be adjusted. For example, quite complex media might be required to predict in vivo performance, and simplifications would be needed to transpose these tests into a design that would be appropriate for routine quality control purposes.

Lipophilic dosage forms present special challenges to the design of release tests. Unlike most immediate release (IR) solid oral dosage forms, the excipients in lipophilic dosage forms often do not lend themselves to easy dispersion in simple aqueous media such as those typically used for dissolution testing (e.g., dilute hydrochloric acid, phosphate buffers, etc.). However, in the gastrointestinal tract, dispersion will occur via emulsification in the stomach and small intestine. Furthermore, for digestible lipids, the excipients will gradually disappear during the digestion process in the small intestine, which will force the active pharmaceutical ingredient (API) to come into contact with the intestinal fluids. Dynamic modelling of release from lipophilic dosage forms resulting from lipolysis of the excipients is discussed elsewhere in this book (Chapter 11) and will not be covered further here.

For APIs that are dissolved in a lipophilic vehicle, some release may occur via partitioning processes prior to and during digestion of the excipients. In this case, it is important to come away from classical notions of dissolution testing and recognize that bulk partitioning processes are dependent on a different set of parameters and that the usual Noyes-Whitney type of model will not be adequate in such cases. For example, in a self-emulsifying system the lipid droplet size formed will have a profound effect on the interfacial area between the lipid and aqueous phases and hence, the kinetics of phase transfer. Other lipophilic vehicles may form micellar phases rather than emulsions upon dispersion in the gastrointestinal fluids, and the kinetics of drug transfer from the micellar phase into the aqueous phase may be rate-determining to the overall release process. Of course, it is quite possible that both emulsion and micellar phases are formed; here the kinetics of transfer will depend on the relative rates of transfer out of the emulsion and from the micellar phase.

Finally, if the API is suspended in the lipophilic vehicle, any one of several processes—dispersion of the vehicle, digestion of the vehicle or dissolution of the API from the particles liberated from the vehicle—could be the rate-determining step to release. In such cases, some effort should be directed to establishing the rate-limiting step and designing the release test primarily around that process.

SPECIAL CONSIDERATIONS FOR DISSOLUTION TESTING OF LIPID-BASED FORMULATIONS

In this section, the considerations specific to designing release tests for lipophilic dosage forms will be addressed. These include the ability of the lipid-based vehicle to disperse into various types of media, whether the API partitions from the vehicle into the aqueous medium from a solution in the lipophilic vehicle or whether it is in suspension, and how to recover the API from the appropriate phases in the release medium.

Dispersability of the Dosage Form into Aqueous Media

The Dosage Form Dissolves into the Aqueous Dissolution Medium

Sometimes vehicles are (somewhat misleadingly) classed as "lipophilic" when they are really just "non-aqueous." A typical example would be the use of poly-ethylene glycol mixtures as vehicles for manufacture of soft gelatine capsule dosage forms. As these excipients are highly water soluble, no special design of

Table 1 Composition of a Medium Biorelevant for Gastric
Conditions in the Fasted State

FaSSGF	Bile salt (sodium taurocholate) (μM)	80
	Lecithin (μM)	10
	Pepsin (mg/mL)	1
	Sodium chloride (mM)	34.2
	Hydrochloric acid	to pH 1.6

Source: From Ref. 2.

the release test is necessary: a simple aqueous buffer solution will suffice unless the API itself is poorly water-soluble. The design of dissolution tests for poorly soluble APIs has been discussed thoroughly elsewhere (1).

The Dosage Form Forms Micelles in the Aqueous Dissolution Medium

Many lipophilic vehicles contain high amounts of surfactants in the formulation and, upon dispersion in the gastrointestinal fluids, these surfactants may form micelles which partly or completely solubilise the API and other components of the formulation. For these formulations as well, a complex media design for the release test is unnecessary. However, it may be worth dispersing such formulations into various biorelevant media to check that micelles are formed as expected and that the API and other components do not separate from the micellar phase. The currently recommended compositions of FaSSGF (2), FaSSIF and FeSSIF are given in Tables 1–3. Care should be taken to use appropriate dilution volumes for such experiments. For FaSSGF and FaSSIF a reasonable volume would be 250 mL, for FeSSIF 500–1000 mL can be used. Measuring the micellar particle size of the resultant fluid may also be useful to forecast the ability of the formulation to form physically stable and reproducible micelles when it comes in contact with the gastrointestinal fluids. For experiments in FaSSGF the particle size distribution of the dispersed phase can be determined by readily available techniques such as laser light scattering or PCS. For FaSSIF and FeSSIF one would look for a change (swelling) in the micellar size associated with dispersion of the dosage form.

The Dosage Form Forms an Emulsion in the Aqueous Medium

Self-emulsifying dosage forms usually contain high levels of surfactant to induce emulsion formation in vivo. For these formulations, it is very likely that dispersion

Table 2 Composition of a Medium Biorelevant for Upper Small
Intestinal Conditions in the Fasted State

NEW FASSIF	Bile salt (sodium taurocholate) (mM)	3
	Lecithin (mM)	0.2
	Phosphate/maleate buffer qs pH	6.5
	Osmolality (mOsm/kg)	180
	Buffer capacity (mEq/L/pH)	10

Source: From Ref. 1.

Table 3   Composition of a Medium Biorelevant for Upper Small Intestinal Conditions in the Fed State

Composition	"NEW-FeSSIF"
Bile salt (mM)	7.5
Lecithin (mM)	2
Glyceryl mono-oleate (mM)	5
Sodium oleate (mM)	0.8
Citrate buffer qs pH	5.80
Osmolality (mOsm/kg)	390
Buffer capacity (mEq/L/pH)	25

Source: From Ref. 1.

in the gastrointestinal fluids will result not only in a fine emulsion but that a micellar phase will be formed either initially or as the dispersion comes in contact with the lipases, bile salts and lecithin secreted into the duodenum from the pancreas and gall bladder, respectively. Here too, attempts to better understand the dispersion process in vivo by diluting the formulation with biorelevant media may aid development of systems which behave robustly under gastrointestinal conditions (see p. 243). Since at least part of the API will initially be located in the emulsion phase, centrifugation and subsequent analysis of the oily and aqueous phases for the API will give some indications of the relative importance of the various phase transfer mechanisms to the overall release rate. If most of the API resides in the emulsion initially, obviously bulk partitioning is going to be more important than if the API has already partly transferred into the aqueous phase as a result of the dilution procedure. A third point to consider is whether the API has remained in solution during the dilution: this can be investigated by comparing turbidometric measurements in formulations with and without API present, in both the oily and aqueous phases obtained after centrifugation.

The Dosage Form Is Already an Emulsion

Sometimes the API is presented in an emulsion, rather than a self-emulsifying formulation. In this case, the question of whether the droplet size of the emulsion will be changed when the formulation comes in contact with the gastrointestinal fluids may well be important to the rate of phase transfer. Interestingly, the motility pattern in the stomach comes into play here. Studies in the food industry indicate that, regardless of the initial droplet size of an emulsion, the droplet size will be adjusted to 15 to 20 μm by the time it is emptied through the pylorus. This phenomenon is observed both with coarse emulsions (>20 μm) and fine emulsions like processed milk, which has a droplet size of about 1 μm (3,4). To study release from ready-made emulsion products with droplet sizes greater than 20 μm under intestinal conditions, shearing the emulsion to produce an appropriate droplet size may improve predictions of in vivo release behaviour. However, for physical stability reasons, most pharmaceutical emulsions aim to have a fine droplet size, far less than

15–20 μm. For such products, one could contemplate breaking the emulsion, though admittedly this might be difficult to achieve with any degree of reproducibility.

Partitioning of the API From the Dosage Form into the Aqueous Phase

The Drug Is in Solution in the Lipid-Based Formulation

If the drug is truly in solution in the lipophilic phase of the dosage form, and the lipid is digested by the gastric and intestinal lipases, release of the API may be governed by the kinetics of lipolysis. Pancreatic juice contains at least three lipolytic enzymes (5).

The first enzyme, usually referred to as lipase, is a glycerol–ester hydrolase that hydrolyses a wide variety of insoluble esters of glycerol at an oil–water interface; it requires the cooperation of surface active agents such as bile salts and of co-lipase which is also secreted by the pancreas. Its pH optimum depends on the substrate and ranges from pH 7 to 9. The rate of reaction will depend on the lipids that are used in the formulation. For example, triglycerides with chain lengths of 16 to 20 are good substrates for lipolysis, but those with longer chain lengths are only slowly, if at all, digested. Long chain triglycerides (C16 and C18) often form the basis for lipophilic formulations, but medium chain triglycerides are being increasingly used for formulation, as well.

The second enzyme hydrolyses esters of secondary and other alcohols, such as those of cholesterol, at an optimal pH of 8.0 and also requires the presence of bile salts. The third enzyme hydrolyzes water-soluble esters.

In addition to hydrolyzing triglycerides, lipase can also remove one of the esterified fatty acid molecules from di-glycerides to form mono-glycerides and the reaction can proceed further, resulting in the formation of free fatty acids and glycerol. Many commercial lipid vehicles contain a mixture of glycerides with varying fatty acid chain length and/or degree of glycerol substitution. For example, soybean oil is a long chain triglyceride, whereas Peceol® consists of long chain mono- and diglycerides, and Capmul® of medium chain mono- and di-glycerides. The monoglycerides, in particular, enjoy some water solubility. For example, glycerol monooleate is soluble in water up to a maximum concentration of about 8–10 mM. Monoglycerides also act as water-in-oil emulsifiers and thus promote generation of interfacial area, which will facilitate both API partitioning into the aqueous phase and hydrolysis of the triglycerides. Thus, their presence will encourage faster release of the API from the lipid vehicle. In addition, many formulations contain one or more additional surfactants such as Labrasol and Softigen 767 [principally macrogol-C8/C10-(partial)glycerides], Gelucire 44/14 (Lauryl macrogol 32 glyceride containing a range of C10 to C18 fatty acid chains), Tweens (e.g., POE-sorbitan-monolaurate and -monooleate) and Vit E TPGS. These additional surfactants can improve the dispersability of the formulation in aqueous systems substantially. This in turn will increase the interface available for both API partitioning and digestion, although the question remains as to whether interactions of the surfactants with co-lipase, lecithin and bile salts favour or hinder the digestive process.

Nondigestible oils for example, paraffin oil, appear not to release lipophilic APIs readily into the aqueous phase. In fact, their continued use has been shown to lead to deficiencies in fat-soluble vitamins. This is a strong indication that digestion of the lipid vehicle is a key factor in the release of the dissolved API from the vehicle.

The Drug Is Suspended in the Lipid-Based Formulation

If the API is suspended rather than dissolved in the lipid vehicle, the slowest of the various processes involved in release from the vehicle will determine the overall rate. Thus, digestion of the lipid vehicle, which enables contact of the solid API with the aqueous medium or dissolution of the API in the aqueous medium after digestion of the lipid surrounding it may determine the overall rate of release. On the other hand, if the drug is very poorly soluble, the particle size of the suspended material may be crucial to the overall rate of release.

APPROACHES TO RELEASE TESTING OF LIPID-BASED DOSAGE FORMS

Compendial Approaches

One approach to release testing of lipid-based dosage forms is to argue that the formulation should be as robust to the gastrointestinal physiology as possible. Following this line of reasoning, the best formulations in terms of reproducibility of performance will be the ones that can release the API into even simple, aqueous media. Common pharmacopieal media such as those described in the United States Pharmacopeia (USP) and International Pharmacopeia (Ph.Int.) of the World Health Organisation (WHO) would be applicable for formulations developed in this context.

Simulated Gastric Fluid

Typically used media for testing robustness of release are simulated gastric fluid (SGF) and simulated intestinal fluid (SIF). Recipes for these vary among the different pharmacopeia, but generally speaking SGF contains a dilute hydrochloric acid solution (mimicking normal gastric pH, although the pH of SGF is a bit on the low side—see the formula for FaSSGF in the tables), some sodium chloride to adjust the osmolarity to a value close to that of gastric aspirates and pepsin, the main digestive enzyme in the stomach. For the purposes of studying release from lipid-based vehicles, the addition of pepsin offers few advantages since it is a protease, not a lipase. Additionally, the amounts of pepsin suggested by the USP are very high compared to those recovered in gastric aspirates from healthy volunteers (6).

Simulated Intestinal Fluid

SIF consists of a phosphate buffer to adjust the pH to 6.8 (a value typical of the mid-jejunum) (7) and pancreatin, which is an extract of the pancreas rich in amylase, proteases and lipase. For lipid-based dosage forms it could obviously be quite important to include the pancreatin in the medium. However, at the USP suggested concentration of 2000 lipase Units/mL, the concentration exceeds, by far, the concentration that would be expected in the fasted state in the intestine of healthy human volunteers.

It should also be taken into consideration that the lipase levels in the fed human small intestine exceed by far the concentration actually required to complete lipolysis, and for release testing purposes it is not necessary to use the fed state physiological concentration. One only needs to make sure there is enough pancreatic lipase added to digest the modest concentrations of lipid in the dosage form to be tested. Moreover, at 2000 Units/mL lipase, the equivalent concentration of pancreatin will not dissolve completely and this can lead to analytical difficulties.

How much lipase is necessary? Assuming that the formulation contributes about one gram of fat/oil, and assuming a density of about 0.9 g/mL, this would correspond to about 900 mg of digestible lipid. Using a molecular weight of just under 900 (e.g., triolein), this corresponds to a concentration of about 1 mMole, which would require 1000 Units of lipase for digestion. Assuming a media volume of 500 mL per vessel in a Biodis (Type III) dissolution apparatus, this will require the addition of about 10 Units/mL. To be on the safe side, a lipase concentration of 100 Units/mL is suggested, which corresponds to one-twentieth of the concentration of pancreatin recommended by the USP for use in SIF.

Addition of Surfactants to Compendial Media

For APIs that have low solubility in aqueous media, it may be useful to consider adding a surfactant to the medium for quality control (QC) testing. Sodium laurylsulphate and Tween 80 are two surfactants that are often used to boost release rates for QC testing. This approach is discussed and elaborated in the new General Chapter on dissolution testing of the USP (8).

Case Example

In some cases, it has been possible to generate in vitro–in vivo correlations (IVIVC) using modified compendial methods. A case example has been described by Schamp et al., who studied a variety of lipid formulations of an experimental Merck API (9). In these studies, lipid semisolid formulations of EMD 50733, a poorly soluble, neutral drug candidate were developed using Gelucire 44/14 and Vitamin E TPGS as the lipid vehicles, and tested both in vitro and in a dog model. The media used in vitro were SGF with a surfactant added to lower the surface tension to physiologically relevant levels (SGF+, the forerunner of FaSSGF), FaSSIF and FeSSIF. Results clearly indicated that the release for the Gelucire formulations is robust—maximum concentrations achieved in SGF+ were similar to those obtained in the biorelevant intestinal media and a supersaturated concentration of the API was sustained for more than an hour. The results in SGF+ also predicted that the API would be better absorbed from the Gelucire than from the other formulations studied (Table 4). The bioavailability of the various formulations in dogs were measured and compared to that of a standard formulation consisting of

Table 4 Solubilities of EMD 57033 in Different Dissolution Media and Maximum Concentrations Resulting from Dissolution of Different Formulations

Media	Solubility of EMD 57033 at 37°C (μg/mL)	C_{max} during dissolution from lactose mixture formulation (μg/mL)	C_{max} during dissolution from Gélucire formulation (μg/mL)	C_{max} during dissolution from vitamin E TPGS formulation (μg/mL)
SGF+	7.8	9.2	26.1	30.9
FaSSIF	6.4	5.7	29.3	not tested
FeSSIF	12.6	12.2	29.3	not tested

Source: From Ref. 9.

a lactose/drug mixture and to i.v. administration in the same dogs. As predicted, the best results with respect to bioavailability were obtained with the Gelucire 44/14 formulation (Fig. 1).

Surface tension measurements showed that the Gelucire 44/14 formulation formed micelles during dissolution in aqueous media: the molecular dispersion of the drug in this self-forming micellar system was postulated to protect the drug from precipitation in vivo as well as in vitro. For other formulations tested, neither the in vitro nor the in vivo performance indicated sufficient drug solubilizing properties. It was concluded that to achieve adequate and reliable dissolution of poorly soluble drugs in vivo, lipid excipients should not only have appropriate solubilizing properties for the drug in the formulation, but should also assist in maintaining drug in solution during release in the GI tract.

From this study it appears that for self-microemulsifying drug delivery systems (SMEDDS) and similar types of formulations, the compendial media, or

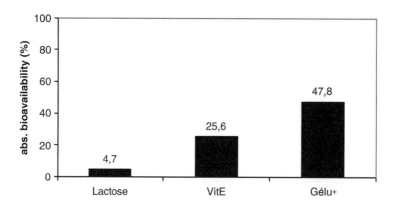

Figure 1 Absolute bioavailability in dogs of an experimental Merck API from three formulations: a lactose/API mixture packed into capsules, a vitamin E TPGS-based formulation and a Gelucire-based formulation. *Source*: From Ref. 9.

slight modifications to them, may be able to adequately address both QC and IVIVC needs, especially when they are used as the basis for formulating APIs with medium lipophilicity. More work is needed to determine how wide the field of application is in terms of both API and formulation type.

Biorelevant Dissolution in Compendial Apparatus

The biorelevant media were conceived to provide better forecasts of oral bioavailability for poorly soluble APIs. The idea was to account for the better wetting and solubilisation of the APIs in presence of bile components. These effects can improve API solubility and dissolution rate by more than an order of magnitude. A prerequisite for the improvement in solubility is that the API has lipophilicity sufficient for interaction with the mixed micelles; typically the logP value should be greater than two to facilitate the partitioning and as the logP increases, so will the extent of solubilization. A more complete discussion of the prediction of absorption of lipophilic APIs with biorelevant dissolution tests can be found in the review article by Dressman and Reppas (10).

Intestinal Biorelevant Media

For many lipid-based formulations, dispersion in the aqueous environment will be aided and abetted by the bile components in the biorelevant media and, if a single phase is formed, characterizing release into the biorelevant media may well be sufficient to forecast the release properties in the intestine. The current composition of the intestinal media is provided in Tables 2 and 3.

Gastric Biorelevant Media

In many cases, dispersion and release will commence in the stomach and it may be worthwhile to study these phenomena under gastric as well as intestinal conditions, especially during the development phase. A suitable, physiologically relevant release-testing medium composition for the fasted state is given in Table 1. Simulation of the fed state in the stomach presents a significantly greater challenge—due to the presence of fats, carbohydrates, and proteins one has to deal with a multiphase medium and the associated problems with separating the phases and analysing each for the API. Various approaches to simulating the fed state conditions in the stomach have been addressed by Klein et al. (11). These authors also proposed viscosified Ensure Plus (a total nutrition drink) as a release medium which would simulate most of the physical properties of the gastric contents in the fed state. In reality, this medium is difficult to work with and efforts are continuing to design a medium which adequately addresses the gastric content composition and yet lends itself to analysis of the API without too much investment of time and effort.

Current research efforts seek to identify a release test medium consisting of a suitable dilution of heat-treated milk with a buffer simulating the gastric secretions to create a kind of "snapshot" composition of the gastric contents corresponding to that observed about one hour after meal ingestion. Although use of such a medium still requires centrifugation and separation of the proteins via precipitation, and is therefore obviously unsuitable for routine QC purposes, it is able to simulate the key processes that can occur in the stomach—partitioning into the lipid phase, incorporation into milk protein (e.g., casein) micelles and dispersion into the aqueous phase. Thus the approach is well suited to studying a wide variety of release mechanisms in a medium that can provide contributions of the different mechanisms in roughly the same proportions as would be experienced by the dosage form when ingested with a usual Western meal.

To summarize, the use of biorelevant dissolution media in a standard compendial dissolution apparatus has the advantages of using well-known media and equipment, and accounting for a range of release mechanisms, but brings with it more work in terms of media preparation and sample analysis. Therefore, this approach is best suited to formulation screening work and evaluating mechanism(s) of release. It is also somewhat limited in range by the fact that not all lipid-based formulations will disperse well in these media.

Adaptation of Biorelevant Dissolution Tests for Screening of Lipid-Based Formulations

An important criterion for selecting a lipid-based formulation to improve API bioavailability is that the solubility of the API is much better in the lipid-based formulation than in aqueous media. The API solubility can be evaluated in a wide variety of lipid-based formulations to determine which is the most favourable to solubility. However, in addition to solubilizing capacity, the chosen formulation must also be able to release the API under physiological conditions. At present, a good screening method for this step in the process appears to be lacking.

To overcome this deficit, a project was initiated between F. Hoffmann-La Roche (Basel) and the Johann Wolfgang University in Frankfurt (12). The approach was to create a medium throughput screening tool based on a 96 well filter plate system (MACA CO2 S5, Millipore). The system consisted of a 96 well receiver plate, with a 96 well filter plate polycarbonate filter (PCF, 0.4 μm) placed on top. Small holes between the wells in the filter plate enabled the removal of samples from the receiver side without having to remove the filter plate from the set-up. Figure 2 shows the configuration of the system, with a donor and a receiver compartment separated by the PCA filter, thus allowing the lipid formulation phase to remain separated from the aqueous phase during the course of the experiment. The concentration in the aqueous receiver compartment can thus be determined without any further phase separation work. Since the filter is hydrophilic, it allows the aqueous phase to equilibrate with the filter and doesn't impede passage of micellar solutions (of the API and/or lipid phase) from the lipid phase into the aqueous receiver compartment. Some key experimental considerations are:

1. To ensure the wettability of the filter membrane and to avoid generation of air bubbles in the system during the experiment, the filter is

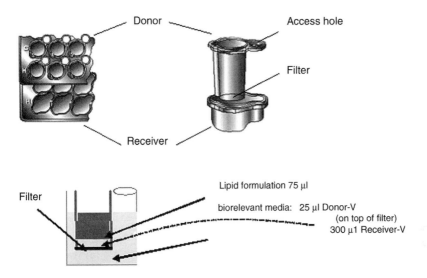

Donor   Access hole

Filter

Receiver

Filter

Lipid formulation 75 μl

biorelevant media: 25 μl Donor-V
(on top of filter)
300 μ1 Receiver-V

Figure 2   Equipment for medium throughput dilution test.

wetted with 25 μL of receiver medium prior to addition of the lipid-based formulation into the donor compartment.

2. A typical volume for the lipid-based formulation in the donor compartment is 100 μL, and a typical volume of 300 μL is used for the receiver compartment.

3. Working with such small volumes, it is prudent to run the experiments at room temperature to reduce evaporation of the media.

4. The receiver compartment is stirred with a miniature magnetic stirrer (300 rpm).

5. Transfer is studied as a function of time, by removing volumes from the receiver compartment at suitable times and replacing with fresh medium.

6. Additionally, 5 μL samples can be removed and examined microscopically to determine whether the receiver phase remains homogeneous or if phase separation occurs. Phase separation may occur if the surfactants in the formulation interact unfavourably with those in the receiver medium (typically, bile components in media such as FaSSIF and FeSSIF). Figure 3 shows examples of lipid-based formulations that form homogenous systems with SGF, FaSSIF, and FeSSIF under these conditions and some which phase separate.

The methodology was applied to an experimental Roche compound. With a clogP value of 5.35, this API is highly lipophilic. Nevertheless, its solubility in triglycerides was very low. Solubility in mono-/diglyceride mixtures was also insufficient to completely solubilize the API dose (anticipated to be 5–20 mg) in

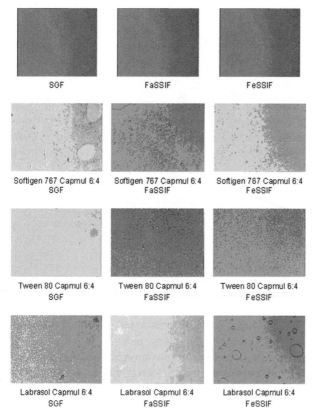

SGF FaSSIF FeSSIF

Softigen 767 Capmul 6:4 SGF | Softigen 767 Capmul 6:4 FaSSIF | Softigen 767 Capmul 6:4 FeSSIF

Tween 80 Capmul 6:4 SGF | Tween 80 Capmul 6:4 FaSSIF | Tween 80 Capmul 6:4 FeSSIF

Labrasol Capmul 6:4 SGF | Labrasol Capmul 6:4 FaSSIF | Labrasol Capmul 6:4 FeSSIF

Figure 3 Comparison of biorelevant media and formulation of Roche compound diluted in biorelevant media (magnification $\times$ 100).

a single-unit dosage form volume of approximately 1 mL. However, the excipient, Capmul, provided somewhat better solubilization (21 mg/mL). Finally, the API solubility in surfactants such as Labrasol and Tween 80 was even higher, with additive effects observed in lipid/surfactant combinations.

Release tests were conducted for several formulations using biorelevant media in the screening method. A typical set of results for the release test are shown in Table 5. Concentrations of the API of about 0.1 mg/mL were achieved within 100 minutes in SGF, FaSSIF, and FeSSIF from the Capmul formulation; with addition of Tween 80 at a ratio of 9:1 the concentration after 100 minutes rose to almost 0.2 mg/mL.

The formulations were subsequently administered to monkeys to determine whether they would perform according to the predictions from the in vitro screening method. The results, shown in Figure 4, confirm the utility of the screening method: the plasma levels of the Roche API were substantially higher with the Tween/Capmul formulation than with Capmul alone. Even more interestingly, a

Table 5   Release of an Experimental Roche Compound from Several Formulations in the 96 Well Plate Screening Model (mg/mL)

Formulation	Medium	Tween 80-Capmul Formulations (starting concentration in the formulation was 20 mg/mL)				
		10min	30min	50min	70min	100min
Capmul	SGF	0.126	0.106	0.136	0.148	0.112
	s.d.	0.018	0.003	0.080	0.004	0.011
	FaSSIF	<0.001	<0.001	<0.001	<0.001	<0.001
	s.d.	—	—	—	—	—
	FeSSIF	0.137	0.131	0.139	0.111	0.103
	s.d.	0.005	0.010	0.036	0.012	0.002
Tween 80-Capmul 3:7	SGF	0.117	0.122	0.119	0.118	0.109
	s.d.	0.003	0.013	0.007	0.008	0.001
	FaSSIF	0.091	0.090	0.085	0.077	0.082
	s.d.	0.001	0.004	0.004	0.001	0.002
	FeSSIF	0.099	0.110	0.097	0.096	0.085
	s.d.	0.002	0.018	0.006	0.003	0.001
Tween 80-Capmul 6:4	SGF	0.109	0.110	0.111	0.113	0.109
	s.d.	0.002	0.002	0.002	0.003	0.004
	FaSSIF	0.078	0.078	0.085	0.073	0.076
	s.d.	0.003	0.005	0.004	0.002	0.004
	FeSSIF	0.114	0.094	0.079	0.076	0.075
	s.d.	0.001	0.003	0.004	0.003	0.002
Tween 80-Capmul 9:1	SGF	0.197	0.231	0.224	0.185	0.180
	s.d.	0.010	0.001	0.029	0.027	0.009
	FaSSIF	0.152	0.172	0.297	0.160	0.209
	s.d.	0.013	0.026	0.014	0.021	0.042
	FeSSIF	0.179	0.183	0.169	0.159	0.197
	s.d.	0.009	0.008	0.008	0.003	0.012

Source: From Ref. 9.

Labrasol/Capmul formulation showed poorer bioavailability (results not presented) than the Tween/Capmul formulation, even though the solubility of the API was better in the Labrasol/Capmul formulation. The screening method was also able to predict this result.

These findings illustrate the need to adequately assess not only solubility improvement of APIs with lipid-based vehicles, but also their compatibility with the gastrointestinal fluids and ability to transfer the API out of the dosage form into the surrounding fluids.

Parallel Digestion and Dissolution

Although the methods described in the foregoing sections can probably be used for a large number of lipid-based formulations, in some cases it will be necessary to use a dynamic lipolysis model to fully characterize release from the dosage

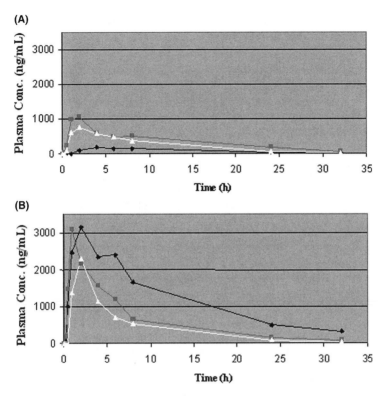

Figure 4 Pharmacokinetic results for the Roche compound formulations in monkeys. (**A**) Administration of the Roche API in a Capmul formulation to three monkeys. (**B**) Administration of the Roche API in a Tween 80/Capmul formulation to three monkeys.

form. The reader is referred to Chapter 11 for a complete discussion of this important topic.

SUMMARY

Since lipid-based formulations are quite diverse in terms of composition and properties, attention must be paid to the specifics of a formulation in order to come up with an appropriate release method. In some cases, simple buffer media (perhaps with addition of a surfactant) might be adequate, in other cases the simulation of the conditions in the gastrointestinal tract must take into account wetting, solubilisation and digestion. Solubility of the API in the formulation, while obviously important, should not be the only criteria in selecting a formulation. Screening for dispersability of the formulation under a variety of conditions seems like a sensible next step for screening potential formulations. Provided the formulation disperses well, the next consideration is the release mechanism and how quickly this occurs. Depending on the type of formulation being contemplated, appropriate methodology should be selected. Following this approach should optimize the bioavailability of the formulation and provide a solid understanding of the behaviour of the formulation under a variety of dosing scenarios, as well as providing the basis for selection of quality control test methodology.

REFERENCES

1. Dressman JB, Klein S. Development of dissolution tests on the basis of gastrointestinal physiology. In: Dressman J, Krämer J, eds., Dissolution Testing of Pharmaceuticals. USA: Taylor&Francis, 2005.
2. Vertzoni M, Dressman J, Butler J, Hempenstall J, Reppas C. Simulation of fasting gastric conditions and its importance for the in vivo dissolution of lipophilic compounds. Eur J Pharm Biopharm 2005; 60:413–417.
3. Armand M, Borel P, Pasquier B, et al. Physicochemical characteristics of emulsions during fat digestion in human stomach and duodenum. Am J Physiol Gastrointest Liver Physiol 1996; 34(1):G172–G182.
4. Armand M, Pasquier B, Andre M, et al. Digestion and absorption of 2 fat emulsions with different droplet sizes in the human digestive tract. Am J Clin Nutr 1999; 70(6):1096–1106.
5. Davenport H. Physiology of the Digestive Tract. USA: Year Book Medical, 1982:170.
6. Kalantzi L, Goumas K, Kalioras V, Abrahamsson B, Dressman J, Reppas C. Characterization of the human upper gastrointestinal contents under conditions simulating bioavailability/bioequivalence studies. Pharm Res 2006; 23:165–176.
7. Gray VA, Dressman JB. Simulated intestinal fluid, TS—change to pH 6.8. USP Pharmacopeial Forum 1996; 22:1943–1945.
8. Gray VA, Brown CK, Dressman JB, Leeson L. A new general information chapter on Dissolution. Pharmacopeial Forum 2002; 27:3432–3439.
9. Schamp K, Schreder S, Dressman J. Development of an in vitro/in vivo correlation for lipid formulations of EMD 50733, a poorly soluble, lipophilic drug substance. Eur J Pharm Biopharm 2006; 62:227–234.
10. Dressman JB, Reppas C. In vitro-in vivo correlations for lipophilic, poorly water-soluble drugs. Eur J Pharm Sci 2000; 11(supp 2):S73-S80.
11. Klein S, Butler J, Hempenstall J, Reppas C, Dressman J. Media to simulate the postprandial stomach. I. Matching the physicochemical characteristics of standard breakfasts. J Pharm Pharmacol 2004; 56:605–610.
12. Karen Beltz. Dissertation: Improvement of Bioavailability using Lipid-Based Formulations. Johann Wolfgang University, Frankfurt am Main, 2007.

11

Using In Vitro Dynamic Lipolysis Modeling as a Tool for Exploring IVIVC Relationships for Oral Lipid-Based Formulations

Dimitris G. Fatouros and Anette Müllertz

Department of Pharmaceutics and Analytical Chemistry, The Danish University of Pharmaceutical Sciences, Copenhagen, Denmark

INTRODUCTION

The development of effective oral dosage forms for hydrophobic new chemical entities (NCE) continues to be a pressing problem for the pharmaceutical industry. Many of these poorly water-soluble NCEs readily permeate biological membranes thus making their maximum solubility and/or dissolution rate in the gastrointestinal tract (GIT) rate-limiting steps to their absorption. These biopharmaceutical properties describe Biopharmaceutics Classification System (BCS) Type II compounds, which usually present with both low and variable bioavailability that is frequently influenced by the dietary status of the patient (fed vs. fasted).

Small intestinal fluid contains various surfactants, including bile salts (BS) and phospholipids (PL), which in combination with dietary or endogenous fats, form mixed micelles with high solubilizing capacity for many BCS 2 compounds (1–6). Several studies have demonstrated a correlation between drug lipophilicity and improved compound in vitro solubility in BS media, relative to the corresponding intrinsic water solubility (7–9).

During the fed state, several changes occur in the GIT, relative to the fasted state, which can significantly impact the absorption of drug substances, particularly BCS 2 compounds. These changes include an increase in the gastric retention time, an increase in pH and ionic strength of the GI fluids, and the secretion of BS and pancreatic juices (10), which catalyze the hydrolysis of dietary lipid to more water-soluble species [e.g., free fatty acids (FFA) and monoglycerides (MG)], which are subsequently emulsified with BS to form mixed micelles. The critical role of the aqueous mixed micellar phase in the efficient absorption of dietary lipids is well accepted and growing evidence has demonstrated a parallel role in facilitating the absorption of concomitantly solubilized drugs (11).

This chapter describes an in vitro method for determining the behavior of poorly soluble compounds under conditions simulating the fluids in the GIT. The dynamic lipolysis model involves BSs, PLs, and generation of lipolysis products (LP), more accurately reproducing the solubilizing environment of the GIT for BCS 2 compounds, with the goal of allowing better prediction of drug absorption under both fasted and fed conditions (12–15).

Liquid dosage forms that rely on the use of lipid and surfactant excipients to fully solubilize the drug in the formulation include simple oil solutions, emulsions, and self-emulsifying drug delivery systems (SEDDS). These formulations are thought to improve the bioavailability of poorly water-soluble drugs by obviating the need for preabsorptive dissolution in the GIT; however, the precise mechanisms by which these formulations increase drug absorption are not fully understood.

Empirical development of lipid-based formulations relies on the following parameters, which are believed to be important to formulation performance:

- the drug solubility in the dosage form and dispersability of the formulation in the GI fluids, and
- for formulations containing a digestible lipid, the digestion rate of the excipient matrix, which controls drug release and subsequent absorption (16), and the solubility of the drug in the digested formulation (17).

At present, a rational formulation development strategy for oral lipid-based formulations has been hampered by not only a lack of understanding of how these formulations enhance drug bioavailability, but also by the lack of reliable in vitro methods for directing formulation development and optimization. The dynamic lipolysis model described in this chapter simulates small intestinal lipid digestion and holds potential for predicting formulation performance in humans in both the fed and fasted states.

SOLUBILIZATION PROCESSES IN THE GASTROINTESTINAL TRACT

While the maximum solubility of a drug in the GIT is probably the most critical parameter controlling its absorption, decades of study have failed to identify a reliable method for consistent and accurate prediction of in vivo drug solubility. The in vivo dissolution rate and maximum solubility of a specific drug substance in the GIT is determined not only by the physicochemical characteristics of the drug substance (e.g., pKa, hydrophilicity, crystal structure, particle size, etc.), but also by the complex interaction of multiple GI physiological factors, each of which is subject to considerable intra- and intersubject variation. Solubilization by BS mixed-micelles, formed during lipid digestion, is thought to play a pivotal role in the absorption of poorly water-soluble hydrophobic drugs. Lipid digestion begins in the stomach, where gastric lipase hydrolyzes approximately 10% to 20% of ingested triglyceride (TG) to FFA and diglyceride (DG), both of which possess surfactant properties and greater water solubility than the parent TG (18). The crude lipid digestate enters the duodenum as a coarse emulsion which, primarily under the influence of pancreatic TG lipase, is almost completely hydrolyzed to 2-monoglyceride (2-MG) and additional FFA, which combine with BS to form mixed micelles. The hydrolytic activity of pancreatic TG lipase is dependent on the presence of colipase, which is essential for promoting its attachment to the relatively hydrophilic surface of the crude TG emulsion formed in the stomach (19–21). In vivo lipolysis is a dynamic process resulting in the formation of multiple colloid phases (22–24). During lipolysis, a lamellar liquid–crystalline phase, which is comprised of a relatively high ratio of LP to BS, forms continuously at the surface of the TG droplets; upon subsequent enrichment in BS, multilamellar vesicles are formed and leave the surface of the TG droplets. Progressive enrichment of these vesicles with BS leads to their transformation into unilamellar vesicles and finally, mixed micelles, which form when the LP:BS ratio decreases to less than unity. The mixed micelles transport the hydrophobic LPs across the intestinal unstirred water layer, where upon arrival at the surface of the intestinal brush border membrane, the acidic microclimate results in micellar disintegration, releasing the hydrophobic LP in close proximity to the lipophilic intestinal epithelium, where they are rapidly absorbed. The remnant BS is returned to the intestinal lumen, where it is incorporated into nascent mixed micelles. Following the completion of lipid absorption, which takes place largely in the duodenum and upper jejunum, the BS is reabsorbed in the ileum by the process of enterohepatic recirculation.

The small intestinal concentrations of BS that control the solubilization of lipids and many hydrophobic drug substances, are not only influenced by dietary status (fed vs. fasted), and by various disease states, but are normally subject to considerable intra- and intersubject variation, as well. Human intestinal BS concentrations reported in the literature are dependent on the method of determination (e.g., site and sampling time with regard to meals and degree of dilution in vivo). But in general, mean fasted state BS concentrations typically range from 1.5 mM to 6 mM (25–28), while mean postprandial concentrations typically range from 8 mM to 20 mM, with values as high as 40 mM having been reported (25,26,29,30). In a recent study, the level of human intestinal BS was found to be 1.8 mM and 8 mM in fasted and fed state respectively (30).

Small intestinal lipase activity in healthy human subjects varies with dietary status and is assumed to be in excess since approximately 95% of ingested dietary lipid is absorbed. It should also be emphasized, however, that lipase activity varies not only with the specific lipid substrate (e.g., compared to long chain TG, short chain, and medium chain TG are better substrates for pancreatic lipase), but also with the physical presentation of the lipid substrate to the GIT. For instance, the lipolysis rate is inversely proportional to the lipid droplet size (31), whereas the presence of certain surfactants used in lipid formulations (32,33), as well as certain drugs themselves (33), have been shown to directly inhibit the rate of lipolysis. And the excipient, Cremophor RH40 (hydrophilic ethoxylated triglyceride surfactant), completely inhibited the lipolysis of medium chain triglyceride (MCT) oil over a 90 minute period when the oil and surfactant were present in equal amounts (32). Subsequent addition of Imwitor 988 (which is a mixture of medium chain mono- and diglycerides) allowed lipolysis to occur, presumably due to a change in the orientation of the surfactant at the oil-water interface. Finally, the lipid excipients Peceol and Gelucire 44/14 have been demonstrated to inhibit pancreatic lipase activity in a concentration-dependent manner (34). The number and complexity of these factors make it difficult to accurately estimate the actual lipase activity in the small intestine (25). However, Armand et al. (35) has reported a 15-fold increase in lipase activity, relative to the fasted state, upon intragastric administration of a test meal containing 48 g triglyceride to healthy human volunteers. In summary, accurate and quantitative in vitro assessment of the solubilization, trafficking, and intestinal absorption of hydrophobic drug substances has remained elusive, emphasizing the need for further work in this area.

THE DYNAMIC LIPOLYSIS MODEL

Description of the Model

Based on the foregoing discussion of intestinal lipid digestion and absorption, the reader should have gained an appreciation for the number and complexity of the parameters which can influence gastrointestinal (GI) absorption of BCS 2 compounds, many of which are absorbed via the same pathways as lipids. The in vitro dynamic lipolysis model developed in our laboratories (Fig. 1), which incorporates many of these parameters, has been used to study the processes governing the absorption of BCS 2 drugs as well as the interactions of formulation and food on these processes. The pH of the media in the lipolysis model was chosen based on the small intestinal pH in the fed (pH 6.5) and fasted (pH 5.5) states (18,36), the pH range for optimal pancreatic lipase activity (between pH 6 and 10) (37) and the average pKa of FFAs (pH 6.4) (38).

Due initially to economic considerations, in vitro lipolysis models have employed crude porcine bile (39–41) and pancreatic extracts (which contain approximately equimolar concentrations of colipase and lipase) (42) in lieu of the more costly purified BSs (43–48) or purified colipase and lipase enzymes, respectively (39,40,49,50). While use of purified BSs and pancreatic lipases allows the researcher to study the mechanism of lipolysis under more controlled conditions, the use of crude extracts will produce a system closer to the in vivo situation due

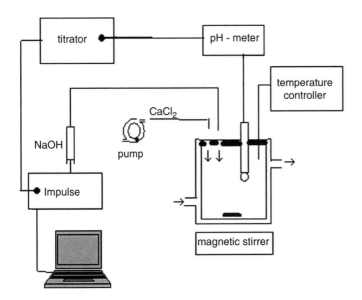

Figure 1 The dynamic lipolysis apparatus consists of a thermostatically controlled, double wall reaction vessel, a computer controlled pH-stat with an auto-burette for the addition of NaOH, and a peristaltic pump for the continuous, controlled addition of calcium chloride. All experiments are performed under continuous agitation via magnetic stirring.

to the presence of phospholipase and other enzymes present in the normal physiological secretions. The pancreatic lipase solution used in our experiments is prepared by dissolving in water, an amount of the crude extract appropriate to the enzymatic activity desired followed by centrifugation to remove insoluble particulate matter. The lipase activity of the resulting solution can be assayed by several different methods; for example, the USP (51) describes a method based on the hydrolysis of a gum arabic/olive oil-in-water emulsion but another assay, based on tributyrin hydrolysis, is also widely used (52). It should be noted that the measured lipase activity is dependent not only on the lipid substrate but also on the oil droplet surface area presented to the lipase enzyme. Therefore, results generated by different experimental methods should not be compared.

The approximate composition of the crude porcine bile extract used in our experiments is glycochenodeoxycholic acid (42.0%), glycocholic acid (23.6%), glycohyocholic acid (16.4%), taurochenodeoxycholic acid (5.2%), chenodeoxycholic acid (5.1%), glycohyodeoxycholic acid (3.2%), taurocholic acid (3.0%), and hyocholic acid (1.4%). The total concentration of BS in the extract is determined colorimetrically and is expressed as the amount of 3α-hydroxy bile acids present (40). Due to a very low PL content in bile extract, egg phosphatidylcholine (PC) is added to the media in a BS:PC ratio of 5:1, to approximate the normal physiological conditions (10). It should be noted that regardless of the source of BS employed, PL must always be added to achieve a physiological BS:PL ratio.

Ionized calcium has been shown to have a significant, positive influence on the lipolysis rate of triglycerides in the presence of BSs, presumably by diminishing the electrostatic repulsion that occurs between enzyme and substrate, thereby facilitating the binding of pancreatic lipase to the TG droplets (12,19,39,40,49,50). In addition, lipolysis is thought to depend on the formation of a catalytically active complex comprised of lipase, mixed micelles, and calcium (49,50). Accumulation of FFA on the surface of the TG droplets during lipolysis will sterically hinder attachment of pancreatic lipase, resulting in a progressive decline in the lipolysis rate (43,50). The FFA chain length has been found to influence the degree of inhibition, with long chain fatty acids (LCFA) being more potent inhibitors of lipolysis than either short or medium chain fatty acids (40). In vivo, solubilization of FFA in BS-PL micelles and subsequent absorption prevents accumulation of FFA in the intestinal lumen thereby preventing inhibition of lipolysis. In the dynamic lipolysis model, continuous addition of calcium chloride solution serves to control accumulation of FFA in the medium by forming insoluble calcium soaps, which precipitate, thus removing FFA from the system and preventing accumulation (32). During in vitro lipolysis experiments, addition of calcium initially results in a relatively high lipolysis rate, which subsequently declines and then stabilizes. This is presumably due to increased concentrations of FFA in the dissolution medium and possibly due to the loss of BS through the formation and precipitation of insoluble calcium-BS complexes (Fig. 2) (24,32,33,39,42,50).

Dynamic lipolysis experiments are conducted in a jacketed thermostatically-controlled reaction vessel maintained at 37°C and agitated continuously with a magnetic stirring device (Fig. 1) (39–41). The reaction medium consists of a mixture of BS, PL, buffer, and lipid substrate (e.g., dietary lipid or lipid-based formulation incorporating the drug substance). Lipolysis is initiated by addition of the lipase solution and the pH and free calcium concentration of the reaction mixture is maintained by the computer-controlled addition of sodium hydroxide and calcium chloride solutions, respectively.

Samples of the reaction medium are withdrawn immediately following addition of the lipase solution and at serial time points subsequent to the initiation of lipolysis. The lipolysis reaction is quenched by addition of the lipase inhibitor, 4-bromobenzene boronic acid, and the samples are subsequently ultracentrifuged, resulting in the formation of three distinct phases:

- a pellet comprised largely of insoluble calcium soaps of fatty acids,
- an intermediate aqueous layer, consisting of BS mixed-micelles and various lipid vesicles, and
- an upper-most, oily layer comprised of DG, and unhydrolyzed TG.

The aqueous phase is of greatest interest in the study of the GI absorption of hydrophobic drugs. This phase has been extensively characterized with regard to its composition and content of LP and solubilized drugs as well as the identity and size of its component micellar and vesicular entities (39,40,53).

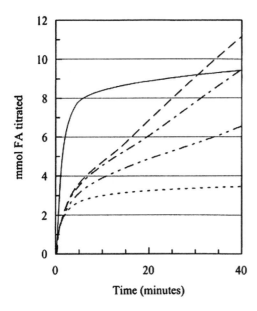

Figure 2 The lipolysis of triglycerides (TG) in the dynamic lipolysis model over 40 minutes, measured as mM fatty acids (FA) titrated, at three different rates of Ca^{2+} addition in the presence of 8 mM bile salts. In this series, 18.3 mM of titrated FA are equivalent to complete hydrolysis of the added TG into FA and monoglycerides. These experiments demonstrate a clear correlation between the lipolysis rate and the rate of Ca^{2+} addition. The initial, high rate of lipolysis declines and remains relatively constant at approximately five minutes after initiation of Ca^{2+} addition. Each line represents a different rate of Ca^{2+} addition, as defined below: (a) 0.072 mmol Ca^{2+}/min, final conc. = 9.4 mM Ca^{2+} (– - - –); (b) 0.135 mmol Ca^{2+}/min, final conc. = 17.4 mM Ca^{2+} (– - –); (c) 0.181 mmol Ca^{2+}/min, final conc. = 23.0 mM Ca^{2+} (– –); (d) 0.0 mmol Ca^{2+}/min, final conc. = 0.0 mM Ca^{2+} (- -); (e) 17.4 mM Ca^{2+} added at the initiation of the experiment (————); this concentration of Ca^{2+} corresponds to the final concentration in (b) and results in a similar rate of lipolysis. All experiments were conducted in duplicate. *Source*: From Ref. 39.

Simulating Fed State Effects Using the Lipolysis Model

During lipid digestion, a drug dissolved in a substrate lipid vehicle will either (*i*) remain in the lipid, (*ii*) be solubilized in the aqueous phase in combination with LPs, or (*iii*) precipitate.

During lipolysis, the trafficking of a particular drug between these various phases will be controlled by multiple factors, many of which are poorly understood, but are thought to include the drug lipophilicity and affinity for the various lipolytic phases.

Zangenberg et al. (41) conducted dynamic lipolysis experiments on the poorly water-soluble drug substances, danazol (Log P 4.5) and probucol (cLog P 11) at up to 75% total lipolysis of the lipid content of model long chain triglyceride

(LCT) emulsion formulations of these drugs. For danazol, the relatively high drug concentration in the aqueous phase was found to be directly correlated with the concentrations of surfactants (BS, PL) and LP (FA, MG) present. In comparison, probucol, which had a relatively high Log P and poor solubility in the aqueous phase, remained largely solubilized in the oil phase, due to its relatively high cLog P. The inverse relationship between Log P of the drug substance and solubilization in the aqueous phase was replicated by Kaukonen et al. (43), who conducted dynamic lipolysis experiments over 30 minutes on five poorly soluble drug substances ranging in log P from 2 to 8.1. At the termination of the experiments, in which only 42% or 61% of the added TG had been hydrolyzed, a considerable amount of undigested oil remained in which the most lipophilic compounds (cinnarizine, log P 5.5 and halofantrine, log P 8.1) were preferentially retained. However, it should be emphasized that in these experiments the entire amount of calcium chloride was added to the lipolysis medium at the initiation of the experiment, in contrast with the controlled, continuous addition of calcium chloride in the dynamic lipolysis model, as it has been described by Zangenberg et al. (41) and this could have influenced the extent of lipolysis.

Christensen et al. (40) employed a lipolysis model to study the solubilization of probucol (Log P 10.9), LU28-179 (Log P 8.5), and flupentixol (Log P 4.5), in media containing 2.8% TG and 20/4 mM BS/PL; lipase-free media was included as a control. The solubility of flupentixol in the lipolysis medium was higher than the added amount, resulting in nearly complete solubilization of the drug prior to the initiation of lipolysis. At 30 minutes subsequent to the initiation of lipolysis, the solubility of flupentixol in the medium was observed to decrease (Fig. 3A). The most likely explanation for this observation is that the continuous addition of Ca^{2+} required to maintain the rate of lipolysis resulted in progressive neutralization of the negative surface charge of the mixed micelles weakening the electrostatic attraction, and subsequently decreasing the solubility of the protonated flupentixol molecules. In contrast, the aqueous concentrations of LU 28-179 and probucol increased as lipolysis progressed, presumably due to the formation of LP in which these drugs had relatively high solubility (Figs. 3B and 3C). During lipolysis, the average micellar size increases, most likely due to the incorporation of newly formed LP. Prior to the initiation of lipolysis, slight increases in micellar size were observed, possibly due to the high concentration of counterions in the media. Immediately following the initiation of lipolysis, a lag phase preceded the incorporation of the drug into the aqueous phase. This may have been due to an initial, preferential association of LP with the undigested oil phase immediately following the initiation of lipolysis or subsequent to the precipitation of insoluble drug-BS complexes prior to the accumulation of solubilizing mixed micelles as lipolysis progressed.

Studies carried out with fed dogs have shown enhanced absorption of the poorly soluble LU 28-179, relative to the fasted state (Internal report, H. Lundbeck). Similar findings have been demonstrated for probucol, administered to mini-pigs (54). The enhancing effect that food has on the absorption of many drugs is due, at least in part, to the generation of LPs with surface-active

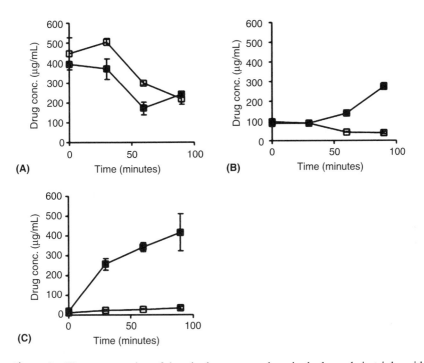

Figure 3 The concentration of drug in the aqueous phase in the long chain triglycerides (LCT) studies with (■) and without (□) addition of lipase ($n \geq 3$, ±S.D). (**A**) Flupentixol (added at 200% (w/w) of the maximum solubility in LCT); (**B**) LU 28-179 (added at 80% (w/w) of the maximum solubility in LCT); (**C**) Probucol (added at 80% (w/w) of the maximum solubility in LCT). *Source*: From Ref. 40.

and solvent properties. The dynamic lipolysis model, employing LCT as a model dietary lipid, has proven valuable for studying food effect in vitro.

Simulating Hydrolysis of Lipid-Based Formulations by Use of the Lipolysis Model

Development of a lipid-based formulation almost always involves the identification of lipid and surfactant excipients in which the drug can be fully solubilized (55). Development of SEDDS formulations requires additional formulation optimization to confer adequate resistance to drug precipitation following dispersion in vivo. Another factor not routinely addressed in formulation development involves the impact of in vivo lipid digestion on drug solubilization and formulation perform-ance. Studies conducted with the dynamic lipolysis model, in the presence of rele-vant amounts of dietary and formulation-derived lipid substrates, can be useful in achieving this objective.

The first attempt to use an in vitro lipolysis model to predict the in vivo per-formance of lipid-based formulations was described in 1988 by Reymond and Sucker

(44,56). However, no in vitro–in vivo correlation (IVIVC) was found, possibly due to an in vitro TG hydrolysis rate that was lower than that occurring in vivo.

An IVIVC has been demonstrated for the oral absorption of LU 28-179 in dogs and the drug release observed in the lipolysis model from a hydroxypropyl-β-cyclodextrin reference solution, a SMEDDS formulation, oil solutions, and dry emulsion formulations containing either LCT or MCT (57). Compared to the reference solution, the absorption of LU 28-179 in dogs was substantially greater for the SMEDDS and dry emulsion formulations, which correlated with the rate and extent of drug release observed in the in vitro lipolysis model.

De Smidt et al. (16) investigated the influence of vehicle dispersion and digestibility on the GI absorption in rats of the poorly soluble drug, penclomedine, in rats administered as either an undispersed solution in MCT and D-α-tocopheryl polyethyleneglycol 1000 succinate or in emulsions prepared to contain oil droplet sizes of 160 or 720 nm. When coadministered with the lipase inhibitor tetrahydrolipstatin (THL), the emulsion droplet size had minimal impact on drug absorption; however, drug absorption from the undispersed solution was substantially reduced in the presence of THL. Although in vitro lipolysis studies were not conducted on these formulations, the influence of in vivo lipolysis on formulation performance is evident from the results.

Porter et al. (47) characterized LC-SMEDDS and MC-SMEDDS formulations of danazol containing comparable amounts of either long (LC) or medium chain (MC) TG. Following approximately 200-fold dilution in 0.1 N HCl, lipid droplet sizes of approximately 40 nm were formed, with the droplet size being independent of the TG fatty acid chain length. In addition, dispersion of these formulations in test media containing 5 mM BS and 1.25 mM PL resulted in minimal drug precipitation. However, 30 minutes after the initiation of lipolysis, 69% of the drug precipitated from the MC-SMEDDS, as compared to only 6% from the LC-SMEDDS. The degree of drug precipitation was inversely correlated with danazol bioavailability in dogs, which was 5.7-fold greater from the LC-SMEDDS formulation relative to the MC-SMEDDS formulation. Studies conducted with the antimalarial drug halofantrine showed a similar relationship between drug precipitation resistance during in vitro lipolysis and superior bioavailability (46).

Several published studies of SEDDS formulations have described an inverse correlation between lipid droplet size and degree of drug absorption (58–61). However, it should be noted that the formulations investigated in these studies were not controlled for either surfactant or lipid type or amount. Since it has been well documented that SEDDS formulations of different qualitative or quantitative composition, but similar lipid droplet size frequently result in different bioavailabilities for a particular drug, no clear-cut conclusion with regard to impact of droplet size on bioavailability can be drawn (47,62,63). To further investigate the effect of droplet size on drug absorption, two SEDDS formulations containing probucol were developed, which differed only in the lipid droplet size. One formulation, a self-nanoemulsifying drug delivery system (SNEDDS), contained lipid droplets of 45 ± 3.4 nm in size, while a SMEDDS formulation contained droplets of $4.58 \pm 0.84\,\mu m$ in size (54). The dynamic lipolysis model was used to evaluate the lipolysis rate and release of probucol from both of these formulations in comparison to a simple oil solution formulation of the drug (64). The solubilization of probucol by the aqueous phase was substantially lower from the oil solution compared to either the SNEDDS or SMEDDS formulations, for which drug solubilization was essentially identical. An in vitro–in vivo relationship was demonstrated between the drug release profiles obtained in vitro using the dynamic lipolysis model, and the drug plasma concentration profiles obtained in a previous bioavailability study conducted in mini-pigs (52). While these initial results are very encouraging, more work is needed in order to further define the lipolysis model with the goal of consistently generating reliable and reproducible projections of formulation performance in man.

CONCLUSIONS

The clear relationship that exists between the GI absorption of many poorly water-soluble, hydrophobic drugs and the solubilization afforded by lipid-based formulations is well accepted by the scientific community. In addition, the frequently observed enhancing effect of the postprandial state on poorly-soluble drug bioavailability suggests important roles for endogenous lipid and surfactant substances and the GI lipid handling pathways in determining the absorption of these drugs. The dynamic lipolysis model described in this chapter was developed to expand upon the utility of earlier biorelevant dissolution media by attempting to more accurately reproduce the process of GI lipid digestion in vitro. Although this technique is relatively unexplored, it has shown great promise as a rapid, cost-effective model for studying and optimizing the performance of lipid-based formulations in vivo as well as for assessing their impact on mitigation of positive food effect seen with many poorly water-soluble drugs.

REFERENCES

1. Bates TR, Gibaldi M, Kanig JL. Solubilizing properties of bile salt solutions. II. Effect of inorganic electrolyte, lipids, and a mixed bile salt system on solubilization of glutethimide, griseofulvin, and hexestrol. J Pharm Sci 1966; 55(2):901–906.
2. Bates TR, Lin SL, Gibaldi M. Solubilization and rate of dissolution of drugs in the presence of physiologic concentrations of lysolecithin. J Pharm Sci 1967; 56(11):1492–1495.
3. Martis L, Hall NA, Thakkar AL. Micelle formation and testosterone solubilization by sodium glycocholate. J Pharm Sci 1972; 61(11):1757–1761.
4. Rosoff M, Serajuddin ATM. Solubilization of diazepam in bile-salts and in sodium cholate-lecithin-water phases. Int J Pharm 1980; 6(2):137–146.
5. Kassem MA, Mattha AG, Elnimr AEM, Omar SM. Study of the influence of sodium taurocholate (Stc) and sodium glycocholate (Sgc) on the mass-transfer of certain drugs—digoxin. Int J Pharm 1982; 12(1):1–9.

6. Serajuddin AT, Sheen PC, Mufson D, Bernstein DF, Augustine MA. Physicochemical basis of increased bioavailability of a poorly water-soluble drug following oral administration as organic solutions. J Pharm Sci 1988; 77(4):325–329.

7. Mithani SD, Bakatselou V, TenHoor CN, Dressman JB. Estimation of the increase in solubility of drugs as a function of bile salt concentration. Pharm Res 1996; 13(1):163–167.

8. Wiedmann TS, Liang W, Kamel L. Solubilization of drugs by physiological mixtures of bile salts. Pharm Res 2002; 19(8):1203–1208.

9. Wiedmann TS, Kamel L. Examination of the solubilization of drugs by bile salt micelles. J Pharm Sci 2002; 91(8):1743–1764.

10. Dressman JB, Amidon GL, Reppas C, Shah VP. Dissolution testing as a prognostic tool for oral drug absorption: immediate release dosage forms. Pharm Res 1998; 15(1):11–22.

11. Porter CJ, Charman WN. In vitro assessment of oral lipid based formulations. Adv Drug Deliv Rev 2001; 50(suppl 1):S127–S147.

12. Kostewicz ES, Brauns U, Becker R, Dressman JB. Forecasting the oral absorption behavior of poorly soluble weak bases using solubility and dissolution studies in biorelevant media. Pharm Res 2002; 19(3):345–349.

13. Dressman JB, Reppas C. In vitro-in vivo correlations for lipophilic, poorly water-soluble drugs. Eur J Pharm Sci 2000; 11(suppl 2):S73–S80.

14. Sunesen VH, Pedersen BL, Kristensen HG, Mullertz A. In vivo in vitro correlations for a poorly soluble drug, danazol, using the flow-through dissolution method with biorelevant dissolution media. Eur J Pharm Sci 2005; 24(4):305–313.

15. Vertzoni M, Dressman J, Butler J, Hempenstall J, Reppas C. Simulation of fasting gastric conditions and its importance for the in vivo dissolution of lipophilic compounds. Eur J Pharm Biopharm 2005; 60(3):413–417.

16. de Smidt PC, Campanero MA, Troconiz IF. Intestinal absorption of penclomedine from lipid vehicles in the conscious rat: contribution of emulsification versus digestibility. Int J Pharm 2004; 270(1–2):109–118.

17. Kossena GA, Charman WN, Boyd BJ, Dunstan DE, Porter CJ. Probing drug solubilization patterns in the gastrointestinal tract after administration of lipid-based delivery systems: A phase diagram approach. J Pharm Sci 2004; 93(2):332–348.

18. Carriere F, Barrowman JA, Verger R, Laugier R. Secretion and contribution to lipolysis of gastric and pancreatic lipases during a test meal in humans. Gastroenterology 1993; 105(3):876–888.

19. Lowe ME. The triglyceride lipases of the pancreas. J Lipid Res 2002; 43(12):2007–2016.

20. Patton JS, Carey MC. Inhibition of human pancreatic lipase-colipase activity by mixed bile salt-phospholipid micelles. Am J Physiol 1981; 241(4):G328–G336.

21. Larsson A, Erlanson-Albertsson C. The importance of bile salt for the reactivation of pancreatic lipase by colipase. Biochim Biophys Acta 1983; 750(1):171–177.

22. Patton JS, Carey MC. Watching fat digestion. Science 1979; 204(13):145–148.

23. Rigler MW, Honkanen RE, Patton JS. Visualization by freeze fracture, in vitro and in vivo, of the products of fat digestion. J Lipid Res 1986; 27(8):836–857.

24. Hernell O, Staggers JE, Carey MC. Physical-chemical behavior of dietary and biliary lipids during intestinal digestion and absorption. 2. Phase analysis and aggregation states of luminal lipids during duodenal fat digestion in healthy adult human beings. Biochemistry 1990; 29(8):2041–2056.

25. Armand M, Borel P, Pasquier B, et al. Physicochemical characteristics of emulsions during fat digestion in human stomach and duodenum. Am J Physiol 1996; 271(1):G172–G183.

26. Tangerman A, van Schaik A, van der Hoek EW. Analysis of conjugated and unconjugated bile acids in serum and jejunal fluid of normal subjects. Clin Chim Acta 1986; 159(2):123–132.

27. Pedersen BL, Brondsted H, Lennernas H, Christensen FN, Mullertz A, Kristensen HG. Dissolution of hydrocortisone in human and simulated intestinal fluids. Pharm Res 2000; 17(7):183–189.

28. Pedersen BL, Mullertz A, Brondsted H, Kristensen HG. A comparison of the solubility of danazol in human and simulated gastrointestinal fluids. Pharm Res 2000; 17(2):891–894.

29. Ladas SD, Isaacs PE, Murphy GM, Sladen GE. Comparison of the effects of medium and long chain triglyceride containing liquid meals on gall bladder and small intestinal function in normal man. Gut 1984; 25(5):405–411.

30. Persson EM, Gustafsson AS, Carlsson AS, et al. The effects of food on the dissolution of poorly soluble drugs in human and in model small intestinal fluids. Pharm Res 2005; 22(12):2141–2151.

31. Armand M, Borel P, Ythier P, et al. Effects of droplet size, triacylglycerol composition, and calcium on the hydrolysis of complex emulsions by pancreatic lipase: an in vitro study. J Nutr Biochem 1992; 3(7):333–341.

32. MacGregor KJ, Embleton JK, Lacy JE, et al. Influence of lipolysis on drug absorption from the gastro-intestinal tract. Adv Drug Deliv Rev 1997; 25(1):33–46.

33. Ljusberg-Wahren H, Seier NF, Brogard M, Troedsson E, Mullertz A. Enzymatic characterization of lipid-based drug delivery systems. Int J Pharm 2005; 298(2):328–332.

34. Subramanian R, Wasan KM. Effect of lipid excipients on in vitro pancreatic lipase activity. Drug Dev Ind Pharm 2003; 29(8):885–890.

35. Armand M, Pasquier B, Andre M, et al. Digestion and absorption of 2 fat emulsions with different droplet sizes in the human digestive tract. Am J Clin Nutr 1999; 70(6):1096–1106.

36. Dressman JB, Berardi RR, Dermentzoglou LC, et al. Upper gastrointestinal (GI) pH in young, healthy men and women. Pharm Res 1990; 7(7):756–761.

37. Gargouri Y, Moreau H, Verger R. Gastric lipases: biochemical and physiological studies. Biochim Biophys Acta 1989; 1006(3):255–271.

38. Shankland W. The ionic behavior of fatty acids solubilized by bile salts. J Coll Int Sci 1970; 34(1):9–25.

39. Zangenberg NH, Mullertz A, Kristensen HG, Hovgaard L. A dynamic in vitro lipolysis model. I. Controlling the rate of lipolysis by continuous addition of calcium. Eur J Pharm Sci 2001; 14(3):115–122.

40. Christensen JO, Schultz K, Mollgaard B, Kristensen HG, Mullertz A. Solubilisation of poorly water-soluble drugs during in vitro lipolysis of medium- and long-chain triacylglycerols. Eur J Pharm Sci 2004; 23(3):287–296.

41. Zangenberg NH, Mullertz A, Gjelstrup KH, Hovgaard L. A dynamic in vitro lipolysis model. II: Evaluation of the model. Eur J Pharm Sci 2001; 14(2): 237–244.

42. Patton JS, Andersson L. Immobilized pancreatic lipase and colipase for purification and binding studies. FEBS Lett 1978; 86(2):179–182.

43. Kaukonen AM, Boyd BJ, Porter CJ, Charman WN. Drug solubilization behavior during in vitro digestion of simple triglyceride lipid solution formulations. Pharm Res 2004; 21(2):245–253.

44. Reymond JP, Sucker H. In vitro model for cyclosporin intestinal absorption in lipid vehicles. Pharm Res 1988; 5(10):673–676.

45. Kaukonen AM, Boyd BJ, Charman WN, Porter CJ. Drug solubilization behavior during in vitro digestion of suspension formulations of poorly water-soluble drugs in triglyceride lipids. Pharm Res 2004; 21(2):254–260.

46. Porter CJ, Kaukonen AM, Taillardat-Bertschinger A, et al. Use of in vitro lipid digestion data to explain the in vivo performance of triglyceride-based oral lipid formulations of poorly water-soluble drugs: studies with halofantrine. J Pharm Sci 2004; 93(5):1110–1121.

47. Porter CJ, Kaukonen AM, Boyd BJ, Edwards GA, Charman WN. Susceptibility to lipase-mediated digestion reduces the oral bioavailability of danazol after administration as a medium-chain lipid-based microemulsion formulation. Pharm Res 2004; 21(8):1405–1412.

48. Kossena GA, Charman WN, Boyd BJ, Porter CJ. Influence of the intermediate digestion phases of common formulation lipids on the absorption of a poorly water-soluble drug. J Pharm Sci 2004; 94(3):481–492.

49. Borel P, Armand M, Ythier P, et al. Hydrolysis of emulsions with different triglycerides and droplet sizes by gastric lipases in vitro. Effect on pancreatic lipase activity. J Nutr Biochem 1994; 5(3):124–133.

50. Sek L, Porter CJ, Charman WN. Characterisation and quantification of medium chain and long chain triglycerides and their in vitro digestion products, by HPTLC coupled with in situ densitometric analysis. J Pharm Biomed Anal 2001; 25(3-4): 651–661.

51. The United States Pharmacopeia/The National Formulary (USP24/NF19) 2000. United states Pharmacopeia Convection, Inc, Rockville, MD, USA, 1254–1255.

52. Alvarez FJ, Stella VJ. The role of calcium ions and bile salts on the pancreatic lipase-catalyzed hydrolysis of triglyceride emulsions stabilized with lecithin. Pharm Res 1989; 6(7):449–457.

53. Borel P, Grolier P, Armand M, et al. Carotenoids in biological emulsions: solubility, surface-to-core distribution, and release from lipid droplets. J Lipid Res 1996; 37(2):250–261.

54. Nielsen FS, Petersen KB, Mullertz A. Bioavailability of Probucol from Lipid and Surfactant Based Formulations in Minipigs: Influence of Particle Size and Dietary State. Submitted for publication.

55. Pouton CW. Lipid formulations for oral administration of drugs: non-emulsifying, self-emulsifying and "self-microemulsifying" drug delivery systems. Eur J Pharm Sci 2000; 11(suppl 2):S93–S98.

56. Reymond JP, Sucker H, Vonderscher J. In vivo model for cyclosporin intestinal absorption in lipid vehicles. Pharm Res 1988; 5(10):677–679.

57. Christensen JO, Schultz K, Mollgaard B, Rohde M, Kristensen HG, Mullertz A. Evaluation of an in vitro digestion model for the prediction of in vivo absorption of poorly water-soluble drug in lipid-based formulations. Submitted for publication.

58. Drewe J, Meier R, Vonderscher J, et al. Enhancement of the oral absorption of cyclosporin in man. Br J Clin Pharmacol 1992; 34(1):60–64.

59. Kovarik JM, Mueller EA, van Bree JB, Tetzloff W, Kutz K. Reduced inter- and intraindividual variability in cyclosporine pharmacokinetics from a microemulsion formulation. J Pharm Sci 1994; 83(3):444–446.

60. Gao ZG, Choi HG, Shin HJ, et al. Physicochemical characterization and evaluation of a microemulsion system for oral delivery of cyclosporin A. Int J Pharm 1998; 161(1):75–86.

61. Odeberg JM, Kaufmann P, Kroon KG, Hoglund P. Lipid drug delivery and rational formulation design for lipophilic drugs with low oral bioavailability, applied to cyclosporine. Eur J Pharm Sci 2003; 20(4-5):375–382.

62. Khoo SM, Humberstone AJ, Porter CJH, Edwards GA, Charman WN. Formulation design and bioavailability assessment of lipidic self-emulsifying formulations of halofantrine. Int J Pharm 1998; 167(1-2):155–164.

63. Holm R, Porter CJ, Edwards GA, Mullertz A, Kristensen HG, Charman WN. Examination of oral absorption and lymphatic transport of halofantrine in a triple-cannulated canine model after administration in self-microemulsifying drug delivery systems (SMEDDS) containing structured triglycerides. Eur J Pharm Sci 2003; 20(1):91–97.

64. Fatouros DG, Nielsen FS, Mullertz A. In Vitro Dynamic Lipolysis Model: A Tool to Predict the In Vivo behavior of Lipid Based Formulations. Presented at the 2004 AAPS Annual Meeting, Baltimore, MD, USA.

12

Case Studies: Rational Development of Self-Emulsifying Formulations for Improving the Oral Bioavailability of Poorly Soluble, Lipophilic Drugs

Ping Gao

Small Molecule Pharmaceutics, Amgen, Inc., Thousand Oaks, California, U.S.A.

Walter Morozowich

Prodrug/Formulation Consultant, Kalamazoo, Michigan, U.S.A.

INTRODUCTION

Oral administration of highly lipophilic, poorly water-soluble drugs often results in poor and highly variable bioavailability due to poor dissolution in vivo. One approach for improving the absorption of these drugs involves the use of self-emulsifying drug delivery systems (SEDDS) (1–6) which rapidly disperse following oral administration yielding an o/w emulsion or microemulsion containing the solubilized drug.

SEDDS formulations are typically developed by an empirical, trial-and-error approach (2,3) although some useful guidelines have emerged from characterization of successful formulations such as the Neoral® formulation of cyclosporine A (7–8). The literature on microemulsion formulations describes a multitude of compositions and functional characteristics producing varying degrees of drug absorption enhancement in both animals and humans (2–4). Formulation scientists are frequently presented with a series of challenging decisions during the development of SEDDS formulations including choice of formulation strategy, excipient selection, solubility and stability assessment, formulation optimization, scale-up and production of the final product.

However, the key consideration in development of a SEDDS formulation involves solubilization of the drug and preventing its precipitation following dilution with aqueous media which requires that the drug molecules remain within the formulation lipid phase following dilution.

Spontaneous generation of a microemulsion following aqueous dilution of a SEDDS requires a high surfactant concentration relative to the other formulation components; an insufficient amount of surfactant can yield a coarse emulsion with increased propensity for drug precipitation. Selection of the lipid component for the SEDDS formulation is commonly based on the physical and/or interfacial characteristics of the resulting formulation (4–5) without understanding the manner in which the lipid influences drug absorption. The selection of a lipid for optimal enhancement of in vivo absorption of the drug is often an iterative, empirical and slow process (2,3).

This chapter describes the design and development of SEDDS formulations with enhanced oral bioavailability as illustrated with two highly lipophilic and poorly soluble drugs, namely, PNU-74006 (Clog P 5.8; water solubility, 50 ng/mL, pH 6.5) and Drug X (Clog P~7, water solubility, ~5 μg/mL, pH 6.5). The influence of the SEDDS formulation variables on the rate and the extent of absorption of lipophilic drugs in animals and in humans is presented along with the in vitro characterization methods employed in determining the emulsification spontaneity and the dispersibility of the SEDDS formulations. This article describes a systematic approach for developing lipid-based formulations of poorly soluble and lipophilic drugs. In addition, a possible mechanism for the enhanced uptake of the drugs from the SEDDS formulations in the intestine is discussed.

IN VITRO EVALUATION OF SEDDS FORMULATIONS

There are a number of physicochemical attributes of SEDDS formulations that are important with respect to oral bioavailability. Although several in vitro test methods have been applied to characterize the performance of SEDDS formulations (9–16), there is a lack of consensus concerning the methodology and the test methods that should be used in their evaluation.

During our exploration and development of SEDDS formulations, in-vitro test methods were developed and these served as a guide in formulation screening and optimization. The three key in vitro performance measures of a SEDDS formulation are:

1. ease of emulsification,
2. dispersibility (i.e., droplet size), and
3. drug solubilization.

These three attributes of SEDDS formulations are conceptually illustrated in Figure 1 and these attributes can be evaluated in vitro with appropriate test methods. The ease of emulsification of a SEDDS formulation in the aqueous medium is important and a number of test methods have been reported (9,12). As shown in Figure 1, the slope of the release profile from the SEDDS formulation observed at the initial stage (e.g., the first 30 minutes) with the use of a conventional drug release test is indicative of its emulsification spontaneity. The emulsification spontaneity of the SEDDS formulation to yield an emulsion or a microemulsion upon contact with an aqueous medium may affect the drug release kinetics and therefore, the extent of drug absorption.

The dispersibility of the SEDDS formulation is evaluated by the droplet size of the resulting emulsion or microemulsion that is generated upon dilution with water. This is considered as a key factor in the performance of SEDDS formulations since the droplet size determines the rate and extent of drug release in vivo and subsequent absorption, as reported by Shah et al. (13). Although the emphasis on generation of a microemulsion is inherent with this technology, the influence of droplet size on the absorption of poorly soluble drugs has not been clearly established (17). It is desirable to assess the lipid droplet size associated with complete drug release in vitro (Fig. 1). However, due to the complexity of the analytical methodologies and instrumentation in the droplet size measurement and corresponding test condition, a reliable droplet size profile from a SEDDS formulation is commonly obtained by multiple analytical methods (the choice of methods is dependent on the range of droplet size) in parallel as a separate test.

The extent of drug solubilization in the test medium upon the release from the SEDDS formulation may change and the drug may precipitate. As indicated

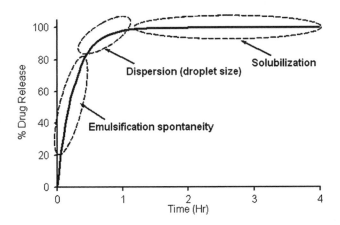

Figure 1   In vitro characterization of the key attributes of an SEDDS formulation is *conceptually* illustrated: emulsification spontaneity, dispersibility (i.e., microemulsion/emulsion droplet size), and the extent of solubilization in a test medium. *Abbreviation*: SEDDS, self-emulsifying drug delivery systems.

in Figure 1, the extent of drug solubilization as a function of time can be conveniently determined as part of an in vitro drug release test. It is worth noting that the choice of a test medium with appropriate composition and volume is a crucial factor since the solubilization capacity of the test medium will inevitably affect the extent of drug solubilization and the precipitation process.

CASE STUDY WITH PNU-74006

Development of SEDDS Formulations

PNU-74006 (Fig. 2) is a potent antioxidant and membrane stabilizing agent with a MW of 607.1, a high CLog P of 5.8, and an extremely low intrinsic aqueous solubility of only 25 ng/mL. With two pKa values of 6.1 and 6.8, the pH-solubility profile of PNU-74006 shows excellent solubility (>10 mg/mL) at pH 3 and below, however, at pH 6.8, the solubility of PNU-74006 is only ~40 ng/mL (Fig. 3).

The oral bioavailability of PNU-74006 is only about 2% in monkeys and 6.7% in humans when dosed as a low pH (pH 3) aqueous micellar (containing polysorbate 80) solution formulation. The low oral bioavailability is probably due to the rapid precipitation of PNU-74006 free base in the duodenum because of the low water solubility at pH 6.

The SEDDS formulation approach was explored for enhancing the oral absorption of PNU-74006. It was anticipated that the drug would be highly soluble in the typical surfactant-lipid vehicles. Upon dilution with water, PNU-74006 should remain partitioned within the resulting emulsion or microemulsion because of the high CLog P value (5.8) of the drug. Three SEDDS formulations (SEDDS-a, SEDDS-b, and SEDDS-c, see Table 2 for compositions) were prepared and contained either medium chain mono-/di-glycerides (Capmul MCM), glyceryl monooleate (GMO-K®) or glyceryl mono-/di-oleate mixture (Maisine®). A description of the aforementioned excipients is provided in Table 1.

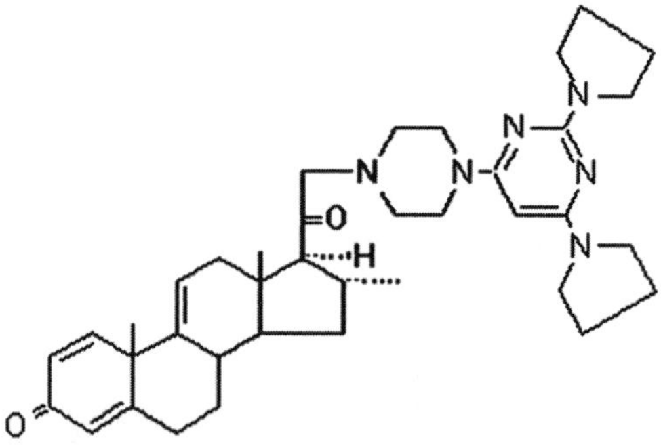

Figure 2 Structure of PNU-74006.

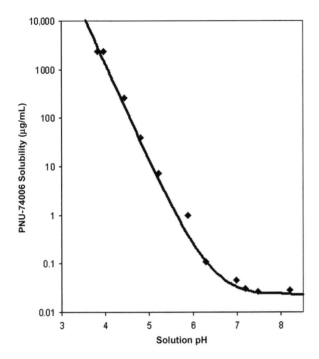

Figure 3 Aqueous solubility of PNU-74006 versus pH. The solid line is fitted to the experimental data and the resulting pKa values are 6.1 and 6.8.

To determine the formulation dispersibility and degree of drug solubilization, the SEDDS formulations were diluted with various aqueous media formulated to simulate the endogenous fluids of the human stomach and duodenum (Table 2). Capmul MCM, which is a mixture of mono- and di-glycerides of C8–C10 fatty acids, was used in the SEDDS-a formulation, whereas GMO-K (mainly glyceryl monooleate, or GMO) was used in the SEDDS-b formulation. Fifty-fold dilution of these two formulations with a simulated gastric fluid (SGF),

Table 1 Lipid Excipients Used in the Case Studies

Excipient	Chemical definition	Vendor
Capmul MCM	C8/C10 Mono-/diglycerides	Abitec
Cremophor EL	Polyoxyethyleneglycerol triricinoleate 35	BASF
Capmul GMO-K	Glycerol mono-oleate	Abitec
GDO	Glycerol di-oleate	Croda
GMO	Glycerol mono-oleate	Croda
Miglyol 812	C8/C10 Triglycerides	Huls America
Maisine	50% GDO, 35% GMO, 10% GTO (Glyceol trioleate) and 5% glycerol (18)	Gattefosse

comprised of 0.01M HCl + 0.15M NaCl, pH = 2.0, followed by an approximate, 10-fold dilution in simulated intestinal fluid (SIF), comprised of 0.05 M phosphate buffer, pH = 6.8, resulted in coarse emulsion formation (10–100 μm droplet size) with no evidence of drug precipitation suggesting that these formulations should prevent PNU-74006 precipitation upon dilution in the GI tract in-vivo. In comparison, the SEDDS-c formulation, which contained Maisine (a mixture of 55% GDO, 50% GMO, and 5% GTO (18) yielded a microemulsion upon dilution with water as evidenced by instantaneous formation of a transparent solution with a faint opalescence.

Table 2 Composition of the PNU-74006 SEDDS Formulations, Behavior in the In Vitro Dilution Test and Oral Bioavailability Data

Ingredient	Aqueous solution (mg/mL)	SEDDS-a (mg/g)	SEDDS-b (mg/g)	SEDDS-c (mg/g)
PNU-74006	25	50	50	50
EtOH 95%	—	—	—	105
PG	200	370	395	105
Polysorbate 80	50	100	—	—
Cremophor EL	—	—	100	400
Capmul MCM	—	400	—	—
Captex 300	—	100	—	—
Capmul GMO-K	—	—	500	—
Maisine	—	—	—	340
Citric acid	78	—	—	—
NaOH	To adjust final solution pH =3.0	—	—	—
Water	q.s.	30	5	—
In vitro dilution test				
Dilution with SGF (1:10)	Solution with turbidity	Coarse emulsion	Coarse emulsion	Microemulsion (p.s. ~130 nm)
Dilution with SIF (1:5)	Solution with turbidity	Coarse emulsion	Coarse emulsion	Microemulsion (p.s. ~21 nm)
In vivo PK data (dose = 80 mg/kg in monkeys, n = 4, fasted)				
C_{max} ± SD (μg/mL)	0.22 ± 0.05	0.26 ± 0.08	0.79 ± 0.17	1.28 ± 0.10
AUC ± SD (μghr/mL)	1.23 ± 0.28	3.00 ± 1.10	7.54 ± 0.91	15.13 ± 0.90
Oral F% (estimated)	2.0	4.9	12.4	24.6
	(Crossover)			(Noncrossover)

Abbreviations: EtOH, ethanol; PG, propylene glycol; SEDDS, self-emulsifying drug delivery systems; SIF, simulated intestinal fluid; SGF, simulated gastric fluid.

Oral Bioavailability of the PNU-74006 SEDDS Formulations

The absolute bioavailability of an 80 mg/kg dose of PNU-74006, administered in the three SEDDS formulations, was determined in fasted cynomolgus monkeys in comparison to an aqueous micellar solution of polysorbate 80 adjusted to pH 3 (Table 2). The pharmacokinetic results are shown in Table 2.

The highest PNU-74006 exposure (Cmax and AUC) was observed with the SEDDS-c formulation, for which the oral bioavailability was 24.6% (approximately 12-fold higher than that for the pH-adjusted aqueous micellar solution.

Extrapolating from the droplet-size determinations made following aqueous dilution in vitro, the superior in vivo performance of the SEDDS-c formulation may be due to the formation of a smaller droplet size following dilution in the GI tract in vivo. However, due to the differing compositions of the SEDDS formulations, this assertion cannot be made with certainty.

The PNU-74006 bioavailability of the SEDDS-a formulation was only ~5%, whereas the bioavailability was ~12% with the SEDDS-b formulation. Relative to the SEDDS-c formulation, the inferior performance of the SEDDS-a and SEDDS-b formulations, which differ from one another in the type of the surfactant (i.e., polysorbate 80 vs. Cremophor EL) and lipid (i.e., Capmul MCM vs. GMO-K) may similarly be due to the relatively poor dispersion of the formulations observed upon aqueous dilution in vitro. However, differing formulation compositions cannot be ruled out as having contributing to the performances of these formulations. First, a much lower level of Cremophor EL was used in SEDDS-b as compared to SEDDS-c. Second, GMO-K was used in SEDDS-b with a higher concentration while the glycerol mono-/di-oleate mixture as a marketed product (Maisine®) was used in the SEDDS-c formulation.

CASE STUDY WITH DRUG X

Development of High Drug Load SEDDS Formulations of Drug X

Drug X is highly lipophilic with an intrinsic Log P of ~7, a MW of ~600 and an aqueous solubility of ~5 µg/mL in the physiologically relevant pH range of pH 2 to 7. Since Drug X has pKa values of ~6 and ~9, a di-sodium salt was prepared and the di-sodium salt bulk drug was filled, as the bulk drug, into hard gelatin capsules for clinical evaluation. SEDDS formulations were developed as an alternate dosage form of Drug X. The solubility of Drug X in the selected pharmaceutically acceptable excipients is shown in Table 3. Since a high dose of Drug X was anticipated, SEDDS formulations containing 300 mg/g Drug X, as the free acid form, is developed.

The SEDDS formulations of Drug X were evaluated and optimized as described below with respect to the following key variables:

1. in-vitro emulsification spontaneity,
2. droplet size upon dilution, and
3. the type of the lipid excipients.

Table 3   Solubility of Drug X in Formulation Excipients

Excipient	Drug X solubility (mg/g excipient)
Ethanol	1950
Propylene glycol	710
PEG 400	670
Glycerol	<10
Polysorbate 80	500
Cremophor EL	430
Capmul MCM	20
GDO/GMO (8:2)	11
Soybean oil	<20
Miglyol 812	20

Abbreviations: EtOH, ethanol; PG, propylene glycol; GDO, glycerol di-oleate; GMO, glycerol mono-oleate.

Influence of Dispersibility of the SEDDS Formulation of Drug X on Oral Absorption

The effect of dispersibility of the 300 mg/g Drug X SEDDS formulation on oral bioavailability was evaluated by two different approaches. In the first approach, the formulation composition was kept constant but the droplet size, upon dilution of the formulation with water, was varied by mechanical reduction of the droplet size using a microfluidizer.

The composition of the 300 mg/g Drug X SEDDS formulation is given in Table 4. In conducting the dispersibility test, the SEDDS formulation was

Table 4   Composition of the 300 mg/g Drug X SEDDS Formulations, Their Properties and Bioavailability in Fasted Rats After an Oral Dose of 20 mg/kg

	Formulation composition (mg/g) Drug X: 300 EtOH/PG (1:1): 200 Cremophor EL: 425 GDO/GMO (8:2): 75	
Processing	Initial emulsion	Microfluidized emulsion
Droplet size ± SD (nm)	~1000	221 ± 115
No. of rats dosed	8	6
Mean AUC/dose [(µg·hr/mL)/(mg/kg)]	2.7 ± 0.4	6.8 ± 4.0
Mean C_{max} ± SD (µg/mL)	14.1 ± 4	33.9 ± 19
Absolute oral F% ± SD	21 ± 3	53 ± 31

Note: The two pre-dispersed emulsions differing in droplet size were obtained from the same lot of the SEDDS formulation wherein a portion of the lot was processed with the microfluidizer.
Abbreviations: GDO, glycerol di-oleate; GMO, glycerol mono-oleate; PG, propylene glycol; SEDDS, self-emulsifying drug delivery systems.

diluted 50-fold with water and subjected to mild agitation. This was achieved by placing 1 g of the SEDDS formulation in 50 mL of water in a 100 mL cylindrical bottle and then gently rocking the container manually back and forth (~90°) about two times per second for a period of about 1 minute.

Dilution of the initial 300 mg/g Drug X SEDDS formulation followed by agitation as described above, resulted in spontaneous generation of an emulsion with a mean droplet size of ~1000 nm. Reduction of the droplet size was achieved by processing the formulation with a microfluidizer (Microfluidics, MFIC Corporation, Newton, Massachusetts, U.S.A.). A portion of the emulsion was passed through the microfluidizer twice with a setting of 3500 psi which reduced the mean droplet size of the emulsion to ~221 nm. The bioavailability of Drug X was determined in fasted rats administered either with the initial emulsion (droplet size of ~1000 nm) or the microfluidizer-processed emulsion (~221 nm).

A summary of the pharmacokinetic parameters of this study is shown in Table 4. The Drug X bioavailability was 21% ± 3% for the crude emulsion and 53 ± 31% for the microfluidizer processed emulsion, which represents ~2.5-fold enhancement attributable to droplet size reduction.

Although variable, the data suggest an inverse correlation between Drug X bioavailability and the lipid droplet size of the emulsion formulations.

Development of a SEDDS formulation that could solubilize 300 mg of Drug X per gram of formulation and spontaneously microemulsify upon dilution was initially challenging because the high drug loading in the excipient matrix resulted in a poorly dispersed emulsion.

In another study, pharmaceutically acceptable amine, diethanolamine (DEA), was added to the SEDDS formulations, and this significantly reduced the lipid droplet size upon dilution with water. The molar ratio between Drug X and DEA investigated during formulation development ranged from 8:1 to 1:1 (0.25–5% total DEA content, respectively).

As shown in Figure 4, the population of the large droplets (>1 μm) upon approximate, 50-fold dilution in SGF was inversely correlated with the amount of DEA in the formulation. In the absence of DEA, a SEDDS formulation containing 300 mg/g Drug X was very poorly dispersed, with greater than 90% of the droplets possessing a droplet size ≥1 μm.

Addition of 0.8% (w/w) or greater amounts of DEA reduced the fraction of large droplets (≥1 μm) to a negligible level. The effect of DEA on the dispersibility of the Drug X SEDDS formulations is rationalized as follows. Drug X is partially neutralized by DEA which, upon dilution of the SEDDS with water, results in a negative surface charge on the dispersed oil droplets, and reduced coalescence as a consequence of electrostatic repulsion.

As shown in Figure 5, the mean droplet size of the emulsions generated from the 300 mg/g Drug X SEDDS formulations upon mixing with water showed a rapid reduction in droplet size as the percentage of DEA increased. The mean droplet size was significantly reduced from ~1000 nm when the amine was absent to ~150 nm with the use of ~0.8% amine. In conclusion, the presence of a small

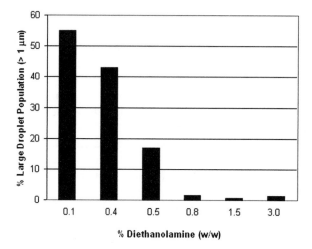

Figure 4 Population of large droplets ($\geqq 1\,\mu m$) after dilution (100-fold) of the 300 mg/g Drug X SEDDS formulation with SIF versus the DEA concentration (w/w) in the formulation. *Abbreviations*: DEA, diethanolamine; SEDDS, self-emulsifying drug delivery systems; SIF, simulated intestinal fluid.

amount of DEA (~1%) effectively reduced the droplet size of the 300 mg/g SEDDS formulation of Drug X to about 150 nm or less.

It was found that other organic amines including primary amines (e.g., tromethamine, ethylenediamine), secondary amines (e.g., diethanolamine,

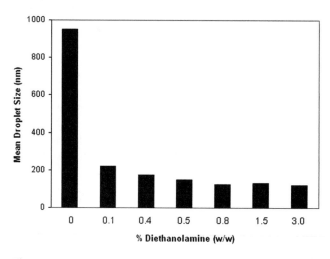

Figure 5 The mean particle size of the 300 mg/g Drug X SEDDS formulations upon dilution with SIF (dilution factor: 100X) versus the DEA concentration (w/w) in the formulation. *Abbreviations*: DEA, diethanolamine; SEDDS, self-emulsifying drug delivery systems; SIF, simulated intestinal fluid.

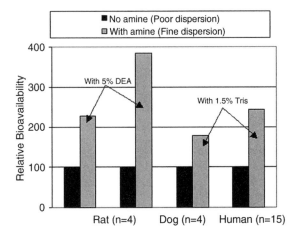

Figure 6   Summary of the relative oral bioavailability of the 300 mg/g Drug X SEDDS formulations in the presence and absence of an amine (either DEA or tris) in the rat, dog (crossover), and human (crossover). *Abbreviations*: DEA, diethanolamine; SEDDS, self-emulsifying drug delivery systems.

diethylamine), tertiary amines (e.g., triethylamine, triethanolamine, dimethylethanolamine), and quaternary ammonium compounds (e.g., choline hydroxide) behaved similarly in the SEDDS formulation by effectively improving the dispersibility and generating a microemulsion on dilution with water.

In the second approach to evaluate the influence of the droplet size of the SEDDS formulations on oral exposure of Drug X, the oral bioavailability of the formulations, with and without an added amine, was determined and compared. The in vivo pharmacokinetic results of these paired 300 mg/g Drug X SEDDS formulations (same composition, differing only with respect to the presence or absence of an amine) were obtained in rats, dogs and humans. The *relative* oral bioavailability of Drug X from the paired SEDDS formulations are normalized and plotted in Figure 6. The relative bioavailability of Drug X in rats (non-crossover), dogs (crossover) and humans (crossover) was consistently improved by approximately two- to three-fold following addition of 1.5% to 5.0% (w/w) of DEA or the primary amine, tromethamine (Tris), to the SEDDS formulation. These results again demonstrate that microemulsion formation following SEDDS formulation dilution, appears to be an important determinant of the extent of absorption of Drug X in animals and humans.

Influence of Lipid Excipient Characteristics on the Absorption of Drug X from SEDDS Formulations

The specific characteristics of the lipid excipients (e.g., degree of esterification of glycerides and fatty acid chain length) chosen for a SEDDS formulation can have a profound effect on the oral bioavailability of poorly soluble drugs and this should be taken into consideration during formulation screening and development (2,5).

In a series of four studies, we systematically evaluated the effect of the following variables on Drug X bioavailability:

1. Is a lipid required for improving bioavailability?
2. If so, what is the optimum amount of lipid excipient required for improving the bioavailability?
3. What effect does the degree of glyceride esterification have on bioavailability?
4. What effect does the glyceride fatty acid chain length have on bioavailability?

These variables were of particular interest since Drug X has relatively low solubility ($\leq$20 mg/g) in the lipid excipients tested (Table 3). Therefore, the lipid was initially considered as an optional component in the SEDDS formulation described below in Examples 1–4.

Example 1

The effect of the long chain mono- and di-glycerides, GDO and GMO (Table 1), on the oral bioavailability of Drug X was evaluated in fasted dogs administered gelatin capsules containing two prototype SEDDS formulations [SEDDS-1 and SEDDS-2, (Table 5)] containing 400 mg Drug X per gram of formulation. The SEDDS-1 formulation contained 70 mg/g of an 8:2 (w/w) mixture of GDO and GMO whereas the SEDDS-2 formulation contained no lipid; both formulations contained 80 mg/g DEA Upon dilution with water, each formulation formed a microemulsion with a mean droplet size of ~100 nm. Although variable, the GDO/GMO-containing SEDDS-1 formulation yielded approximately two-fold greater Drug X exposure (as determined by the AUC) than that associated with

Table 5 Bioavailability of Two 400 mg/g Drug X SEDDS Formulations in Dogs at a Single Dose of 20 mg/kg ($n = 4$, Crossover)

	SEDDS-1	SEDDS-2
Composition (mg/g)	Drug X 400	Drug X 400
	EtOH/PG (1:1) 120	EtOH/PG (1:1) 160
	Cremophor EL 330	Cremophor EL 360
	GDO/GMO (8:2) 70	GDO/GMO (8:2) 0
	DEA 80	DEA 80
Droplet size after dilution with water (100X)	~100 nm	~100 nm
Mean AUC ± SD (μm · hr)	54.8 ± 38.8	21.7 ± 16.0
Mean C_{max} (μM)	18.7	7.4

Abbreviations: EtOH, ethanol; GDO, glycerol di-oleate; GMO, glycerol mono-oleate; PG, propylene glycol; SEDDS, self-emulsifying drug delivery system.

the SEDDS-2 formulation (Table 5). The results of this study suggest that, despite similar dispersibility, presence of a solubilizing glyceride excipient in the formulation may improve Drug X absorption.

Example 2

To examine the effect of glyceride fatty acid chain length on the absorption of Drug X, a bioavailability study was conducted in dogs comparing SEDDS formulations that contained either Capmul MCM (C8–C10 mono-/di-glycerides) or an 8:2 mixture of GDO/GMO, at concentrations of 75 mg/g or 180 mg/g (Table 6). At the 75 mg/g lipid concentration (SEDDS-1a and SEDDS-1b), Drug X bioavailability was similar; however, at the 180 mg/g lipid concentration, the SEDDS formulation containing the GDO/GMO mixture (SEDDS-1c) produced greater Drug X exposure (AUC and Cmax) than the formulation containing an equal concentration of Capmul MCM (SEDDS-1d).

Example 3

Medium chain mono- and di-glycerides (e.g., Capmul MCM) and tri-glycerides (MCT) are commonly used in oral SEDDS formulations where they may promote more facile drug absorption than long chain glyceride excipients (19). To investigate the effect of the degree of glyceride esterification on Drug X absorption, two SEDDS formulations of similar fractional composition, differing only in the lipid excipient used, were administered to fasted rats as predispersed emulsions (200–300 nm lipid droplet size), prepared by 50-fold dilution in water (Table 7). The lipids employed were Capmul MCM (a mixture of medium chain mono- and

Table 6 Bioavailability of the 300 mg/g Drug X SEDDS Formulations at a Single Dose of 20 mg/kg in Dogs ($n = 4$, Crossover)

	SEDDS-1a	SEDDS-1b	SEDDS-1c	SEDDS-1d
Composition (mg/g)	Drug X 300	Drug X 300	Drug X 300	Drug X 300
	EtOH/PG	EtOH/PG	EtOH/PG	EtOH/PG
	(1:1) 190	(1:1) 190	(1:1) 200	(1:1) 200
	Cremophor	Cremophor	Cremophor	Cremophor
	EL 420	EL 420	EL 280	EL 280
	GDO/GMO	MCM 75	GDO/GMO	MCM 180
	(8:2) 75	Tris 15	(8:2) 180	DMAE 45
	Tris 15		DMAE 45	
Droplet size after dilution with SIF, pH 2	~150 nm	~140 nm	~120 nm	~160 nm
Mean AUC ± SD (μm · hr)	50.3 ± 18.8	43.6 ± 20.7	50.7 ± 18.7	36.5 ± 20.2
Mean C_{max} ± SD (μM)	9.7 ± 4.4	9.0 ± 4.1	11.1 ± 2.0	5.3 ± 4.3

Abbreviations: EtOH, ethanol; GDO, glycerol di-oleate; GMO, glycerol mono-oleate; SEDDS, self-emulsifying drug delivery systems; SIF, simulated intestinal fluid.

Table 7 Composition of the 300 mg/g Drug X SEDDS Formulations and Oral
Bioavailability in Fasted Rats at a Single Dose of 20 mg/kg

	Miglyol 812 SEDDS	Capmul MCM SEDDS
Composition (mg/g)	Drug X 300	Drug X 300
	EtOH/PG (1:1) 200	EtOH/PG (1:1) 200
	Cremophor EL 275	Cremophor EL 275
	Miglyol 812 180	Capmul MCM 180
	DMAE 45	DMAE 45
Droplet size (nm) in water	~300 nm	~200 nm
No. of rats dosed	5	6
Mean AUC /Dose (μg · hr/mL/mg/kg)	2.9 ± 1.6	6.6 ± 1.5
Mean C_{max} ± SD (μg/mL)	20.4 ± 10.8	30.2 ± 13
Absolute oral bioavialability ± SD	22 ± 12	51 ± 11

Abbreviations: EtOH, ethanol; GDO, glycerol di-oleate; GMO, glycerol mono-oleate;
PG, propylene glycol; SEDDS, self-emulsifying drug delivery system.

di-glycerides) or Miglyol 812 (a mixture of medium chain tri-glyerides) and each
animal received a total dose of 6 mg Drug X from formulations containing
300 mg/g of the drug.

The Miglyol 812-containing formulation produced less than half the bioavailability of the Capmul MCM-containing formulation ($p < 0.05$, paired t-test).
In conclusion, the absorption of Drug X was improved with the SEDDS formulation
containing medium chain *mono-/di-* glycerides (Capmul MCM) as compared to
that of the SEDDS containing the medium chain *tri*-glycerides (Miglyol).

Example 4

To evaluate the effect of the administered lipid volume on Drug X absorption, three
SEDDS formulations containing 300 mg/g Drug X were prepared which were identical in composition (see inset in Fig. 7) with the exception of the quantity of the lipid
excipient (an 8:2 mixture of GDO:GMO), which ranged from 50 to 180 mg/g; a
fourth SEDDS, from which GDO/GMO had been omitted, was prepared and administered as a control. Addition of 45 mg/g DEA to the formulations resulted in a mean
lipid droplet size of ~120–150 nm, which was independent of the lipid content. This
observation suggests that (*i*) the dispersion performance of these SEDDS formulations is dictated by the presence of a small amount of an organic amine (vide supra)
and (*ii*) the presence of a substantial amount of lipid in the formulation does not alter
the droplet size significantly. The Drug X exposure was determined in fasted rats
administered a 20 mg/kg dose of the drug as the predispersed microemulsion of each
SEDDS formulation (prepared by 50-fold dilution in water followed by manual agitation). The mean, dose-normalized (AUC/dose) Drug X exposures were positively
correlated with the amount of GDO/GMO in the formulation between 50 and

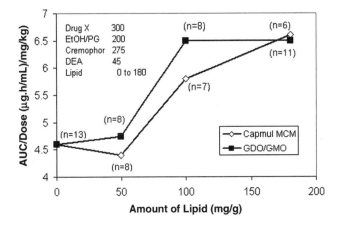

Figure 7   Normalized AUC/dose ratios obtained in fasted rats with the Drug X SEDDS formulations where the amount of lipid [either GDO/GMO (8:2) mixture or Capmul MCM] is varied. The number of the rats is given in parenthesis.

100 mg of GDO/GMO; however, there is virtually no difference in the dose-normalized Drug X exposures when the GDO/GMO concentrations in the SEDDS formulation range from 0 to 50 mg/g or from 100 to 180 mg/g (Fig. 7).

The study was repeated in fasted rats in a similar manner, except an equivalent amount of Capmul MCM was substituted for GDO/GMO in the SEDDS formulations described above. As with GDO/GMO, a positive correlation was seen between the mean dose-normalized Drug X exposure and the amount of Capmul MCM present in the formulation (Fig. 7). Again, there was little change in the dose normalized Drug X exposure when the Capmul MCM concentrations ranged from 0 to 50 mg/g. An increase in the dose-normalized Drug X exposure was observed when the Capmul MCM concentration was increased to 180 mg/g from 100 mg/g (Fig. 7). The difference in the dose-normalized Drug X exposures between the two SEDDS formulations containing 0 and 180 mg/g mono-/di-glycerides (in both series) is statistically significant ($p < 0.05$, paired t-test).

Both GDO/GMO and Capmul MCM are mono- and di-glyceride mixtures but they differ in the chain lengths of the esterified fatty acids. GDO and GMO consists of C18 fatty acid esters (oleate) whereas Capmul MCM consists of C8–C10 fatty acid glyceride esters (octanoate–decanoate). The dose-normalized exposures to Drug X from SEDDS formulations containing 180 mg/g of either GDO/GMO or Capmul MCM are essentially the same in rats, indicating that the excipient fatty acid chain length dose not appear to influence drug absorption (Fig. 7).

In summary, the bioavailability data with the GDO/GMO and the Capmul MCM SEDDS formulations indicates that the bioavailability of Drug X in rats is dependent on the amount of mono-/di-glyceride present in the formulation. The small difference in the dose-normalized exposure of Drug X between the SEDDS formulations containing 100 and 180 mg/g GDO/GMO or Capmul MCM (Fig. 7) indicates that ~100 mg/g of the mono-/di-glycerides is the optimal quantity required for enhancing oral absorption.

Influence of Ethanol and Propylene Glycol Level on the Emulsification Spontaneity with the SEDDS Formulations of Drug X

Ethanol (EtOH) and propylene glycol (PG) are commonly employed as cosolvents in SEDDS formulations, where they promote spontaneous emulsification of SEDDS formulations, which was observed in the following studies. Eight SEDDS formulations of Drug X were prepared with their compositions reported in Table 8. In four of the SEDDS formulations (2a–2d), the concentration of PG was held constant at 73 mg/g while the ethanol content was varied between 0 and 100 mg/g. In the other four formulations (2e–2h), the EtOH concentration was held constant at 100 mg/g while the PG level was varied between 0 and 75 mg/g.

An in vitro release test was conducted in 900 mL SIF (0.05 M phosphate buffer, pH 6.8) at 37°C using a VanKel 7010 dissolution apparatus with a paddle rate of 50 rpm. Since the presence of a solubilizing agent in the test medium would affect the drug release profile and thus, reduce the differentiation of the performance among the SEDDS formulations, no surfactant was added which resulted in nonsink conditions for Drug X due to its poor solubility at pH 6.8. Analytical samples were manually collected, without filtration, from the test medium at predetermined times and assayed for apparent drug concentration.

The drug release profiles from the four SEDDS formulations containing 73 mg/g PG and in which the ethanol concentrations were varied from 0 to 100 mg/g (SEDDS-2a to SEDDS-2d, Table 8) are shown in Figure 8. The initial slope and the shape of the profiles indicate that an increase in the ethanol concentration gives an

Table 8 Composition of 250 mg/g Drug X SEDDS Formulations with Variation in the EtOH and PG Concentrations

SEDDS formulation	Amount of excipient (mg)							
	2a	2b	2c	2d	2e	2f	2g	2h
Drug X				250				
Propyl gallate				2				
EtOH	0	30	60	100	100	100	100	100
PG	73	73	73	73	0	20	40	75
Cremophor EL				455				
Capmul MCM				75				
Tris/water (1:2)				45				
Total weight (mg)	900	930	980	1000	927	947	967	1002

Abbreviations: EtOH, ethanol; PG, propylene glycol; SEDDS, self-emulsifying drug delivery systems.

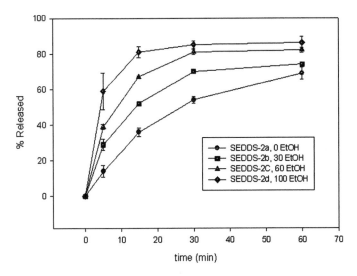

Figure 8 Effect of EtOH concentration (mg/g) on the release profile of Drug X from the SEDDS formulations containing 73 mg/g PG. *Abbreviations*: EtOH, ethanol; PG, propylene glycol.

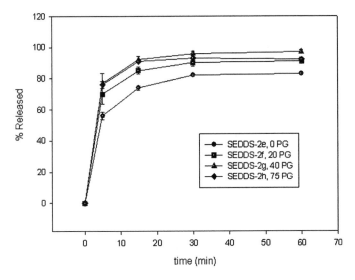

Figure 9 Effect of PG concentration (mg/g) on the release profile of Drug X from the SEDDS formulations containing 100 mg/g EtOH. *Abbreviations*: EtOH, ethanol; PG, propylene glycol; SEDDS, self-emulsifying drug delivery systems.

increase in the emulsification spontaneity with a concomitant increase in the extent of drug release.

The drug release profiles from the four SEDDS formulations in which the ethanol concentration was held constant at 100 mg/g but the PG content was varied from 0 to 75 mg/g (SEDDS-2e to SEDDS-2h, Table 8) are shown in Figure 9. In contrast to the studies in which the SEDDS EtOH content was varied, the profiles indicate little impact of the PG concentration on the initial percent of drug released. In all cases described above, less than 100% release of Drug X from SEDDS formulations was observed which was attributed to both the high viscosity of the formulation and high drug loading.

In conclusion, the release test for evaluating emulsification spontaneity and dispersibility (i.e., droplet size) is useful in formulation optimization. During the encapsulation of SEDDS formulations in soft gelatin capsules, a significant reduction in the PG and EtOH solvent concentration in the fill solution was found. This was due to a combination of solvent (PG and EtOH) migration into the gelatin shell and EtOH evaporation during the soft gelatin capsule drying process. Loss of solvent from the fill solution in the final soft gelatin capsules can have a significant effect on the in vitro dispersibility and the resulting oral bioavailability as described below.

CLINICAL EVALUATION OF THE SEDDS FORMULATIONS OF DRUG X AND DEVELOPMENT OF IN VITRO–IN VIVO RELATIONSHIPS (IVIVR)

Clinical Evaluation of the SEDDS Formulations of Drug X

The di-sodium salt of Drug X was formulated as a wet-granulation tablet (WG-tablet), a bulk drug filled capsule (HFC), a coated bead (CB) formulation, a bead mixed with apple sauce (AS) (CB–AS) formulation and a prototype SEDDS formulation. A total dose of 1200 mg of Drug X was administered to fasted human subjects and the plasma profiles for each formulation are shown in Figure 10. The four solid dosage forms produced very similar plasma profiles. In comparison, the mean AUC and the Cmax values obtained with the 300 mg/g Drug X SEDDS formulation was ~2.5-fold higher than those of the solid formulations.

Subsequently, three additional Drug X SEDDS formulations (containing 300 mg/g Drug X) were developed for further clinical evaluation in fasted subjects (Table 9). The objective of this study was to explore the relationship between the in-vitro performance (e.g., release profile and droplet size distribution) and Drug X absorption from the SEDDS formulations.

The in vitro release of Drug X from the SEDDS formulations was evaluated in a VanKel 7010 dissolution apparatus in 900 mL of SIF (pH 6.8) at 37°C with 50 rpm paddle speed. As shown in Figure 11, the "Tris/MCM" SEDDS HFC showed the highest release value (60% at $t = 60$ minutes). The "No Tris" SEDDS soft gelatin capsules performed poorly with a maximum Drug X release of only 13% at 60 minutes. The "Tris/GDO/ GMO" SEDDS soft gelatin capsules showed an intermediate release value of 25% at 60 minutes.

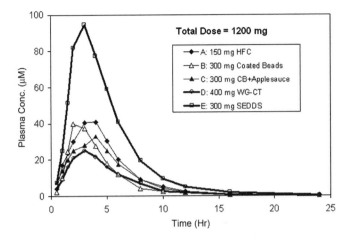

Figure 10 Plasma concentration profiles of Drug X observed from four solid dosage forms of the di-sodium salt of Drug X (150 mg HFC, 300 mg CB, 300 mg CB with applesauce, 400 mg WG-CT) and the 300 mg/g Drug X SEDDS formulation after a single total dose of 1200 mg in fasted human subjects (*n* = 12). *Abbreviations*: CB, coated beads; SEDDS, self-emulsifying drug delivery systems; WG-CT, wet granulation compressed tablet.

The results of the clinical studies with these SEDDS formulations and a total Drug X dose of 1200 mg are shown in Figure 12. The "No Tris" SEDDS soft gelatin capsules showed the lowest AUC and Cmax values among the three SEDDS formulations tested and the AUC was slightly lower than the AUC observed with the hard filled capsule (HFC) containing the di-sodium salt of Drug X. The "Tris/GDO/ GMO" SEDDS soft gelatin capsules showed a two-fold higher C_{max} and AUC as compared to that of the "No Tris" SEDDS soft gelatin capsules formulation. It is worth noting that these two SEDDS formulations differ only in

Table 9 Composition of the Three 300 mg/g Drug X SEDDS Formulations of Drug X Evaluated in the Clinical Study

Ingredients	SEDDS formulation composition (mg/g)		
	"No Tris"	"Tris/GDO/GMO"	"Tris/MCM"
Drug X	300	300	300
Ethanol/PG (1:1, w/w)	175	180	180
Cremophor EL	453	428	428
GDO/GMO (8:2)	70	75	—
Capmul MCM	—	—	75
Tris (tromethamine)	—	15	15
Propyl gallate	2	2	2
Dosage form	Soft gelatin capsules	Soft gelatin capsules	Hard filled capsules (HFC)

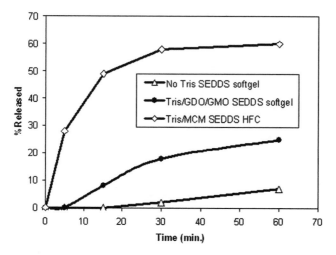

Figure 11 Drug release profiles from three 300 mg/g Drug X SEDDS dosage forms (i.e., "No Tris" softgel, "Tris/GDO/GMO" softgel and "Tris/MCM" HFC. The formulation compositions are reported in Table 9). The test medium was 900 mL SIF (pH 6.5) with a stirring speed of 50 rpm. *Abbreviation*: SEDDS, self-emulsifying drug delivery systems.

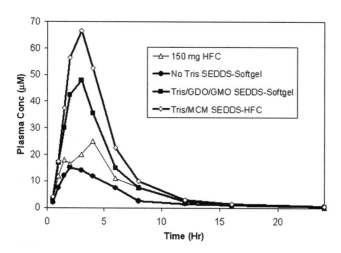

Figure 12 Plasma concentration profiles of Drug X from three 300 mg/g Drug X SEDDS dosage forms (compositions are reported in Table 9) along with the Drug X di-sodium salt powder formulation in a HFC (control) with a single total dose of 1200 mg in fasted human subjects ($n = 15$). *Abbreviation*: SEDDS self-emulsifying drug delivery systems.

the presence of 15 mg/g Tris in the former formulation (Table 9), confirming the critical role of a small amount of amine in the formulation. The highest bioavailability and C_{max} were achieved with the "Tris/MCM" SEDDS HFC formulation.

Preliminary In Vitro–In Vivo Relationship (IVIVR)

The enhanced absorption of Drug X from the Tris containing formulations may be due to the more rapid emulsification and the smaller droplet size upon dilution, as described earlier in this chapter. Although the Tris/GDO/GMO SEDDS and Tris/MCM SEDDS formulations of Drug X are very similar in composition, there is a noticeable difference between the release profiles of these two dosage forms (Fig. 11) as well as the droplet size upon dilution with water. Further investigation revealed that both *liquid* formulations, without the use of the gelatin capsule, showed little difference in emulsification spontaneity and release profile. This suggests that the emulsification spontaneity of the SEDDS formulation is influenced by soft gelatin encapsulation. After encapsulation of the Tris/GDO/GMO SEDDS formulation in soft gelatin capsules, there was a substantial reduction of the solvent levels (EtOHand PG) in the fill due to solvent migration into the shell and ethanol evaporation during the drying process. In contrast, there was very little loss of the solvent when the Tris/MCM SEDDS formulation was filled into hard gelatin capsules with appropriate packaging and storage conditions. These findings suggest that the reduction of the solvent level (both EtOH and PG) in the fill solution associated with soft gelatin capsules manufacturing process inevitably affects the drug release profile. This is an important factor that should be taken into consideration during formulation design and optimization.

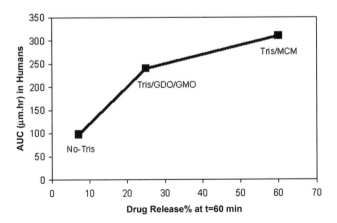

Figure 13 In vivo AUC values obtained from the clinical trial results (shown in Fig. 12) are plotted against the in vitro percentage of drug release using three 300 mg/g Drug X SEDDS formulations at $t = 60$ minutes (in vitro release profiles shown in Fig. 11). *Abbreviation*: SEDDS, self-emulsifying drug delivery systems.

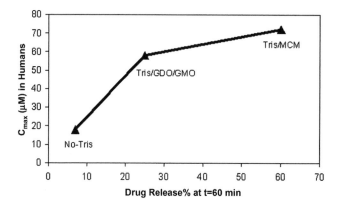

Figure 14   In vivo C_{max} values obtained from the clinical trial results (shown in Fig. 12) plotted against the in vitro percentage of drug release using three 300 mg/g Drug X SEDDS formulations at $t = 60$ minutes (in vitro release profiles shown in Fig. 11). *Abbreviation*: SEDDS, self-emulsifying drug delivery systems.

Figures 13 and 14 show the IVIVR plots of the mean in vivo AUC and C_{max} values with the three SEDDS dosage forms of Drug X observed in the clinical trial against the percent of drug released at 60 minutes in the in vitro test. A rank order correlation was observed between the in vitro release and the oral exposure of Drug X among the three SEDDS dosage forms. In addition, there is a rank order correlation between the bioavailability data and the population of large droplets (>1 μm) formed upon dispersion in vitro. The in vitro dispersibility test showed that the "Tris/MCM" SEDDS HFC yielded the smallest amount (~2.3%) of large droplets (>1 μm) while the "No Tris" SEDDS soft gelatin capsules showed the highest amount (~70%). The "Tris/GDO/GMO" SEDDS soft gelatin capsules had an intermediate amount of large droplets (~12%, >1 μm). These results concur with the Drug X bioavailability results in rats and dogs, as discussed above.

The IVIVR observed in the clinical trial is in agreement with previously described nonclinical studies in which drug absorption was correlated directly with in vitro emulsification spontaneity and inversely with droplet size formed upon dilution in water. These combined results suggest that the in vitro release test method described herein may be a useful tool in the development, optimization and evaluation of SEDDS formulations.

POSSIBLE MECHANISM FOR ENHANCED PRESENTATION OF DRUGS TO THE INTESTINAL ENTEROCYTE BRUSH BORDER WITH SEDDS FORMULATIONS

The enhanced oral bioavailability observed with SEDDS formulations of poorly soluble lipophilic drugs as compared to the bioavailability of a simple aqueous suspension or the bulk drug in a capsule indicates that SEDDS formulations present the drug more efficiently to the intestinal enterocyte brush border. This section suggests that the enhanced oral bioavailability seen with the SEDDS formulations might be due to improved presentation of the poorly soluble drug to the enterocyte brush border membrane.

Drugs with water solubility less than about 1 to 50 μg/mL frequently show incomplete oral absorption. However, there are many other extremely insoluble, highly lipophilic compounds that have solubilities orders of magnitude less than 1 to 50 μg/mL and, yet, they are absorbed orally.

The pioneering work of Borgstrom et al. (25–26) and later, Carey et al. (27–29), as well as many others (30–61) contributed to the finding that the bile acid mixed micelle (BAMM) in the fed state and the bile acid (BA) micelle in the fasted state constitute the endogenous surfactant system that is responsible for the delivery or presentation of extremely lipophilic drugs to the enterocyte brush border region.

Cholesterol with a ClogP of 12 and a water solubility of ~10 ng/mL is efficiently absorbed from the intestine by presentation of cholesterol dissolved in the BAMM droplets to the enterocyte brush border mucosa with subsequent collisional transfer to the glycocalyx (25–30). Many other extremely insoluble and lipophilic compounds are absorbed more efficiently in the fed state where the BAMM is present. The BAMM system is more effective that the BA system because of the higher micellar concentration in the fed as compared to the fasted state.

Lipophilic drugs can partition into the BA/BAMM system (61–64) and predictive relationships have been reported (64).

Highly lipophilic compounds can equilibrate between size populations of liposomes by collisional contact while less lipophilic compounds equilibrate between populations of liposomes via the compound that is dissolved in the aqueous medium (73).

Based on the above, it appears that drugs could be delivered to the intestinal enterocyte brush border region by the aqueous diffusional pathway as well as by the BA/BAMM pathway. The delivery of cholesterol from the BAMM to the enterocyte surface occurs via collisonal transfer (50–52,55,56,58–60,67–73,75).

SEDDS formulations generate emulsions (E) or microemulsions (ME) upon contact with water and they can undergo size reduction through a number of phenomena such as the hydrolytic action of the pancreatic or membrane bound enzymes or by the removal of the E/ME components by collisional transfer with other lipophilic or solid materials in the intestine. Thus, drugs or other compounds in the E/ME or the remnant E/ME can either dissolve in the aqueous medium or they can undergo collisional transfer to the enterocyte brush border (24,52–75).

Based on this background, Figure 15 shows a possible scheme for the presentation of poorly soluble lipophilic drugs in SEDDS formulations to the intestinal enterocyte brush border by:

1. the aqueous pathway, or by,
2. equilibrating with the BA/BAMM pathway, or by,
3. mimicking the BA/BAMM pathway.

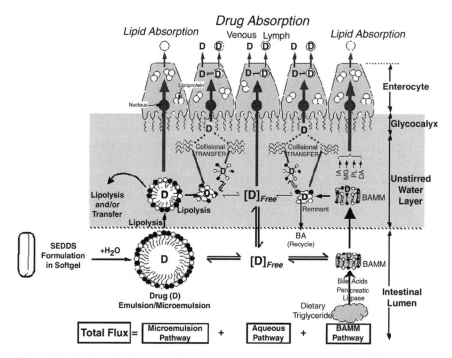

Figure 15 Proposed scheme for the enhanced oral absorption seen with poorly soluble lipophilic drugs in SEDDS formulations. The drug (D) from the SEDDS formulation could be presented to the interstinal enterocyte brush border region by either simulating or equilibrating with the BAMM pathway with collisional transfer to the brush border or by the aqueous diffusional pathway. *Abbreviation*: SEDDS, self-emulsifying drug delivery systems.

After absorption into the enterocyte, the drug could diffuse across the enterocyte or, if the drug is highly lipophilic, the drug could partition into the chylomicrons in the fed state with subsequent transfer to the lymphatics and ultimately to the systemic venous circulation (3,6,65,66). Moderately lipophilic drugs could escape from the chylomicrons by partitioning or collisional transfer with entry into the venous system.

The implication from the above proposal is that the selection of the excipients in the SEDDS formulation could have a profound effect on oral bioavailability by affecting the delivery of the drug to the enterocyte brush border or by affecting the transport across the enterocyte. Lipophilic drugs such as cyclosporin in the emulsion generating Sandimmune® formulation show a strong food effect with enhanced absorption in the fed state whereas the microemulsion-generating formulation, Neoral®, shows virtually no food effect. This is attributed to the use of glycerol mono-/di-oleate (Maisine®) in the Neoral® formulation (8,18) and it is likely that this microemulsion or a remnant of this, delivers cyclosporin efficiently to the enterocyte brush border and, in effect, this mimics the BAMM system. It is difficult to predict the effect of lipid excipients in SEDDS formulations on oral bioavailability and, therefore, the selection (and optimization) of the key ingredients (e.g., lipid and surfactant) in the SEDDS formulations must be guided by in vivo evaluation in animals and humans.

CONCLUSIONS

1. SEDDS formulations are useful in enhancing the oral bioavailability of poorly soluble drugs. The highly lipophilic drug PNU-74006 (Log p = 5.8) and Drug X (Log P ~ 7) show a substantial increase in oral bioavailability by use of appropriately designed SEDDS formulations. The clinical evaluation of the a high drug load (300 mg/g) Drug X SEDDS formulations revealed significantly enhanced oral bioavailability relative to the solid dosage forms.
2. The in vitro test methods demonstrated with the Drug X SEDDS formulations are useful in guiding the development of the SEDDS formulations. The emulsification spontaneity, the resulting droplet size, and the extent of drug solubilization in the aqueous medium are key attributes that are critical in achieving optimal oral exposure. Generation of microemulsion from the 300 mg/g Drug X SEDDS formulation upon in vitro dilution is proven to be crucial in improving the oral absorption of Drug X in animals and humans. An agreement between the in vivo oral bioavailability of Drug X from the SEDDS formulation and the percentage of drug release at 60 minutes is observed.
3. The enhanced oral absorption of poorly soluble drugs with the SEDDS formulation approach is presumably due to more efficient presentation of rug to the enterocyte brush border region by:

    a. Equilibration of the drug with the aqueous medium and subsequent enterocyte uptake by the aqueous diffusional pathway or, alternatively.
    b. Simulating or equilibrating with the BAMM system with transfer by collisional contact with the brush border glycocalyx.

ACKNOWLEDGMENTS

Sincere appreciation is extended to J. W. Skoug, P. R. Nixon, M. J. Hageman, F. J. Schwende, B. R. Rush, S. R. Davio, M. Borin, J. Ferry, S. Turner, J. T. Baldwin, R. J. Haskell, T. J. Raub, M. Antman, J. R. Shifflett, J. B. Berimach, K. M. Zamora, J. M. Bauer, T. Huang, S. Douglas, M. M. McGlinchy, M. Murphy, and J. Chen for collaboration in conducting the case studies reviewed herein and for many valuable discussions on formulation excipients and the mechanism of drug absorption.

REFERENCES

1. Bagwe RP, Kanicky JR, Palla BJ, Patanjali PK, Shah DO. Improved drug delivery using microemulsions: rationale, recent progress, and new horizons. Critical Rev in Therap Drug Carrier Syst 2001; 18(1):77–140.
2. Charman CH. Lipids, lipophilic drugs and oral drug delivery—some emerging concepts. J Pharm Sci 2000; 89:967–978.
3. Humberstone AJ, Charman WN. Lipid-based vehicles for oral delivery of poorly soluble drugs. Adv Drug Deliv Rev 1997; 25:103–128.
4. Pouton CW. Lipid formulations for oral administration of drugs: non-emulsifying, self-emulsifying and 'self-microemulsifying' drug delivery systems. Eur J Pharm Sci. 2000; 11(suppl 2)S93–S98.
5. Pouton CW. Formulations of self-emulsifying drug delivery systems. Adv Drug Dele Rev 1997; 25:47–48.
6. Hause D. Lipid based systems for oral drug delivery: enhancing the bioavailability of poorly soluble drugs. Am Pharm Rev 2002; Nov/Dec:22–26.
7. Vonderscher J, Meinzer A. Rationale for the development of sandimmune neoral. Transplant Proc 1994; 26(5):2925–2927.
8. Meinzer A, Mueller E, Vonderscher J. Microemulsion—a suitable galenical approach for the absorption enhancement of low soluble compounds? B T Gattefosse 1995; N88:21–27.
9. Pouton CW. Self-emulsifying drug delivery systems: assessment of the efficiency of emulsification. Int J Pharm 1996; 27:335–348.
10. Gao ZG, Choi HG, Shin HJ. Physicochemical characterization and evaluation of a microemulsion system for oral delivery of cyclosporin A. Int J Pharm 1998; 161: 75–86.
11. Devani M, Ashford M, Craig DQM. The emulsification and solubilization properties of polyglycolyzed oils in self-emulsifying formulations. J Pharm Pharmacol 2004; 56(3):307–316.
12. Nazzal S, Smalyukh II, Lavrentovich DO, Khan MA. Preparation and in vitro characterization of an eutectic based semisolid self-nanoemulsified drug delivery system (SNEDDS) of ubiquinone: mechanism and progress of emulsion formation. Int J Pharm 2002; 235:247–265.
13. Shah NH, Carvajal MT, Patel CI, Infeld MH, Malick AW. Self-emulsifying drug delivery systems (SEDDS) with polyglycolyzed glycerides for improving in vitro dissolution and oral absorption of lipophilic drugs. I J Pharm 1994; 106:15–23.
14. Porter CJH, Charman WN. In vitro assessment of oral lipid based formulations. Adv Drug Del Rev 2001; 50:S127–S147.
15. Wasan KM. Formulations and physiological and biopharmaceutical issues in the development of oral lipid-based drug delivery systems. Drug Devel Ind Pharm 2001; 27(4):267–276.
16. MacGregor KJ, Embleton JK, Lacy JE, Perry EA, Solomon LJ, Seager H, Pouton CW. Influence of lipolysis on drug absorption from the gastro-intestinal tract. Adv Drug Deliv Rev 1997; 25:33–46.
17. Odeberg JM, Kaufmann P, Kroon KG, Hoglund P. Lipid drug delivery and rational formulation design for liphilic drugs with low oral bioavailability, applied to cyclosporine. Europ J Pharm Sci 2003; 20:375–382.
18. UK Patent GB 2257359 B Cyclosporin compositions for oral administration.

19. Armand M, Borel P, Ythier P, et al. Effects of droplet size, triacylglycerol composition, and calcium on the hydrolysis of complex emulsions by pancreatic lipase: an in vitro study. J Nutri Biochem 1992; 3(7):333–341.

20. Pouton CW, Charman WN. The potential of oily formulations for drug delivery to the gastro-intestinal tract. Adv Drug Deliv Rev 1997; 25:1–2.

21. O'Driscoll CM. Lipid-based formulations for intestinal lymphatic delivery. Europ J Pharm Sci 2002; 15:405–415.

22. Bach A, Babayan VM. Medium chain triglycerides: an update. Am J Clin Nutr 1982; 36:950–962.

23. Bachynsky MO, Shah NH, Patel CI, Malick AW. Factors affecting the efficiency of a self-emulsifying oral delivery system. Drug Dev Ind Pharm 1997; 23(8): 809–816.

24. Corsico B, Cistola DP, Frieden C, Storch J. The helical domain of intestinal fatty acid binding protein is critical for collisional transfer of fatty acids to phospholipid membranes. Proc Natl Acad Sci USA 1998; 95:12174–12178.

25. Börgstrom B, Dahlquist A, Lundh G, Sjövall J. Studies of intestinal digestion and absorption in the human. J Clin Invest 1957; 36:1521–1529.

26. Borgström B, Patton JS. Luminal events in gastrointestinal lipid digestion. In: Schultz SG, ed. Handbook of Physiology Section 6. The Gastrointestinal System IV, Bethesda: American Physiological Society, 1991:475–504.

27. Staggers JE, Hernell O, Stafford RJ, Carey MC. Physical–chemical behavior of dietary and biliary lipids during intestinal digestion and absorption. 1. Phase behavior and aggregation states of model lipid systems patterned after aqueous duodenal contents of healthy adult human beings. Biochemistry 1990; 29: 2028–2040.

28. Hernell O, Staggers JE, Carey MC. Physical–chemical behavior of dietary and biliary lipids during intestinal digestion and absorption. 2. Phase analysis and aggregation states of luminal lipids during duodenal fat digestion in healthy adult human beings. Biochemistry 1990; 29:2041–2056.

29. Carey MC, Small DM. The characteristics of mixed micellar solutions with particular reference to bile. Am J Med 1970; 49:590–598.

30. Hofmann AF, Borgström B. The intraluminal phase of fat digestion in man: the lipid content of the micellar and oil phases of intestinal content obtained during fat digestion and absorption. J Clin Invest 1964; 43:247–257.

31. Mattson FH, Volpenhein RA. The digestion and absorption of triglycerides. J Biol Chem 1964; 239:2772–2777.

32. Simmonds WJ, Hofmann AF, Theodor E. Absorption of cholesterol from a micellar solution: intestinal perfusion studies in man. J Clin Invest 1967; 874–890.

33. Wilson FA, Dietschy JM. Characterization of bile acid absorption across the unstirred water layer and brush border of the rat jejunum. J Clin Invest 1972; 51(12):3015–3025.

34. Mattson FH, Nolen GA. Absorbability by rats of compounds containing one to eight ester groups. J Nutr 1972; 102:1171–1176.

35. Groves MJ, Mustafa RMA. Measurement of the "spontaneity" of self-emulsifiable oils. J Phar Pharmacol 1974; 26:671–681.

36. Mansbach CM, Cohen RS, Leff PB. Isolation and properties of the mixed lipid micelles present in intestinal content during fat digestion in man. J Clin Invest 1975; 56:781–791.

37. Westergaard H, Dietschy JM. The mechanism whereby bile acid micelles increase the rate of fatty acid and cholesterol uptake into the intestinal mucosal cell. J Clin Invest 1976; 58:97–108.
38. Ho NFH, Park JY, Morozowich W, Higuchi WI. In: Roche EB ed. Design of Biopharmaceutical Properties Through Prodrugs and Analogs. Washington: APHA, 1977:35–75
39. Montet C, Reynier MO, Montet AM, Gerolami A. Distinct effects of three bile salts on cholesterol solubilization by oleate–monoolein–bile salt micelles. Biochim Biophys Acta 1979; 575(2):289–294.
40. Shiau YF, Levine GM. pH dependence of micellar diffusion and dissociation. Am J Physiol 1980; 239:G177–G182.
41. Higuchi WI, Ho NFH, Park JY, Komiya I. Rate-limiting steps and factors in drug absorption. In: Prescott LF, Nimmo WS, eds. Drug Absorption. Edinburgh: MTP Press, 1981:35–90.
42. Thomson ABR, O'Brien BD. Uptake of cholesterol into rabbit jejunum using three in vitro techniques: importance of bile acid micelles and unstirred layer resistance. Am J Physiol 1981; 241:G270–G274.
43. Iranloye TA, Pilpel N, Groves MJ. Some factors affecting the droplet size and charge of dilute oil-in-water emulsions prepared by self-emulsification. J Disp Sci Tech 1983; 4(2):109–121.
44. Shiau YF. Lipid digestion and absorption. In: Johnson LR, ed. Physiology of the Gastrointestinal Tract. 2nd ed. New York: Raven Press, 1987:1527–1556.
45. Reynier MO, Crotte C, Montet JC, Sauve P, Gerolami A. Intestinal cholesterol and oleic acid uptake from solutions supersaturated with lipids. Lipids 1987; 22(1), 28–32.
46. Poelma FGJ, Tukker JJ, Crommelin DJA. Intestinal absorption of drugs. I. The influence of taurocholate on the absorption of dantrolene in the small intestine of the rat. J Pharm Sci 1989; 78:285–289.
47. Thurnhofer H, Hauser H. Uptake of cholesterol by small intestinal brush border membrane is protein-mediated. Biochemistry 1990; 29:2142–2148.
48. Poelma FG, Breas R, Tukker JJ, Crommelin DJ. Intestinal absorption of drugs. The influence of mixed micelles on the disappearance kinetics of drugs from the small intestine of the rat. J Pharm Pharmacol 1991; 43(5):317–24.
49. Small DM. The effects of glyceride structure on absorption and metabolism. Annu Rev Nutr 1991; 11:413–434.
50. Thurnhofer H, Schnabel J, Betz M, Lipka G, Pidgeon C, Hauser H. Cholesterol-transfer protein located in the intestinal brush border membrane. Partial purification and characterization. Biochim Biophys Acta 1991; 1064:275–286.
51. Lipka G, Imfeld D, Schulthess G, Thurnhofer H, Hauser H. Protein mediated cholesterol absorption by small intestinal brush border membranes. In: Structural and Dynamic Properties of Lipids and Membranes. London, UK: Portland Press, 1992:7–18.
52. Thomson ABR, Schoeller C, Keelan M, Smith L, Clandinin MT. Lipid absorption: passing through the unstirred layers, brush-border membrane, and beyond. Can J Physiol Parmacol 1993; 71:531–555.
53. Tso P. Intestinal lipid absorption. In: Johnson LR, ed. Physiology of the Gastrointestinal Tract. 3rd ed. New York: Raven Press, 1994:1867–1907.
54. Schoeller SC, Keelan M, Mulvey G, Stremmel W, Thomson ABR. Oleic acid uptake into rat and rabbit jejunal brush border membranes. Biochim Biophys Acta 1995; 1236:51–64.

55. Narayanan VS, Storch J. Fatty acid transfer in taurodeoxycholate mixed micelles. Biochemistry 1996; 35:7466–7473.
56. Dawson A, Rudel LL. Intestinal cholesterol absorption. Curr Opin Lipidol 1999; 10:315–320.
57. Bosner SM, Lange LG, Stenson WF, Ostlund RE. Percent cholesterol absorption in normal women and men quantified with dual stable isotopic tracers and negative ion mass spectrometry. J Lipid Res 1999; 40:302–308.
58. Wang DQH. New concepts of mechanism of intestinal cholesterol absorption. Ann Hepatol 2003; 2(3):113–121.
59. Kramer W, Girbig F, Corsiero D, et al. Intestinal cholesterol absorption: identification of different binding proteins for cholesterol and cholesterol absorption inhibitors in the enterocyte brush border membrane. Biochim Biophys Acta 2003; 1633(1):13–26.
60. Mel'nikov SM, Seijen T, Hoorn JW, Eijkelenboom AP. Effect of phytosterols and phytostanols on the solubilization of cholesterol by dietary mixed micelles: an in vitro study. Chem Phys Lipids 2004; 127(2):121–141.
61. Wiedmann TS, Liang W, Kamel L. Solubilization of drugs by physiological mixtures of bile salts. Pharm Res 2002; 19(8):1203–1208.
62. Bakatselou V, Oppenheim RC, Dressman JB. Solubilization and wetting effects of bile salts on the dissolution of steroids. Pharm Res 1991; 8(12):1461–1469.
63. TenHoor CN, Bakatselou V, Dressman JB. Solubility of mefenamic acid under simulated fed- and fasted-state conditions. Pharm Res 1991; 8(9):1203–1205.
64. Mithani SD, Bakatselou V, TenHoor CN, Dressman JB. Estimation of the increase in solubility of drugs as a function of bile salt concentration. Pharm Res 1996; 13(1):163–167.
65. Constantinides PP, Scalart JP. Formulation and physical characterization of water-in-oil microemulsions containing long- versus medium-chain glycerides. Int J Pharm 1997; 158:57–68.
66. Hauss DJ, Fogal SE, Ficorilli JV, et al. Lipid-based delivery systems for improving the bioavailability and lymphatic transport of a poorly water-soluble LTB4 inhibitor. J Pharm Sci 1998; 87:164–169.
67. Cho MJ, Chen FJ, Huczek DL. Effects of inclusion complexation on the transepithelial transport of a lipophilic substance in vitro. Pharm Res 1995; 12(4):560–564.
68. Ho SY, Storch J. Common mechanisms of monoacylglycerol and fatty acid uptake by human intestinal Caco-2 cells. Amer J Physio 2001; 281(4 Pt 1): C1106–C1117.
69. Schulthess G, Lipka G, Compassi S, et al. Absorption of monoacylglycerols by small intestinal brush border membrane. Biochemistry 1994; 33(15):4500–4508.
70. Hsu KT, Storch J. Fatty acid transfer from liver and intestinal fatty acid-binding proteins to membranes occurs by different mechanisms. J Biol Chem 1996; 271(23):13317–13323.
71. Trotter PJ, Ho SY, Storch J. Fatty acid uptake by Caco-2 human intestinal cells. J Lipid Res 1996; 37(2):336–46.
72. Ho SY, Delgado L, Storch J. Monoacylglycerol metabolism in human intestinal Caco-2 cells: evidence for metabolic compartmentation and hydrolysis. J Biol Chem 2002; 277(3):1816–1823.
73. Storch J, Kleinfeld AM. Transfer of long chain fluorescent free fatty acids between unilamellar vesicles. Biochemistry 1986; 25(7):1717–1726.

74. Dressman JB, Reppas C. In vitro–in vivo correlations for lipophilic poorly water soluble drugs. Europ J Pharm Sci 1986; 11(suppl 2):S73–S80.
75. Austgen L, Bowen RA, Rouge M. Pathophysiology of the Digestive System. Colorado State University, http://arbl.cvmbs.colostate.edu/hbooks/contrib.html (2004). See statement: "As the ingesta is mixed, the bile salt mixed micelles *bump* into the brush border and the lipids, including monoglyceride and fatty acids, are absorbed."

13

Design and Development of Supersaturatable Self-Emulsifying Drug Delivery Systems for Enhancing the Gastrointestinal Absorption of Poorly Soluble Drugs

Ping Gao

Small Molecule Pharmaceutics, Amgen, Inc., Thousand Oaks, California, U.S.A.

Walter Morozowich

Prodrug/Formulation Consultant, Kalamazoo, Michigan, U.S.A.

INTRODUCTION

Background on Conventional Self-Emulsifying Drug Delivery Systems and the Supersaturatable Formulations

Low water solubility is widely recognized as the main reason for the poor oral absorption of many new chemical entities. Conventional solubilization approaches such as salt formation, cosolvents and, more recently, surfactant-based micellar systems, are now widely employed in enhancing the oral absorption of drugs, primarily poorly soluble drugs. In particular, self-emulsifying drug delivery systems (SEDDS) are commonly employed in improving the oral exposure of poorly soluble, lipophilic drugs (1–5). However, a high surfactant level is needed in the conventional SEDDS formulations in order to prevent precipitation of the drug on dilution with water in the gastrointestinal (GI) tract. The surfactants that are commonly employed in SEDDS formulations can increase the incidence of

GI side-effects (6,7) and, therefore, a reduced amount of surfactant in the formulations should minimize the surfactant-induced GI side-effects (8–10).

The potential of increasing the thermodynamic activity of drug formulations and, thereby, increasing the bioavailability of poorly soluble drugs through supersaturation was recognized by Higuchi more than four decades ago (11). Since then, a number of publications have appeared in the literature employing supersaturated formulations as a means of enhancing bioavailability. While most work on supersaturation reported in the literature has been devoted to topical delivery (11–22), less attention has been focused on the use of supersaturation for improving oral delivery of poorly soluble drugs (23–29).

Polyvinylpyrrolidone (PVP) was found useful in generating a supersaturated state with a number of poorly soluble drugs (12–16,23,24,30). Other studies reported the use of the water soluble cellulosic polymers such as HPMC (17–20,22,25,26,31), methylcellulose (20), hydroxypropyl methylcellulose phthalate (28,29), and sodium carboxymethylcellulose (32). The cellulosic polymers are excellent crystal growth inhibitors and they are effective in maintaining the supersaturated state of the drugs (16,18,31,32).

One of the most promising approaches for enhancing the oral bioavailability of poorly soluble drugs is the use of the principle of supersaturation in the development of supersaturatable formulations (33,34). It should be clearly recognized that *supersaturatable* formulations differ from supersaturated formulations. Supersaturated formulations are not thermodynamically stable and drugs in supersaturated formulations can crystallize on storage. Therefore, the physical stability of such formulations is fundamentally challenging and this limits their practical utility. In contrast, supersaturatable formulations are thermodynamically stable dosage forms; they yield a supersaturated state only after administration in vivo.

Development of Supersaturatable Self-Emulsifying Drug Delivery Systems

To take advantage of supersaturation, the generation and maintenance of a supersaturated system in vivo from supersaturatable dosage forms is a prerequisite. In our studies, we found that reducing the amount of surfactant in a SEDDS formulation in order to generate a supersaturated state on dilution of the formulation with an aqueous medium can result in rapid precipitation of the poorly soluble drug. However, we found that incorporation of hydroxypropyl methyl cellulose (HPMC) or other cellulosic polymeric excipients in the SEDDS formulations can sustain the supersaturated state by preventing precipitation of the drug. These formulations are termed supersaturatable SEDDS or S-SEDDS formulations.

This chapter describes the development of supersaturatable S-SEDDS formulations using three poorly soluble drugs, namely, PNU-91325, paclitaxel, and Drug X along with the behavior of these S-SEDDS formulations in an in vitro dissolution/precipitation test. These studies show that the S-SEDDS formulations containing a reduced amount of surfactant along with a supersaturation promoting polymer can generate a supersaturated drug solution on contact with water and the resulting supersaturated state can be maintained sufficiently long to achieve enhanced absorption. These S-SEDDS formulations of poorly soluble drugs have the potential of improving the tox/safety profile of the product due to a reduced amount of surfactant and they can show higher oral bioavailability as compared with the corresponding conventional SEDDS formulation of the same drug. The studies described below clearly demonstrate that the supersaturatable S-SEDDS formulation approach is a powerful approach for improving the oral absorption of poorly soluble, lipophilic drugs.

TESTS FOR IN VITRO EVALUATION OF THE SUPERSATURATABLE FORMULATIONS

Prompted by the biorelevant dissolution system reported by Tang et al. (35), we developed a small-scale in vitro *dissolution/precipitation test* for evaluating the S-SEDDS formulations and the related formulations of our poorly soluble drugs. The biorelevant in vitro dissolution/precipitation test method employed herein consists of a simulated gastric fluid (SGF) containing 0.01 M HCl and 0.15 M NaCl (pH 2.0) stirred at 50 revolutions per minute (rpm) at 37°C with the use of a VanKel 7010 dissolution apparatus. The total volume of the medium chosen was 50 to 100 mL which is the approximate combined volume of the residual stomach fluid (~20–50 mL) and the amount of water (~30–60 mL) coadministered commonly during dosing in the fasted dog or human. No surfactants were added in the test medium to improve the solubility of the drug and, therefore, the composition and the limited volume of the test medium provide nonsink conditions for the poorly soluble drugs under investigation.

A unit dose of the S-SEDDS formulation or related formulation was placed in the aforementioned test medium and samples were withdrawn from the test medium as a function of time followed by filtration (0.8 μm) and determination of the total drug concentration in solution by assaying with high-performance liquid chromatography (HPLC). The apparent solution concentration of drug thus obtained is a measure of the total concentration of the drug in the filtrate present in various states (i.e., emulsion, solid particle less than 0.8 μm, and free drug) in the test medium (33,34).

The aforementioned in vitro dissolution/precipitation test and the resulting apparent drug concentration versus time plots were employed in guiding the development of the S-SEDDS formulations as illustrated with the three case studies described below. This simple in vitro dissolution/precipitation test was valuable in formulation screening and optimization as well as in developing in vitro/in vivo relationships (IVIVR).

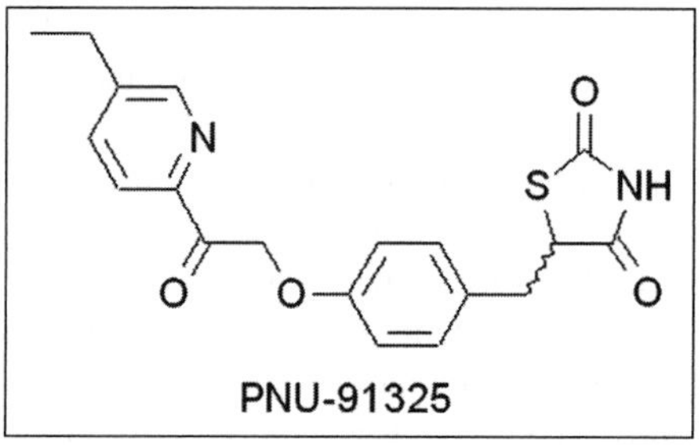

Figure 1 Stucture of PNU-91325.

CASE STUDY WITH PNU-91325

Physicochemical Properties of PNU-91325

PNU-91325 (Fig. 1) is an insulin-enhancing agent that is poorly water soluble with a CLog P of 2.8 (33). The aqueous solubility of the PNU-91325 shows a U-shaped pH-solubility profile with pKa_1 (base) = 2.61 ± 0.04 and pKa_2 (acid) = 6.85 ± 0.06 and an intrinsic solubility, S_0, of 3 μg/mL. The solubility of PNU-91325 is essentially constant at approximately 3 μg/mL within the physiological pH range of 3 to 6.

In Vitro Dissolution/Precipitation Test with Four Formulations of PNU-91325

PEG400 Formulation

PNU-91325 (25 mg/g) was dissolved in PEG400 and this formulation is referred to as the PEG400 formulation (Table 1). This formulation was filled into a hard

Table 1 Composition of the PNU-91325 Formulations

Ingredients	Tween 80 (mg)	PEG400 (mg)	S-SEDDS (mg)	Propylene glycol + 2% HPMC (S-cosolvent) (mg)
PNU-91325	25	25	40	25
PEG400		975	90	
Propylene glycol				860
Water			80	95
HPMC (grade)			200 (E50LV)	20 (E5LV)
Tween 80	975			
Cremophor EL (EL)			300	
Dimethylacetamide			50	
Pluronic-L44			180	
Glyceryl dioleate/ glyceryl monooleate (8:2, w/w)			60	
Total	1000 mg/g	1000 mg/g	1000 mg/g	1000 mg/g

Abbreviation: S-SEDDS, supersaturatable self-emulsifying drug delivery systems.

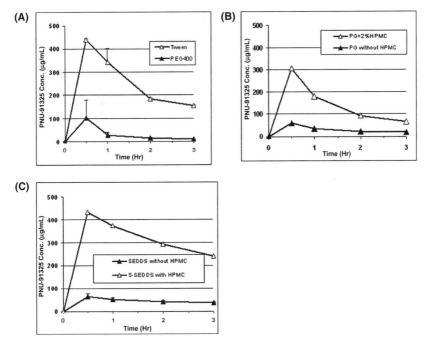

Figure 2 Apparent concentration-time profiles of PNU-91325 observed in the in vitro dissolution/precipitation test using formulations with or without HPMC.

gelatin capsule just before the in vitro dissolution test. The PEG400 formulation was readily miscible with water upon opening of the gelatin capsule in the dissolution medium (0.01 M HCl) and immediate precipitation of the drug was visually apparent as evidenced by an increase in the solution turbidity. The apparent concentration of PNU-91325 in the test medium was determined as a function of time and the data are plotted in Figure 2A. Based on the dilution factor (50X), the theoretical concentration of PNU-91325 was 0.5 mg/mL if the complete drug is dissolved. The observed apparent concentration of PNU-91325 was approximately 0.10 mg/mL at $t = 0.5$ hours (the first sampling time) and this decreased rapidly to about 0.02 mg/mL at $t = 1$ hour as a result of drug precipitation.

Propylene Glycol + 2% HPMC Formulation

A supersaturatable cosolvent (S-cosolvent) formulation was prepared by dissolving 25 mg/g of PNU-91325 in propylene glycol (PG) with 20 mg/g (2%, w/w) of HPMC suspended in the solution (Table 1). This formulation of PNU-91325, referred to as the PG + 2% HPMC formulation, showed a unique concentration versus time plot in the in vitro dissolution/precipitation test (Fig. 2B) with a peak in the PNU-91325 concentration at 0.3 mg/mL observed at $t = 0.5$ hours (the first time point) and the concentration gradually decreased to about 0.06 mg/mL at

$t = 3$ hours. The drug concentrations were much higher in this case as compared with those observed before with the PEG400 formulation during the three-hour time course (Fig. 2A).

To determine the effect of 2% HPMC on drug precipitation, a PG formulation was prepared identical to the previous formulation but without HPMC and this was evaluated in the in vitro dissolution/precipitation test. Without HPMC, the PNU-91325 concentrations were very low as shown in Figure 2B, and these were similar to those observed with the PEG400 formulation (Fig. 2A). This was anticipated because both the PEG400 and the PG formulations are simple cosolvent formulations and they did not contain supersaturation-promoting polymers. The higher drug concentration in the in vitro dissolution/precipitation test with the PG + 2% HPMC formulation clearly indicates that a small amount of HPMC is remarkably effective in generating and maintaining a high solution concentration with PNU-91325 by retarding drug precipitation.

Tween 80 Formulation

A formulation of PNU-91325, 25 mg/g, was prepared by dissolving the drug in neat Tween 80 (polysorbate 80) (Table 1). The PNU-91325 concentration versus time profile observed in the in vitro dissolution/precipitation test (Fig. 2A) was approximately 0.43 mg/mL at $t = 0.5$ hours and the concentration of PNU-91325 gradually decreased to approximately 0.16 mg/mL at $t = 3$ hours due to precipitation of the drug. Precipitation of the drug from the neat Tween 80 formulation was slower than precipitation with the PEG400 formulation. This was presumably due to partitioning of the drug into the Tween 80 micelles, thereby reducing the degree of supersaturation.

Supersaturatable Self-Emulsifying Drug Delivery Systems

An S-SEDDS formulation of PNU-91325 was prepared containing cremophor EL as the surfactant along with the additional excipients and containing 20% (200 mg/g) HPMC (Table 1). This S-SEDDS formulation of PNU-91325 was initially predispersed by contact with water (10 mL) using gentle hand shaking for 30 seconds and then, the in vitro dissolution/precipitation test was conducted. The resulting drug concentration–time profile for the PNU-91325 S-SEDDS formulation (Fig. 2C) was similar to that of the Tween 80 formulation (Fig. 2A).

A similar PNU-91325 SEDDS formulation was prepared containing the same excipients but without HPMC. The apparent concentration of PNU-91325 from the SEDDS formulation (without HPMC) (Fig. 2C) was approximately 10-fold lower than the PNU-91325 concentration obtained with the S-SEDDS formulation containing HPMC during the time course of three hours.

In Vivo Evaluation of PNU-91325 Formulations in Dogs

The *mean* plasma concentrations of PNU-91325 in beagle dogs ($n = 4$, crossover) are plotted in Figure 3 as obtained upon oral dosing with the Tween 80

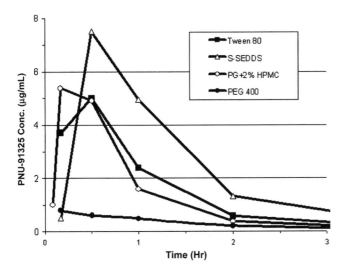

Figure 3 Mean plasma concentration-time profiles of PNU-91325 in dogs (n = 4, crossover) using four PNU-91325 formulations.

formulation, the PEG400 formulation, the S-SEDDS formulation, and the PG + 2% HPMC (S-cosolvent) formulation (Table 1). The mean dose, mean $AUC_{0 - \infty}$, $C_{max,}$ and the estimated absolute bioavailability ($F\%$) observed with each of the formulations are summarized in Table 2. The estimated oral bioavailability ($F\%$) of PNU-91325 in dogs was based on the actual dose of the drug from each of the formulations along with the area under the curve (AUC) observed after oral administration to the dogs and the mean AUC obtained from a separate intravenous study (10 mg/kg) of PNU-91325 (33).

The PEG400 solution formulation showed the lowest absolute bioavailability, namely, 12% (Table 2). As described before, the rapid precipitation of PNU-91325 observed with the PEG400 solution formulation in simulated gastric fluid (SGF) and the generation of large aggregates ($>50\,\mu$m) were due to the high degree of supersaturation. Thus, the low oral bioavailability observed with the PEG400 solution of PNU-91325 is due to the rapid precipitation of the drug in vivo.

As indicated by the in vitro dilution/precipitation tests, the PG + 2% HPMC (S-cosolvent) formulation of PNU-91325 yielded a significantly higher apparent drug concentration (Fig. 2B). This formulation resulted in an approximately sevenfold higher C_{max} (6.04 μg/mL) and fivefold higher oral bioavailability (~60%) as compared with the PEG400 formulation that showed a lower C_{max} (0.88 μg/mL) and a lower oral bioavailability (~12%). These studies clearly demonstrate the key role of supersaturation in enhancing the absorption of PNU-91325 and the utility of HPMC in achieving and stabilizing the supersaturated state.

Table 2 Oral Bioavailability of PNU-91325 Administered to Dogs as Four Different Formulations[a]

Formulation	Mean dose (mg/kg)	Mean C_{max} ± SD (μg/mL)	Mean AUC ± SD (μg hr/mL)	Mean % bioavailability (%F ± SD)
S-SEDDS	15.96	8.19 ± 4.09	9.15 ± 3.17	76 ± 26
PG + 2% HPMC	10.75	6.04 ± 3.53	4.88 ± 1.86	60 ± 23
Tween 80	10.81	5.94 ± 2.20	5.54 ± 0.69	68 ± 8
PEG400	11.82	0.88 ± 0.12	1.03 ± 0.21	12 ± 2

[a]Values are the means ± SD ($n = 4$).
Abbreviations: HPMC, hydroxy propyl methyl cellulose; PG, propylene glycol; SD, standard deviation; S-SEDDS, supersaturatable self-emulsifying drug delivery systems.

The PNU-91325 S-SEDDS formulation showed an oral bioavailability of approximately 76% which is higher than the bioavailability of approximately 68% observed with the Tween 80 formulation (Table 2). The weight ratio of drug:cremophor EL is 1:7.5 in the S-SEDDS formulation while the weight ratio of drug:Tween 80 is 1:39 in the Tween 80 formulation. Clearly, the surfactant level is about fivefold higher in the Tween 80 formulation as compared with that in the S-SEDDS formulation. Thus, it is likely that, on dilution, a lower free drug concentration of PNU-91325 in the test medium occurs with the Tween 80 formulation as compared with that of the S-SEDDS formulation. The S-SEDDS formulation yielded a supersaturated state on dilution as evidenced by the decline in the apparent drug concentration with respect to time (Fig. 2C) and by the observation of crystal formation in the in vitro dissolution/precipitation test medium.

In conclusion, the S-cosolvent and the S-SEDDS formulations containing HPMC generate a supersaturated state with PNU-91325 with higher concentrations in the in vitro dissolution/precipitation test and, as a result, the oral bioavailability is significantly increased as compared with the same SEDDS formulation without HPMC (33).

In Vitro–In Vivo (Dog) Relationship with the PNU-91325 Formulations

The AUC values observed in the dog with each of the four formulations of PNU-91325 were normalized with respect to the dose. The dog AUC/dose ratios observed with each of the four PNU-91325 formulations were obtained over the time interval of 0 to 2 and 0 to 3 hours and the corresponding AUC/dose values were used in developing an IVIVR. The in vitro AUC of each formulation was obtained by integrating the in vitro dissolution/precipitation profile over the 0 to 2- and the 0 to 3-hour time periods (Fig. 2). The corresponding in vivo AUC/dose values for the four formulations examined are plotted against the in vitro AUC values as shown in Figure 4A and 4B.

The current in vitro dissolution/precipitation test method is simple, however, other factors that occur in the GI lumen such as the lipid/surfactant lipolysis or

(A)

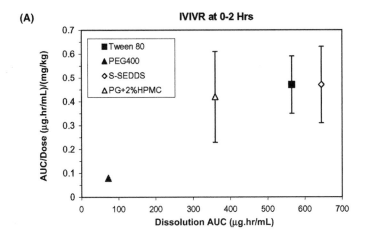

(B)

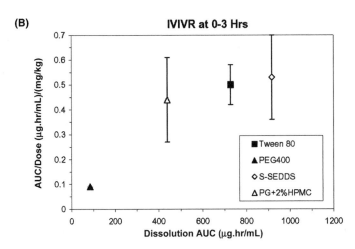

Figure 4 Plot of the oral AUC data in dogs obtained with the four PNU-91325 formulations against the AUC values obtained from the in vitro dissolution/precipitation profiles. Both in vivo and in vitro AUC values are integrated from 0 to 2 hours in Figure 4A (IVIVR at 0–2 hours) and from 0–3 hours in Figure 4B (IVIVR at 0–3 hours).

digestion and the presence of the bile acid or salts are not considered. These factors could affect the oral exposure of lipophilic, poorly soluble drugs as indicated in the literature (4,36,37). The observed IVIVR trend suggests that the enhanced bioavailability of PNU-91325 is related to the supersaturating effects of HPMC as demonstrated in vitro. These results imply that, in this case, the other biological factors encountered in vivo are not critical. Therefore, the IVIVR obtained in this case justifies the use of our simple biorelevant in vitro dissolution/precipitation test method in formulation screening and optimization.

CASE STUDY WITH PACLITAXEL

Properties of Paclitaxel and Marketed Formulations Thereof

Paclitaxel is an antitumor agent that is widely used in the treatment of advanced breast and ovarian cancer. Paclitaxel (Fig. 5) has a molecular weight of 853 and a low solubility in water (<1 μg/mL) as well as a low solubility in common pharmaceutical vehicles (38–40). The currently marketed intravenous (IV) formulation of paclitaxel (Taxol®, Bristol-Meyers Squibb, BMS) contains 6 mg/mL of paclitaxel, 527 mg/mL of cremophor EL (polyoxyethylenated castor oil), and 49.7% (v/v) of dehydrated ethanol (41). IV administration of paclitaxel using this formulation is associated with severe side-effects that are attributed to the surfactant, cremophor EL (39,42–44). The oral bioavailability of paclitaxel using the Taxol® formulation is extremely low (<2%) in rats and in humans (45–48). Coadministration of the Taxol® formulation orally along with cyclosporin A (CsA), an inhibitor of P-gp and CYP3A enzymes, resulted in a sevenfold increase in the plasma AUC value for paclitaxel in humans (45–48).

In Vitro Evaluation of the Supersaturatable Self-Emulsifying Drug Delivery Systems of Paclitaxel

In an effort to examine the applicability of the S-SEDDS technology, paclitaxel was selected as a model drug and prototype S-SEDDS formulations were prepared. The in vitro and in vivo performance of the paclitaxel SEDDS formulations without HPMC and the paclitaxel formulations with HPMC (S-SEDDS) were evaluated and compared with the commercial Taxol® formulation. In addition, the in vivo oral bioavailability of paclitaxel from the S-SEDDS formulation coadministered with CsA was also assessed in rats in order to assess the maximal exposure possible and the potential role of P-gp inhibition when the transporter is exposed to the supersaturated concentrations of paclitaxel.

A prototype S-SEDDS solution formulation containing approximately 60 mg/g of paclitaxel and 5% (w/w) HPMC (formulation A) was prepared with the composition reported in Table 3. The apparent paclitaxel solution concentrations in SGF (e.g., 0.01 M HCl + 0.15 M NaCl, pH 2.0) after dilution of the

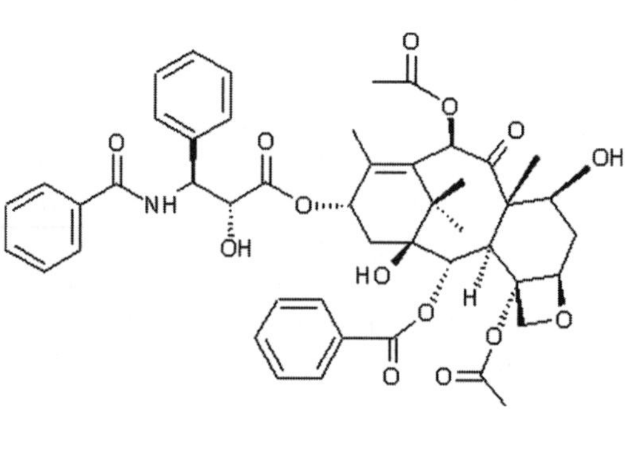

Figure 5   Structure of paclitaxel.

Table 3 Composition of the Paclitaxel Formulations Employed in the Dissolution/Precipitation Test and in the Dog Oral Bioavailability Study

Composition	Formulation A (mg/g)	Formulation B (mg/g)	Formulation C (mg/g)	Formulation D (mg/g)
Brief description	S-SEDDS (with HPMC)	Taxol® (BMS)	SEDDS (without HPMC)	S-SEDDS + cyclosporin A
Paclitaxel	57	6.8	62.5	60
Cyclosporin A	—	—	—	30
Absolute EtOH	151.5	423.2	156.25	150
PEG400	151.5	—	156.25	150
Cremophor EL	400	570	417	400
Glyceryl dioleate	190	—	208	160
HPMC-E5LV	50	—	—	50
Total	1000	1000	1000	1000
In vivo treatment	A	B and E	C	D

Abbreviations: BMS, Bristol-Meyers Squibb; EtOH, ethanol; S-SEDDS, supersaturatable self-emulsifying drug delivery systems.

SEDDS formulation without HPMC (formulation C) and the S-SEDDS formulation with 5% HPMC (formulation A) are shown in Figure 6. The theoretical concentration of paclitaxel in the test medium with these formulations, differing only in the presence or absence of HPMC, was 1.2 mg/mL based on the dilution factor of 50 (i.e., 60 mg paclitaxel in 50 mL).

Immediately on dilution of the SEDDS formulation in the SGF test medium, an opalescent solution characteristic of a microemulsion was formed.

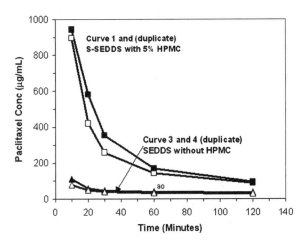

Figure 6 Apparent concentration-time profiles of paclitaxel observed from the in vitro dissolution/precipitation test using the S-SEDDS formulation containing 5% HPMC (curves 1 and 2) and the SEDDS formulation without HPMC (curves 3 and 4).

However, turbidity developed by the first sampling time (10 minutes) and was confirmed to be crystalline paclitaxel. The formation of paclitaxel crystals in the test medium indicates that the system was supersaturated with respect to crystalline paclitaxel. The apparent paclitaxel concentration provided by this formulation was about 0.12 mg/mL at the first sampling point (10 minutes) and this decreased to approximately 0.03 mg/mL at $t = 30$ minutes and afterwards, due to rapid precipitation of the drug. The apparent paclitaxel concentration (~0.03 mg/mL) observed in the test medium from the SEDDS formulation over the two-hour course was close to the equilibrium solubility of the drug in this medium indicating the absence of appreciable supersaturation.

Similarly, the S-SEDDS formulation with HPMC (formulation A) initially showed a transparent, translucent solution, indicating the formation of a microemulsion with a small particle size (presumably <50 nm). The apparent paclitaxel concentration produced by this formulation was high (~0.95 mg/mL) at $t = 10$ minutes (Fig. 6) and this gradually decreased to approximately 0.12 mg/mL over two hours. The fact that the S-SEDDS formulation yielded an apparent solution concentration much higher than the aqueous equilibrium solubility of paclitaxel (~0.030 mg/mL) in the in vitro test medium suggests that this formulation should produce and maintain a supersaturated drug solution in vivo.

These in vitro studies clearly show that the presence of a small amount of HPMC (5%, w/w) in the S-SEDDS formulation is remarkably effective in suppressing precipitation of paclitaxel and in generating a supersaturated state that is maintained for longer than two hours.

Rat Oral Bioavailability of the Supersaturatable Self-Emulsifying Drug Delivery Systems of Paclitaxel

The mean plasma concentration of paclitaxel obtained in rats with the four oral treatment groups (formulation A, S-SEDDS with HPMC; formulation B, Taxol®; formulation C, SEDDS without HPMC; and formulation D, S-SEDDS with HPMC and CsA) are plotted in Figure 7 and the pharmacokinetic parameters corresponding to these treatment groups are summarized in Table 4. The rank order of the mean total exposure as given by the $AUC_{0-\infty}$ for the four formulations is:

S-SEDDS + CSA	> S-SEDDS	>> Taxol®	> SEDDS
(Treatment D)	(Treatment A)	(Treatment ʃB)	(Treatment C)

The difference in the pharmacokinetic profiles exhibited by the SEDDS and S-SEDDS (with HPMC) formulations in Figure 7 is impressive because these two formulations differ only in the content of HPMC (0% vs. 5%), respectively. The SEDDS formulation (without HPMC) showed a very low C_{max} of only 13.1 ng/mL and an oral bioavailability of 0.9% whereas the S-SEDDS formulation (with HPMC) resulted in a 20-fold increase in C_{max} (~277 ng/mL) and an oral bioavailability of 9.5%. The S-SEDDS formulation with CsA and HPMC showed similar absorption kinetics but slower elimination kinetics, resulting in a twofold increase in the oral bioavailability over that of the S-SEDDS formulation with HPMC only. The rat

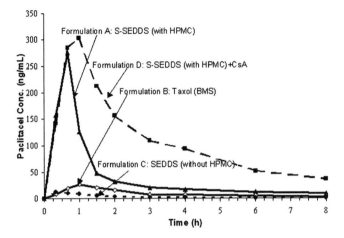

Figure 7 Mean plasma concentration-time profiles of paclitaxel in rats after oral administration using four formulations.

bioavailability results indicate that the higher paclitaxel solution concentration generated by the S-SEDDS formulation in the in vitro dissolution/precipitation test as a result of supersaturation is responsible for the enhanced oral bioavailability of paclitaxel from the S-SEDDS formulation.

Table 4 Pharmacokinetic Parameters for Paclitaxel in Rats Following Intravenous (Dose = 2.5 mg/kg) and Oral Administration (Dose = 10 mg/kg) of Four Different Formulations[a]

	Treatment group				
	A	B	C	D	E
Brief description	S-SEDDS (with HPMC)	Taxol® (BMS)	SEDDS (without HPMC)	S-SEDDS+ cyclosporin A	Taxol® (BMS)
Route of administration			Oral		Intravenous
Target dose (mg/kg)			10		2.5
$AUC_{0-\infty}$ (ng hr/mL)	443 ± 202	94.2 ± 35.1	42.1 ± 54.7	1050 ± 545	1160 ± 230
C_{max} (ng/mL)	277 ± 104	26.3 ± 10.3	13.1 ± 14.2	312 ± 150	n/a
T_{max} (hr)	0.63 ± 0.12	1.02 ± 0.23	0.42 ± 0.15	0.79 ± 0.17	n/a
Bioavailability (%)	9.5	2.0	0.9	22.6	n/a

[a]Values are the means ± SD ($n = 8$) except the intravenous dose ($n = 2$).
Abbreviations: BMS, Bristol-Meyers Squibb; n/a, not available; SD, standard deviation; S-SEDDS, supersaturatable self-emulsifying drusg delivery systems.

The Taxol® formulation (formulation B) generated a microemulsion as evidenced by the formation of a nearly transparent solution on dilution with water and no precipitation of paclitaxel was observed for several days after dilution of the formulation with water. The inhibition of precipitation of the drug on dilution of this formulation with water is due to the high cremophor EL content in the formulation (weight ratio of cremophor EL:paclitaxel = 88:1) and this results in complete solubilization of paclitaxel by the cremophor micelles. However, it is noteworthy that the Taxol® (formulation B, Fig. 7) produced a low mean C_{max} (~30 ng/mL) and a low oral bioavailability (F~2%). The poor oral exposure of paclitaxel from the Taxol® formulation in rats is probably due to the excess cremophor in the formulation and this is consistent with the literature (49,50).

Significance of the Supersaturatable Self-Emulsifying Drug Delivery Systems of Paclitaxel

The failure to provide high oral exposure of paclitaxel with the Taxol® formulation is significant in that the common practice of formulating poorly soluble drugs with high concentrations of surfactants inevitably results in reduction in the free drug concentration and the thermodynamic activity. As revealed in the case of Taxol®, a high content of surfactant in the formulation can prevent drug precipitation but this can also reduce oral bioavailability.

It is well known that micelle solubilization of poorly soluble, lipophilic drugs can result in a low free drug concentration and this can reduce the rate and possibly the extent of absorption (8–10). The work by Poelma et al. (8,9) is especially noteworthy in that the kinetics of the intestinal absorption of griseofulvin in rats was found to be directly related to the concentration of the free griseofulvin in the aqueous solutions containing Tween 80 (8). These workers also showed a reduction in the absorption of griseofulvin from the small intestine of rats in the presence of 10 to 20 mM of taurocholate and they attributed this to micellar solubilization with subsequent reduction in the free drug level (9). Likewise, Amidon et al. (10) recently showed that the presence of surfactants (cremophor EL, RH40, and VE-TPGS with surfactant concentrations at 0.02% w/v or higher) significantly decreased the apparent permeability of CsA in Caco-2 cells and the magnitude of the decrease in permeability (2- to 12-fold) was clearly dependent on the surfactant concentration. Again, the reduction in the apparent permeability of CsA in the presence of surfactants was attributed to the decrease in the free drug content of CsA in the solution as a result of micellar solubilization.

CASE STUDY WITH DRUG X

Physicochemical Properties of Drug X

Drug X was under development for preclinical and clinical evaluation. Drug X has a log P of approximately 3.5, a water solubility of only approximately 5 μg/mL in the physiological pH range of 2 to 7 and it is nonionizable in this pH range. A human oral pharmacokinetic study using Drug X showed slow and incomplete oral absorption using a powder formulation of the bulk drug in a gelatin capsule, whereas rapid and more complete absorption was found with a small particle aqueous suspension of Drug X. These data suggest that the absorption of Drug X is most likely dissolution-rate limited. To improve the rate and the extent of the oral absorption of Drug X, a S-SEDDS formulation containing HPMC along with a reduced amount of a nonionic surfactant was designed and developed for evaluation in the clinic.

In Vitro Evaluation of Supersaturatable Self-Emulsifying Drug Delivery Systems of Drug X and Relevance to Oral Bioavailability

Supersaturatable Self-Emulsifying Drug Delivery Systems Containing Suspended HPMC Powder

The in vitro dissolution/precipitation test was used to evaluate the apparent Drug X concentration profile on dilution of the prototype S-SEDDS formulations with SGF (pH 2.0). Optimizing the effectiveness of HPMC in suppressing the precipitation of Drug X and in prolonging the supersaturated state was the main objective in the development of the S-SEDDS formulation. The in vitro dissolution/precipitation test using 50 mL of SGF fluid (0.01 M HCl + 0.15 M NaCl, pH 2) was employed in evaluating the performance of 1 g of the S-SEDDS formulations containing 200 mg of Drug X filled into two hard gelatin capsules (0.5 g per capsule). Based on a dilution factor of 50, the theoretical concentration of Drug X in the test medium is 4 mg/mL.

The apparent Drug X concentration found with the SEDDS formulation (without HPMC) in the in vitro dissolution/precipitation test is plotted in Figure 8A. The concentration of Drug X in the medium was about 0.3 mg/mL at the first time point (0.5 hours) and this remained unchanged over the six-hour test period. A white precipitate of Drug X was observed with the SEDDS formulation in the dissolution/precipitation test medium at 0.5 hours and the precipitate was found to be crystalline as shown by polarized light microscopy. The formation of drug crystals in the test medium indicates that the solution was supersaturated with respect to the crystalline form of Drug X.

In contrast, a markedly higher concentration of Drug X (~2.7 to 3.5 mg/mL) was observed with the same SEDDS formulation in the in vitro dissolution/precipitation test that contained 12.5 mg (0.025%, w/v) of HPMC dissolved in the 50-mL test medium (Fig. 8A). Comparison of the apparent concentration–time profiles from these two SEDDS formulations shows that the presence of HPMC in the test medium results in a markedly higher apparent concentration of Drug X (~2.7 to 3.5 mg/mL) as compared with that of the test medium without HPMC (Drug X concentration, ~0.3 mg/mL). A supersatuarated state is generated, clearly shown by the fact that the Drug X concentration decreases with time. The presence of HPMC in the S-SEDDS formulation leads to a higher and a more extended time period for the supersaturated state. The presence of HPMC at the remarkably low

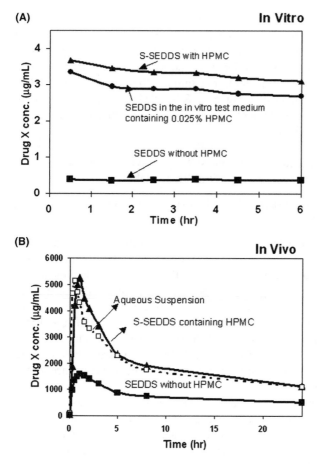

Figure 8 (**A**) Apparent concentration-time profiles of Drug X observed from the in vitro dissolution/precipitation test using the same SEDDS formulation with and without HPMC. All formulations were filled into gelatin hard capsules. (**B**) Mean plasma concentration profiles of Drug X in the dogs (n = 6, crossover) using the two SEDDS formulations with and without HPMC (*solid line*) as compared to an aqueous suspension formulation (*dashed line*).

concentration of only 0.25 mg/mL in the test medium is sufficient to generate and maintain the supersaturated state for at least six hours.

In an attempt to evaluate the effect of HPMC on the bioavailability of Drug X when HPMC is suspended in the SEDDS formulation, the following study was conducted. HPMC powder (44 mg) was suspended in the same SEDDS formulation (1 g) as before and the resulting suspension formulation was filled into hard gelatin capsules for evaluation in the in vitro dissolution/precipitation test under the same conditions. This is referred to as an S-SEDDS formulation. The apparent Drug X concentration observed with this S-SEDDS formulation containing HPMC is plotted versus time in Figure 8A. The resulting concentration of HPMC in the dissolution/precipitation test medium is 0.88 mg/mL assuming that all of the HPMC in the formulation is dissolved. This concentration (0.88 mg/mL) is higher than the HPMC concentration of 0.25 mg/mL that was predissolved in the test medium as discussed before. Little precipitation of Drug X was observed over the six-hour test period and the Drug X concentration was approximately 3 to 3.5 mg/mL which is similar to that in the previous case where the HPMC was predissolved in the SGF medium. The apparent Drug X concentration from the S-SEDDS formulation in the dissolution/precipitation test was about 10-fold higher than the SEDDS formulation without HPMC in the dissolution medium.

The in vivo pharmacokinetics of both the SEDDS and the S-SEDDS formulations of Drug X were evaluated after oral administration in dogs as compared with an aqueous suspension. Figure 8B shows that the mean plasma concentration profile of Drug X obtained after dosing the S-SEDDS formulation (with 4.4% HPMC) is about threefold higher in the C_{max} and the AUC is 2.5-fold larger as compared with that of the same SEDDS formulation without HPMC. This clearly indicates that the S-SEDDS formulation containing HPMC results in an increase in both the rate and the extent of absorption of Drug X. The aqueous suspension and the S-SEDDS formulation showed a similar pharmacokinetics profile in dogs. However, the next section shows that the oral bioavailability of the S-SEDDS formulation of Drug X is greater than that of the aqueous suspension in the human.

Supersaturatable Self-Emulsifying Drug Delivery Systems in a HPMC Capsule

The use of a HPMC capsule was explored as an alternate approach for incorporating HPMC into the S-SEDDS formulation. The same SEDDS liquid fill that was used in the previous studies was filled into HPMC capsules (Size "00" Quali-V capsules, Shionogi; capsule weight ~90 mg) and the capsules were manually sealed with a HPMC solution. The in vitro dissolution/precipitation test was conducted with these HPMC capsules. In this study, the volume of the in vitro dissolution/precipitation test medium was 100 mL rather than the 50 mL employed before.

Three dosage forms were selected for comparison in the in vitro dissolution/precipitation test. The formulations consisted of:

1. the SEDDS liquid formula filled in hard gelatin capsules,
2. the SEDDS liquid formula containing 44 mg of HPMC powder suspended in a hard gelatin capsule and,
3. the SEDDS liquid formula filled into an HPMC capsule.

The SEDDS liquid formula in all three formulations was identical. Figure 9A shows the apparent drug concentrations of Drug X as a function of time obtained with these three dosage forms in the in vitro dissolution/precipitation test. As expected, the SEDDS liquid in the hard gelatin capsule showed a low Drug X concentration of approximately 1 mg/mL initially (15 minutes) in the dissolution test. However, the Drug X solution concentration rapidly decreased to approximately 0.2 mg/mL within 30 minutes and the concentration remained unchanged. In con-

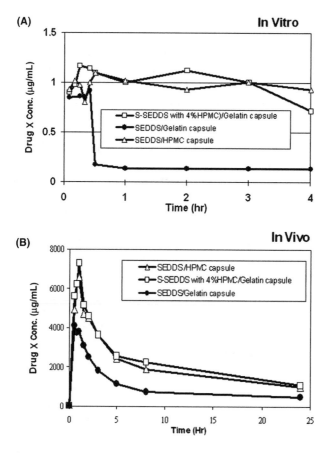

Figure 9   (**A**) Apparent concentration-time profiles of Drug X observed from the in vitro dissolution/precipitation test using the three formulations with different capsule shells as indicated. (**B**) Mean plasma concentration profiles of Drug X in the dogs from the three formulation (n = 6, crossover).

trast, the 1-g SEDDS formulation containing 44 mg of HPMC suspended in hard gelatin capsules showed an almost constant drug concentration of approximately 1 mg/mL over the entire four-hour period (Fig. 9A). The SEDDS liquid filled into an HPMC capsule showed essentially the same concentration–time profile as the SEDDS formulation containing suspended HPMC powder filled into gelatin capsules. In both cases, wherein HPMC is present either as suspended powder in the SEDDS liquid or HPMC provided by the capsule shell, the Drug X concentration was maintained at a level approximately five-fold higher than that of the SEDDS liquid in a hard gelatin capsule. This set of data clearly indicate that an HPMC capsule acts similar to HPMC powder suspended within the SEDDS liquid with respect to maintaining the supersaturated state with Drug X.

The oral bioavailability study was determined in dogs ($n = 6$, cross-over) with the three SEDDS formulations described previously. The mean plasma concentration–time profiles of Drug X are plotted in Figure 9B. As expected, the SEDDS formulation in the gelatin capsule showed a low C_{max} and a low AUC. However, the plasma concentration–time profiles observed for the SEDDS formulation containing HPMC and the SEDDS formulation filled into HPMC capsules were almost superimposable and the resulting C_{max} and AUC values were approximately two-fold higher than that of the SEDDS liquid without HPMC in the gelatin capsule. The in vivo behavior of the three formulations is in accord with the in vitro test results.

In summary, Drug X in S-SEDDS formulations containing HPMC either as suspended powder or as HPMC in the capsule shell generates and sustains a supersaturated Drug X solution on contact with water and this results in higher in vivo oral bioavailability in dogs. Further evaluation in the clinic is discussed in the following section.

Clinical Evaluation of the Supersaturatable Self-Emulsifying Drug Delivery Systems

With the exciting proof-of-concept from the in vivo dog study, a human clinical trial was designed to evaluate the oral bioavailability of an S-SEDDS softgel formulation of Drug X in comparison with two other formulations, namely a powder formulation in a gelatin capsule and an aqueous suspension with fine particles of Drug X. A S-SEDDS formulation of Drug X containing suspended

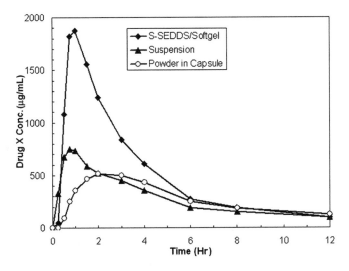

Figure 10 Human bioavailability study with three formulations of Drug X: formulated powder filled in a hard gelatin capsule, an aqueous suspension, and a S-SEDDS formuation with HPMC in a softgel (n = 23).

Table 5 Oral Bioavailability of Drug X in Humans Administered a 200-mg Dose as Three Different Formulations ($n = 23$, Crossover)

Pharmacokinetic parameters	Formulations		
	Formulated powder in gelatin capsule	Aqueous suspension	S-SEDDS softgel
C_{max} (ng/mL)	621 (45)	804 (45)	2061 (34)
T_{max} (hr)	2.15 (42)	0.97 (43)	1.03 (36)
AUC [(ng/mL)^{a}hr]	5060 (45)	4892 (45)	7004 (41)

^{a}Values are the means (% CV).
Abbreviation: S-SEDDS, supersaturatable self-emulsifying drug delivery systems.

HPMC was encapsulated in softgels and these softgels were orally administered to fasted humans (23 subjects, cross-over).

The plasma concentration versus time profiles for Drug X administered as each of these formulations are shown in Figure 10 and the mean C_{max}, T_{max}, and AUC values are reported in Table 5. The conventional powder formulation in the gelatin capsule showed the lowest C_{max} (621 ng/mL) and the aqueous suspension showed a slightly higher C_{max} (804 ng/mL). In contrast, the S-SEDDS softgel showed the highest C_{max} (2061 ng/mL) and this is an impressive 300% increase in the C_{max} and a 40% increase in the AUC as compared with that of the powder formulation. The highest C_{max} and the largest AUC along with the shortest T_{max} (~1 hour) were observed with the S-SEDDS softgel containing suspended HPMC indicating rapid and more complete absorption. It is interesting to note that in the dog, the same S-SEDDS formulation performed similar to the aqueous suspension (Fig. 8B) whereas in the human the S-SEDDS formulation of Drug X was clearly superior with respect to C_{max} and AUC (Fig. 10).

The remarkable improvement in the oral bioavailability of Drug X in the S-SEDDS formulation containing HPMC in the clinical study is attributed to the generation and the maintenance of a supersaturated state in the GI tract. A proposed mechanism for enhanced oral absorption of poorly soluble drugs in S-SEDDS formulations is described next.

PROPOSED MECHANISM FOR ENHANCED ORAL BIOAVAILABILITY WITH SUPERSATURATABLE SELF-EMULSIFYING DRUG DELIVERY SYSTEMS

In Chapter 12 of this book, which deals with SEDDS formulations of poorly soluble lipophilic drugs (1), it was suggested that the enhanced oral bioavailability seen with the SEDDS formulations can be explained by improved presentation of the poorly soluble drug to the enterocyte brush border region. This could be achieved by equilibration of the emulsion/microemulsion (E/ME) arising from contact of the SEDDS formulation with water or by equilibration of the drug in the remnant E/ME with the aqueous medium. The drug in the aqueous medium could become absorbed by the aqueous diffusional pathway or the drug could equilibrate with the BAMM with delivery to the enterocyte brush border membrane by collisional contact. Alternatively, the E/ME remnant could simulate the behavior of the BAMM in delivering the poorly soluble drug to the enterocyte brush border region.

In this chapter, it was found that the S-SEDDS formulations containing a small amount of HPMC (~40 mg/g of formulation) can result in generation of a supersaturated state that can be maintained for a few hours and this leads to enhanced absorption of poorly soluble, lipophilic drugs. The following discussion supports this proposed mechanism.

The existence of the supersaturated state was shown in our in vitro dissolution test where the drug filtrate concentration for a S-SEDDS formulation of PNU-91325 showed a maximum value of about 420 μg/ml at 30 minutes (Fig. 2C, S-SEDDS with HPMC). However, the SEDDS formulation of PNU-91325, without HPMC, gave a drug filtrate concentration of only about 30 μg/ml at three hours in the dissolution/precipitation test and thus, the approximate degree of supersaturation with the S-SEDDS formulation of PNU-91325 is 420/30 or about 14.

The approximately 10-fold (and higher) degree of supersaturation observed with the S-SEDDS formulation of PNU-91325, paclitaxel, and Drug X suggests that intestinal absorption should be markedly increased as a result of the supersaturated state. Based on intestinal flux theory, a drug with an aqueous solubility of only approximately 5 μg/ml or less and a 200-mg dose would be expected to be incompletely absorbed in humans assuming a maximum permeability (plateau region) and a particle size of the drug in the micron range (51–55). The 10-fold improvement of the aqueous concentration of the drug from the supersaturatable formulations should allow complete absorption of 200 mg under the same circumstances.

The ability to generate a supersaturated state with HPMC with the S-SEDDS formulations is probably associated with the formation of a widely spaced cellulosic polymer network created by the HPMC chains in water, which, according to the literature, consists of "cellulosic bundles resulting in a tenuous network of swollen clusters with hydrophobic substituents surrounded by sheaths of structured water" (56,57). Studies on the mechanism responsible for inhibiting crystallization of drugs in aqueous solutions containing HPMC suggest that the HPMC polymer chain may inhibit nucleation as well as crystal growth by adsorption of the HPMC molecules onto the surface of the nuclei or on to the surface crystals (15,23,58). The general applicability of the cellulosic polymers in inhibiting crystallization of many pharmaceutical substances is widely reported (16–18,20,22,26,28,29,31).

In conclusion, the mechanism responsible for the enhanced intestinal absorption of poorly soluble drugs from S-SEDDS formulations containing HPMC is probably due to enhanced presentation of the drug to the enterocyte brush border region by the aqueous pathway due to the increased free drug levels achieved by supersaturation, and along with enhanced presentation of the drug to the enterocyte brush border by mimicking or equilibrating with the BA/BAMM pathway (1).

CONCLUSIONS

Raising the thermodynamic activity of a drug substance by the supersaturated state and thereby improving topical drug absorption was proposed four decades ago and now it is possible to achieve enhanced absorption by means of supersaturatable formulations. Increasing the free drug concentration by generating and sustaining a temporarily supersaturated state in vivo with S-SEDDS formulations is the fundamental concept in this approach. The S-SEDDS formulation approach may be useful in overcoming the solubility- and dissolution-limited absorption of other poorly soluble drugs. The three case studies including PNU-91325, paclitaxel, and Drug X discussed in this chapter demonstrate the utility of the S-SEDDS formulation approach in improving the oral bioavailability of poorly soluble, lipophilic drugs. The other main advantage of the S-SEDDS approach is the reduction in the amount of surfactant in the formulation, thereby achieving an improved tox/safety profile with the S-SEDDS formulations.

We are exploring further applications of the supersaturatable formulation technology and acquiring a scientific understanding of the precipitation kinetics and the mechanism of supersaturation with the use of the polymeric substances. The advances in this area will allow a better control of the supersaturated state and improved oral delivery of poorly soluble drugs.

ACKNOWLEDGMENTS

Appreciation is extended to our colleagues including J. W. Skoug, P. R. Nixon, M. J. Hageman, B. R. Rush, S. R. Davio, W. P. Pfund, M. E. Guyton, M. T. Kuo, T. Huang, Q. Lu, J. M. Bauer, R. J. Haskell, J. R. Shifflett, R. J. Dalga, and for collaboration on the case studies that were reviewed herein.

REFERENCES

1. Gao P, Morozowich W. Case studies: rational development of self-emulsifying formulations for improving the oral bioavailability of poorly soluble, lipophilic drugs. Chapter 12.
2. Bagwe RP, Kanicky JR, Palla BJ, Patanjali PK, Shah DO. Improved drug delivery using microemulsions: rationale, recent progress, and new horizons. Critical Rev Therap Drug Carrier Syst 2001; 18(1):77–140.
3. Wasan KM. Formulations and physiological and biopharmaceutical issues in the development of oral lipid-based drug delivery systems. Drug Devel Ind Pharm 2001; 27(4):267–276.
4. Charman WN. Lipids, lipophilic drugs and oral drug delivery—some emerging concepts. J Pharm Sci 2000; 89:967–978.

5. Pouton CW. Lipid formulations for oral administration of drugs: non-emulsifying, self-emulsifying and "self-microemulsifying" drug delivery systems. Eur J Pharm Sci 2002; 11(suppl):S93–S98.

6. Wignot TM, Stewart RP, Schray KJ, Das S, Sipos T. In vitro studies of the effects of HAART drugs and excipients on activity of digestive enzymes. Pharm Res 2004; 21(3):420–427.

7. Sherman DS, Fish DN. Management of protease inhibitor associated diarrhea. Clin Infec Dis 2000; 30:908–914.

8. Poelma FGJ, Breas R, Tukker JJ, Crommelin DJA. Intestinal absorption of drugs. The influence of mixed micelles on the disappearance kinetics of drugs from the small intestine of the rat. J Pharm Pharmacol 1991; 43(5):317–324.

9. Poelma FGJ, Breas R, Tukker JJ, Josef J. Intestinal absorption of drugs. III. The influence of taurocholate on the disappearance kinetics of hydrophilic and lipophilic drugs from the small intestine of the rat. Pharm Res 1990; 7(4):392–397.

10. Chiu YY, Higaki K, Neudeck BL, Barnett JL, Welage LS, Amidon GL. Human jejunal permeability of cyclosporin A: influence of surfactants on P-glycoprotein efflux in Caco-2 cells. Pharm Res 2003; 20(5):749–756.

11. Higuchi T. Physical chemical analysis of the percutaneous absorption process. J Soc Cosmetic Chem 1960; 11:85–97.

12. Megrab NA, Williams AC, Barry BW. Oestradiol permeation through human skin silastic membrane: effects of propylene glycol and supersaturation. J Control Rel 1995; 36:277–294.

13. Ma X, Taw J, Chiang C. Control of drug crystallization in transdermal matrix systems. Int J Pharm 1996; 142:115–119.

14. Schwarb FP, Imanidis G, Smith EW, Haigh JM, Surber C. Effect of concentration and degree of saturation of topical fluocinonide formulations on in vitro membrane transport and in vivo availability on human skin. Pharm Res 1997; 16:909–915.

15. Raghavan SL, Trividic A, Davis AF, Hadgraft J. Crystallization of hydrocortisone acetate: influence of polymers. Int J Pharm 2001; 212:213–221.

16. Raghavan RL, Kiepfer B, Davis AF, Kazarian SG, Hadgraft J. Membrane transport of hydrocortisone acetate from supersaturated solutions: the role of polymers. Int J Pharm 2001; 221:95–105.

17. Pellet MA, Davis AF, Hadgraft J. Effect of supersaturation on membrane transport: 2. Piroxicam. Int J Pharm 1994; 111:1–6.

18. Pellet MA, Castellano S, Hadgraft J, Davis AF. The penetration of supersaturated solutions of piroxicam across silicone membranes and human skin in vitro. J Control Rel 1997; 46:205–214.

19. Pellet MA, Roberts MS, Hadgraft J. Supersaturated solutions evaluated with an intro stratum corneum tape stripping technique. Int J Pharm 1997; 151:91–98.

20. Raghavan RL, Trividic A, Davis AF, Hadgraft J. Effects of cellulose polymers on supersaturation and in vitro membrane transport of hydrocortisone acetate. Int J Pharm 2000; 193:231–237.

21. Iervolino M, Raghavan RL, Hadgraft J. Membrane penetration enhancement of ibuprofen using supersaturation. Int J Pharm 2000; 198:229–238.

22. Iervolino M, Cappello B, Raghavan RL, Hadgraft J. Penetration enhancement of ibuprofen from supersaturated solutions through human skin. Int J Pharm 2001; 212:131–141.

23. Simonelli AP, Mehta SC, Higuchi WI. Inhibition of sulfathiazole crystal growth by polyvinylpyrrolidone. J Pharm Sci 1970; 59:633–638.

24. Sekikawa H, Fujiwara J, Naganuma T, Nakano M, Arita T. Dissolution behaviors and gastrointestinal absorption of phenytoin in phenytoin–polyvinylpyrrolidone coprecipitate. Chem Pharm Bull 1978; 26;3033–3039.

25. Suzuki H, Sunada H. Comparison of nicotiamide, ethylurea and polyethylene glycol as carriers for nifedipine solid dispersion systems. Chem Pharm Bull 1997; 45(10):1688–1693.

26. Suzuki H, Sunada H. Some factors influencing the dissolution of solid dispersions with nicotiamide and hydroxypropylmethycellulose as combined carriers. Chem Pharm Bull 1998; 46(6):1015–1020.

27. Yamada T, Saito N, Imai T, Otagiri M. Effect of grinding with hydroxypropyl cellulose on dissolution and particle size of a poorly water-soluble drug. Chem Pharm Bull 1999; 47(9):1311–1313.

28. Kohri N, Yamayoshi Y, Xin H, et al. Improving the oral bio-availability of albendazole in rabbits by the solid dispersion technique. J Pharm Pharmacol 1999; 51:159–164.

29. Hasegawa A, Nakagawa H, Sugimoto I. Application of solid dispersions of nifedipine with enteric coating agent to prepare a sustained-release dosage form. Chem Pharm Bull 1985; 33(4):1615–1619.

30. O'Driscoll KM, Corrigan OI. Chlorothiazide-polyvinylpyrrolidone (PVP) interactions: influence on membrane permeation (everted rat intestine) and dissolution. Drug Dev Ind Pharm 1982; 8(4):547–564.

31. Usui F, Maeda K, Kusai A, Nishimura K, Yamamoto K. Inhibitory effects of water soluble polymers on precipitation of RS-8359. Int J Pharm 1997; 154:59–66.

32. Hasegawa A, Taguchi M, Suzuki R, Miyata T, Nakagawa H, Sugimoto I. Supersaturation mechanism of drugs from solid dispersions with enteric coating agents. Chem Pharm Bull 1988; 36(12):4941–4950.

33. Gao P, Guyton ME, Huang T, Bauer JM, Stefanski KJ, Lu Q. Enhanced oral bioavailability of a poorly water soluble drug PNU-91325 by supersaturatable formulations. Drug Dev Ind Pharm 2004; 30(2):221–229.

34. Gao P, Rush RD, Pfund WP, et al. Development of a supersaturatable SEDDS (S-SEDDS) formulation of paclitaxel with improved oral bioavailability. J Pharm Sci 2003; 92(12):2395–2407.

35. Tang L, Khan SU, Muhammad NA. Evaluation and selection of bio-relevant dissolution media for a poorly water soluble new chemical entity. Pharm Dev Tech 2002; 6(4):531–540.

36. Humberstone AJ, Charman WN. Lipid-based vehicles for the oral delivery of poorly water soluble drugs. Adv Drug Dev Rev 1997; 25:103–128.

37. Sek L, Porter CJH, Kaukonen AM, Charman WN. Evaluation of the in vitro digestion profiles of long and medium chain glycerides and the phase behaviour of their lipophilic products. J Phar Pharmaco 2002; 54:29–41.

38. Lee J, Lee SC, Acharya G, Chang C, Park K. Hydrotropic solubilization of paclitaxel: analysis of chemical structures for hydrotropic property. Pharm Res 2003; 20(7):1022–1030.

39. Straudinger RM. Biopharmaceutics of paclitaxel (Taxol®): formulation, activity, and pharmacokinetics. In: Suffness M, ed., Taxol Science and Applications. Chap. 9. New York: CRC Press Inc., 1995.

40. Mathew AE, Mejillano MR, Nath JP, Himes RH, Stella VJ. Synthesis and evaluation of some water-insoluble prodrugs and derivatives of Taxol with antitumor activity. J Med Chem 1992; 35:145–149.

41. Trissel LA, ed. Handbook on Injectable Drugs. 8th ed. Bethesda, MD: Am Soc Hosp Pharm Inc., 1994:808.

42. Nuijen B, Bouma M, Schellens JHM, Beijnen JH. Progress in the development of alternative pharmaceutical formulations of taxanes. Inv New Drugs 2001; 19:143–153.

43. Zuylen LV, Verweij J, Sparreboom A. Role of formulation vehicles in taxane pharmacology. Inv New Drugs 2001; 19:125–141.

44. Lassus M, Scott D, Leyland JB. Allergic reactions associated with cremophor containing antineoplastics. Proc Am Soc Clin Oncol 1985; 4:268.

45. Malingre MM, Beijnen JH, Schellens JHM. Oral delivery of taxanes. Inv New Drugs 2001; 19:155–162.

46. Bardeleijer HA, Tellingen OV, Schellens JHM, Beijnen JH. The oral route of the administration of cytotoxic drugs: strategies to increase the efficiency and consistency of drug delivery. Inv New Drugs 2000; 18:231–241.

47. Terwogt JMM, Malingre MM, Beijnen JH, et al. Coadministration of oral cyclosporin A enables oral therapy with paclitaxel. Clin Cancer Res 1999; 5:3379–3384.

48. Malingre MM, Beijnen JH, Rosing H, et al. A phase I and pharmacokinetic study of bi-daily dosing of oral paclitaxel in combination with cyclosporin A. Cancer Chemother Pharmacol 2001; 47:347–354.

49. Woo JS, Lee CH, Shim CK, Hwang SJ. Enhanced oral bioavailability of paclitaxel by coadministration of the P-glycoprotein inhibitor KR30031. Pharm Res 2003; 20:24–30.

50. Montaseri H, Jamali F, Micetich RG, Daneshtalab M. Improving oral bioavailability of Taxol. Pharm Res 1995; 12:S-429.

51. Lennernaes H, Fagerholm U, Raab Y, Gerdin B, Haellgren R. Regional rectal perfusion: a new in vivo approach to study rectal drug absorption in man. Pharm Res 1995; 12(3):426–432.

52. Takamatsu Narushi, Welage Lynda S, Idkaidek Nasir M, et al. Human intestinal permeability of piroxicam, propranolol, phenylalanine, and PEG400 determined by jejunal perfusion. Pharm Res 1997; 14(9):1127–1132.

53. Ho NFH, Day JS, Barsuhn CL, Burton PS, Raub TJ. Biophysical model approaches to mechanistic transepithelial studies of peptides. J Cont Rel 1990; 11(1–3):3–24.

54. Amidon GL, Lennernas H, Shah VP, Crison JR. A theoretical basis for a biopharmaceutic drug classification: the correlation of in vitro drug product dissolution and in vivo bioavailability. Pharm Res 1995; 12(3):413–420.

55. Amidon GE, Higuchi WI, Ho NF. Theoretical and experimental studies of transport of micelle-solubilized solutes. J Pharm Sci 1982; 71(1):77–84.

56. Haque A, Morris ER. Thermogelation of methylcellulose. Part I. Molecular structures and processes. Carbohydrate Polymers 1993; 22:161–173.

57. Haque A, Richardson RK, Morris ER, Gidley MJ, Caswell DC. Thermogelation of methylcellulose. Part II. Effect of hydroxypropyl substituents. Carbohydrate Polymers 1993; 22:175–186.

58. Ziller KH, Rupprecht H. Control of crystal growth in drug suspensions. Drug Dev Ind Pharm 1988; 14:2341–2370.

Index